Clinical Problems in Gastroenterology

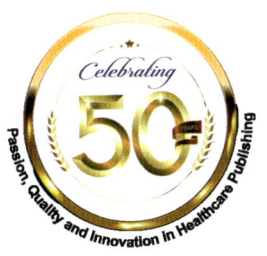

Clinical Problems in Gastroenterology

Editor

Her Hsin Tsai MD FRCP FECG
Consultant Gastroenterologist
Inflammatory Bowel Disease Unit
Department of Gastroenterology
Hull and East Yorkshire Hospitals
NHS Trust, Hull, UK

Foreword

Jonathan Rhodes

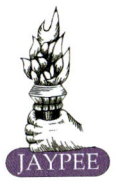

JAYPEE BROTHERS MEDICAL PUBLISHERS
The Health Sciences Publisher
New Delhi | London | Panama

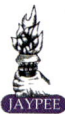 **Jaypee Brothers Medical Publishers (P) Ltd**

Headquarters

Jaypee Brothers Medical Publishers (P) Ltd
4838/24, Ansari Road, Daryaganj
New Delhi 110 002, India
Phone: +91-11-43574357
Fax: +91-11-43574314
E-mail: jaypee@jaypeebrothers.com

Overseas Offices

J P Medical Ltd
83 Victoria Street, London
SW1H 0HW (UK)
Phone: +44 20 3170 8910
Fax: +44 (0)20 3008 6180
E-mail: info@jpmedpub.com

Jaypee-Highlights Medical Publishers Inc
City of Knowledge, Bld. 235, 2nd Floor, Clayton
Panama City, Panama
Phone: +1 507-301-0496
Fax: +1 507-301-0499
E-mail: cservice@jphmedical.com

Jaypee Brothers Medical Publishers (P) Ltd
Bhotahity, Kathmandu, Nepal
Phone: +977-9741283608
Email: kathmandu@jaypeebrothers.com

Website: www.jaypeebrothers.com
Website: www.jaypeedigital.com

© 2019, Jaypee Brothers Medical Publishers

The views and opinions expressed in this book are solely those of the original contributor(s)/author(s) and do not necessarily represent those of editor(s) of the book.

All rights reserved. No part of this publication may be reproduced, stored or transmitted in any form or by any means, electronic, mechanical, photocopying, recording or otherwise, without the prior permission in writing of the publishers.

All brand names and product names used in this book are trade names, service marks, trademarks or registered trademarks of their respective owners. The publisher is not associated with any product or vendor mentioned in this book.

Medical knowledge and practice change constantly. This book is designed to provide accurate, authoritative information about the subject matter in question. However, readers are advised to check the most current information available on procedures included and check information from the manufacturer of each product to be administered, to verify the recommended dose, formula, method and duration of administration, adverse effects and contraindications. It is the responsibility of the practitioner to take all appropriate safety precautions. Neither the publisher nor the author(s)/editor(s) assume any liability for any injury and/or damage to persons or property arising from or related to use of material in this book.

This book is sold on the understanding that the publisher is not engaged in providing professional medical services. If such advice or services are required, the services of a competent medical professional should be sought.

Every effort has been made where necessary to contact holders of copyright to obtain permission to reproduce copyright material. If any have been inadvertently overlooked, the publisher will be pleased to make the necessary arrangements at the first opportunity. The **CD/DVD-ROM** (if any) provided in the sealed envelope with this book is complimentary and free of cost. **Not meant for sale.**

Inquiries for bulk sales may be solicited at: jaypee@jaypeebrothers.com

Clinical Problems in Gastroenterology

First Edition: **2019**

ISBN: 978-93-5270-585-6

Printed at: Samrat Offset Pvt. Ltd.

Dedicated to
*The loving memory of
My Father, My Inspiration*

Contributors

Barry Taylor FRCS
Consultant Surgeon
Surgery Division
Warrington and Halton Hospitals
NHS Foundation Trust
Warrington, UK

Benjamin Chan
MBChB (Hons) MRes MRCS
Hepatobiliary Research Fellow
University of Liverpool
Department of Hepatobiliary Surgery
Aintree University Hospital
Liverpool, UK

Her Hsin Tsai MD FRCP FECG
Consultant Gastroenterologist
Inflammatory Bowel Disease Unit
Department of Gastroenterology
Hull and East Yorkshire Hospitals
NHS Trust, Hull, UK

Lynsey Corless MBChB PhD FRCP
Consultant Hepatologist
Liver Unit
Department of Gastroenterology
Hull and East Yorkshire Hospitals
NHS Trust
Hull Royal Infirmary
Hull, UK

Foreword

There are many reviews and guidelines on the management of specific conditions available on the internet, but they are often blocked by paywalls and are of varying clarity and currency. Moreover, it can be hard to find good quality guidance to help in diagnosis. In *Clinical Problems in Gastroenterology*, Her Hsin Tsai and his colleagues have done a really great job in writing with great clarity and accuracy about the current management of gastrointestinal and liver conditions. The problem-based structure also makes this an excellent guide to diagnosis. Whilst increasing attention is paid to training in practical skills such as endoscopy, acquisition of diagnostic skills has in the past too often been left to chance—to be accrued by experience—too often by "trial and error". A good-read of this book by clinicians, who are either relatively new to the specialty or simply in need of some educational refreshment should go a long way to providing valuable "virtual" experience.

Jonathan Rhodes MA MD FRCP FMed Sci
Emeritus Professor
Department of Medicine
University of Liverpool, UK
Past-President
British Society of Gastroenterology

Preface

In 1995 Professor Jonathan M Rhodes and I wrote a book of the same title, now long out of print. There has been many changes and advances in the specialty and the book is now completely rewritten, and all the clinical images and illustrations are new and fresh, thanks in no small part to the excellent graphics team at Jaypee Brothers Medical Publishers, New Delhi, India.

Many medical textbooks follow a traditional format of organ-based layout or by disease headings. While this may work in some specialties, it is quite unhelpful in a clinical specialty like gastroenterology. Here, patients present with a symptom, not with a disease. It is not always evident with the clinical presentation which organ may be the cause of the problem.

In this book I, with my specialty contributors, shall attempt to approach the subject from a practical problem-orientated manner. Each chapter is major clinical problem and the reader is led up a path of rational clinical decision making in arriving at the right diagnosis or choosing the right diagnostic test or imaging modality to make the right diagnosis. Hence, most chapters will be in two parts. The first section will be "Reaching a Diagnosis" and the second section will be on "Conditions Causing" the problem. However, this basic model is adapted for each clinical problem.

We live in an age when information is freely available at a click of a mouse or a swipe of a mobile device's screen. However, it is still the clinicians' role to make the necessary decisions to arrive at the right diagnosis in a timely manner with the efficient use of the diagnostic tools. Some investigations are unpleasant and not without risks. It is hoped that this approach will amply equip the gastroenterology trainee or fellow. It should also contain the bulk of the knowledge base required by the European Section and Board of Gastroenterology and Hepatology examination.

It is the publisher's policy to have all their medical titles published with American spellings. I apologise to UK readers but it is beyond my control. It is hoped it does not offend those who prefer standard English spellings.

Her Hsin Tsai
Beverley, UK
18/08/2018

Acknowledgments

I am grateful to my contributors, Dr Lynsey Corless, who wrote the hepatology chapters and Mr Benjamin Chan and Mr Barry Taylor, who wrote the chapter on the acute abdomen. I would also like to thank Drs Corinna Hauff, James Cast, and Christopher Keegan, for providing radiological images and Dr Laszlo Karsai for providing some of the histological images. Finally, to my patients for their support of this project and giving free consent to the publication of clinical images.

I am grateful for the constant support and encouragement of Shri Jitendar P Vij (Group Chairman) and Mr Ankit Vij (Managing Director), M/s Jaypee Brothers Medical Publishers (P) Ltd, New Delhi, India, in publishing this book and also their associates, particularly Ms Chetna Malhotra Vohra (Associate Director—Content Strategy) and Ms Prerna Bajaj (Development Editor) who have been prompt, efficient and most helpful.

Contents

1. **Chronic or Recurrent Abdominal Pain** 1
   Her Hsin Tsai
   - Reaching A Diagnosis   1
   - Conditions Causing Chronic or Recurrent Abdominal Pain: Natural History and Management   21

2. **Acute Abdomen** 55
   Benjamin Chan, Barry Taylor
   - Reaching a Diagnosis   55
   - A Step-by-step Approach to Acute Abdominal Pain   58
   - Conditions Causing Acute Abdominal Pain: Natural History and Management   73
   - Intestinal Obstruction   88
   - A Step-by-step Approach to Intestinal Obstruction   88
   - Vascular Abnormalities   94

3. **Diarrhea** 102
   Her Hsin Tsai
   - Reaching a Diagnosis   102
   - Conditions Causing Diarrhea: Natural History and Management   127
   - Secretory Diarrhea   178

4. **Constipation** 182
   Her Hsin Tsai
   - What is Constipation?   182
   - Is it Primary Constipation?   185
   - Is it Constipation-predominant Irritable Bowel Syndrome?   185
   - Is it Slow-transit Constipation?   186
   - Is it Pelvic Floor Dysfunction?   187
   - Is it Secondary Constipation?   188
   - Is there Hirschsprung's Disease?   189
   - Solitary Rectal Ulcer Syndrome   189

5. **Anorectal Problems** 191
   Her Hsin Tsai
   - Diagnosis   191
   - Natural History and Management of Anorectal Conditions   195

6. **Gastrointestinal Bleeding and Anemia** 205
   Her Hsin Tsai
   - Reaching a Diagnosis and Management   205

- Conditions Causing GI Bleeding: Natural History and Management *213*
- Other Causes of Non-variceal Upper GI Bleeding *219*
- Rarer Causes of Small Intestinal Bleeding *233*
- Colonic Bleeding *235*
- Other Colonic Malignancies *253*

7. **Nausea and Vomiting** 256
   Her Hsin Tsai
   - Neurophysiology of Nausea and Vomiting *256*
   - Diagnosis *257*
   - Drug Therapy of Vomiting *264*

8. **Eating Disorders and Weight Loss** 265
   Her Hsin Tsai
   - Physiology of Appetite *265*
   - Anorexia and Weight Loss *267*
   - Anorexia Nervosa *269*
   - Obesity *270*

9. **Wind** 274
   Her Hsin Tsai
   - Belching *274*
   - Flatus *274*
   - Bloating *276*

10. **Gastrointestinal Complications of Obesity Surgery and Other Gastric Operations** 279
    Her Hsin Tsai
    - Abdominal Pain *281*
    - Vomiting *283*
    - Dysphagia *283*
    - Diarrhea *284*

11. **Esophageal Pain and Difficulty with Swallowing** 288
    Her Hsin Tsai
    - Diagnosis *288*
    - Natural History and Management *300*

12. **Jaundice** 319
    Lynsey Corless
    - Reaching a Diagnosis *320*
    - Specific Conditions Causing Jaundice *326*

Contents

13. Abdominal Masses and Swelling 334
Her Hsin Tsai
- Generalized Swelling *334*
- Hepatomegaly *336*
- Splenomegaly *339*
- Renal Mass *340*
- Other Localized Masses *341*
- Liver Tumors *343*
- Hepatic Cysts and Abscesses *347*

14. Liver Failure 351
Lynsey Corless
- Acute Liver Failure *351*
- Cirrhosis as a Consequence of Chronic Liver Disease *356*
- LT and Transjugular Intrahepatic Portosystemic Shunt *370*

15. Abnormal Liver Biochemistry 375
Lynsey Corless
- Reaching a Diagnosis *375*
- Abnormal LFT in Pregnancy *384*
- Guidance on Specific Conditions *385*

16. Enteral and Parenteral Nutrition 399
Her Hsin Tsai
- Is the Patient at Risk of Malnutrition? *399*
- Does the Patient have Dysphagia? *400*
- Is the Patient at Risk of Refeeding Syndrome? *401*
- Types of Feeds *403*
- Parenteral Nutrition *405*

Index *407*

CHAPTER 1

Chronic or Recurrent Abdominal Pain

Her Hsin Tsai

■ REACHING A DIAGNOSIS

Is the Pain Functional or Organic?

The vast majority of patients who consult a doctor, especially in the primary care sector, with chronic abdominal pain, will have a functional rather than organic cause for the pain. Over-investigation of such patients is often counterproductive. Many of these investigations are unpleasant, even painful and associated with considerable cost and patients often get alarmed by the number of investigations and they tend to equate that to serious illness. It is therefore essential that the physician identifies those patients positively rather than negatively by excluding a whole lot of organic diseases.

Based on the UK general practitioner studies, the UK general practitioner with an average patient list will encounter over 25 new cases of functional bowel problems compared to a probability of 1 incidental case of colorectal cancer and the average general practitioner will encounter inflammatory bowel disease like a new case of Crohn's disease once every 7 years or more. Identifying the individuals who are likely to have an organic disease rather than a functional disease is therefore very important. Probably the single most important consideration is the patient's age. It is unsafe to label any chronic abdominal pain developing for the first time in a patient over 40 years of age as functional without further investigation. If the patient is under 40 years of age, then it is important to try to make a positive diagnosis of functional pain, such as irritable bowel syndrome (IBS), from the history and ask specific questions if the answers are not provided spontaneously. These questions include:
- Is the pain associated with gaseous distention?
- Is the pain associated with constipation or diarrhea?
- Is the pain relieved by defecation?
- Is the pain an intermittent pain and interspersed with episodes of trouble-free days or weeks?

A positive answer to the above questions usually suggests functional abdominal pain. Conversely, the pain is usually more likely to be organic and warrants further investigation regardless of the age if:
- It awakes the patient at night.
- It persists for weeks or many months.
- It is associated with persistent rather than intermittent alteration of bowel habit.
- It is accompanied by weight loss or rectal bleeding.

Thorough general examination including rectal examination and a few blood tests should usually suffice. A blood test should include full blood count, erythrocyte sedimentation rate (ESR) or plasma viscosity and liver function tests (LFTs) as found in many automated serum profiles. Even if these are normal one can miss inflammatory bowel diseases, particularly Crohn's disease, especially if the patient comes from a high-prevalence country. Serum acute phase reactant test like C-reactive protein (CRP) can also be quite useful as it does reflect an inflammatory process. More recently, fecal calprotectin has been shown to be useful in differentiating between inflammatory bowel conditions and those with normal or IBS (Fig. 1.1). The prevalence of the conditions and incidental cases per year, per general practitioner, is given in Table 1.1.

A simple diagnostic algorithm to differentiate between IBS and other causes of abdominal pain is illustrated in Figure 1.2. When a physician encounters a patient with abdominal pain with some bowel symptoms, it is important to try to make a positive diagnosis of IBS early. This will reassure the patient, enable early implementation of treatments and prevent unnecessary and painful investigations.

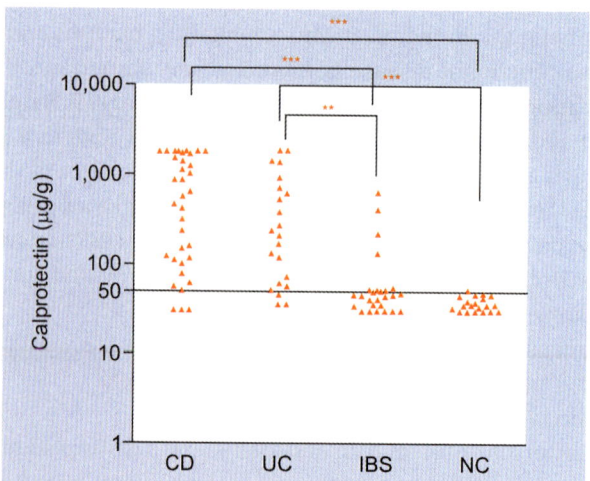

Fig. 1.1: Fecal calprotectin IBS or IBD. **$p<0.01$, ***$p<0.001$. (CD: Crohn's disease; UC: Ulcerative colitis; IBS: Irritable bowel syndrome; NC: Normal controls.)

Chronic or Recurrent Abdominal Pain

Table 1.1: Likelihood of general practitioner (GP) episode.		
Condition	Prevalence (%)	Incidence cases/year/GP
Crohn's disease	0.15	0.12
Ulcerative colitis	0.2	0.4
Ovarian cancer	0.14	0.18
Celiac disease	0.8–1	0.25
Colorectal cancer	0.24	1.17
Irritable bowel syndrome	10.5	4–27

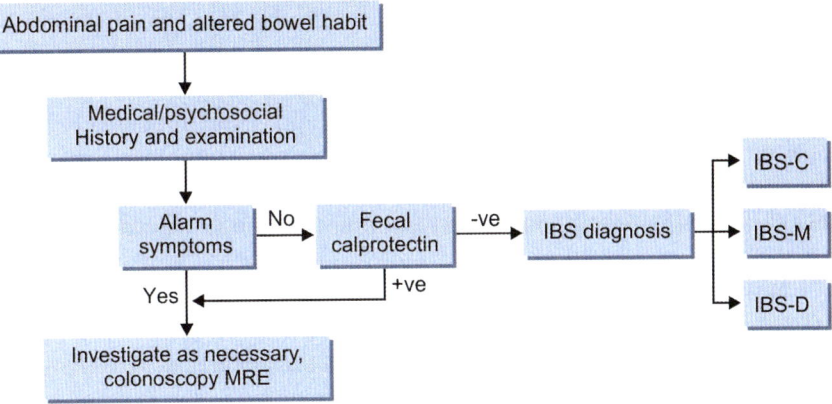

Fig. 1.2: Diagnostic algorithm for IBS.
(**IBS:** Irritable bowel syndrome; IBS-C: IBS-constipation; IBS-M: IBS-mixed; IBS-D: IBS-diarrhea; MRE: Magnetic resonance enteroclysis)

Symptoms that should concern the physician are:
- Age over 40 years
- A strong family history of colorectal cancer or inflammatory bowel disease, any rectal bleeding
- Anemia
- Weight loss or
- Palpable abdominal mass.

If they do not have these symptoms, then the physician should proceed to obtain fecal calprotectin and, if that is negative, a firm diagnosis of IBS can be made. For the case of predominant diarrhea, refer to Chapter 3 for reaching a diagnosis.

Is it Due to Gastric or Duodenal Disease?

When pain is due to gastric or duodenal disease, it is usually in the epigastric region. Sometimes with posterior duodenal ulcers, the pain can radiate through to the back, but in general the pain is often poorly localized. A typical history would be of a patient being awakened at night with these symptoms and this is usually in the early hours of the morning. It is often periodic, it may last several weeks separated by weeks or months without pain.

Patients taking nonsteroidal anti-inflammatory drugs (NSAIDs) may have duodenal ulcer disease with little or no symptoms at all, probably due to the analgesic effects of non-steroidal drugs themselves. As a result, they may present late and perhaps with a complication like bleeding or perforation. A history of drug use is important, therefore as part of the work-up for these patients.

The best way of diagnosing patients with upper gastrointestinal (GI) abdominal pain is to perform an endoscopy (Figs. 1.3 and 1.4). In patients under the age of 40 years, it is not unreasonable to carry out non-invasive investigations before considering an endoscopy. This could be a *Helicobacter pylori* fecal antigen test which is a simple and low-cost investigation. If the patient is young and presents with predominantly dyspeptic symptoms, it is also not unreasonable to give a trial of a proton pump inhibitor (PPI) like lansoprazole or omeprazole to see if it alleviates the symptoms. However, in areas where there is a high incidence of gastric cancer, it is not unreasonable to perform a prompt endoscopy in order to detect early cases of gastric cancer.

Duodenal ulcer disease is associated with *Helicobacter* infection in the majority of patients without a history of non-steroidal use. The easiest and cheapest method of detecting *H. pylori* with a high degree of sensitivity and specificity is the fecal antigen test. However, other tests such as blood serum antigen testing and urea-based breath tests are also available.

Endoscopy remains the investigation of choice when there is a suspicion of gastroduodenal disease. A well performed endoscopy can be done without sedation or under light sedation and is usually very well tolerated. This would also be able to pick up suspicious pathology like early gastric cancer. If the endoscopist encounters an ulcer in the stomach, it would be mandatory to biopsy it and also to review it at an interval of 6–8 weeks after treatment

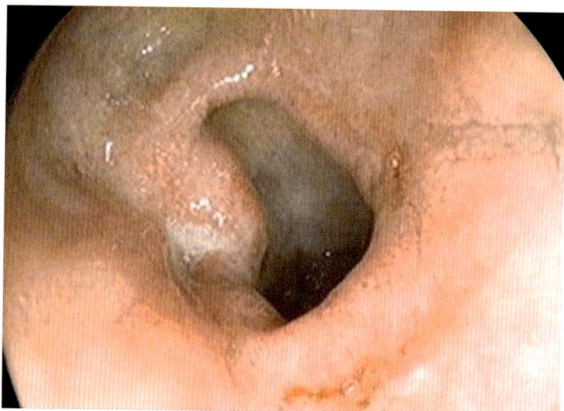

Fig. 1.3: Pre-pyloric ulcer: This ulcer sits at the pyloric opening.

Chronic or Recurrent Abdominal Pain

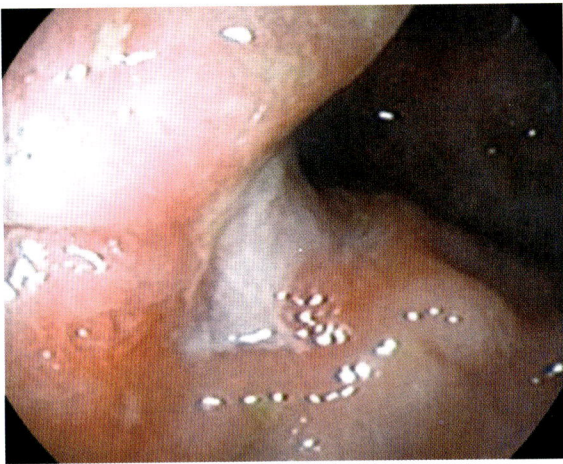

Fig. 1.4: Duodenal ulcer: The most common location is the first part of the duodenum.

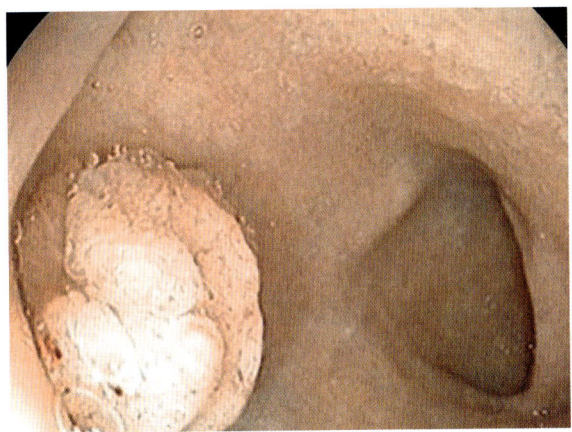

Fig. 1.5: Duodenal adenoma: This is a benign lesion with malignant potential and can be removed endoscopically. Usually found around the papilla, this one in the first part of the duodenum is rare. May be associated with colonic polyposis syndromes hence colonoscopy should be offered.

to make sure it is healed completely. This is to make absolutely sure that we are not dealing with gastric cancer. Ulcers in the first part of the duodenum are almost always benign, but malignant lesions can occur in the duodenum but tend to be in the second or third part of the duodenum or associated with the ampulla of Vater. A well-performed endoscopy should exclude all these possible lesions (Figs. 1.5 to 1.7).

A diagnosis of Zollinger–Ellison syndrome (gastrin-producing tumor) should be considered if there are extensive multiple duodenal ulcers or patients with ulcers resistant to treatment with PPIs, patients with extensive ulcers who are *Helicobacter* negative or continue to have ulcers after

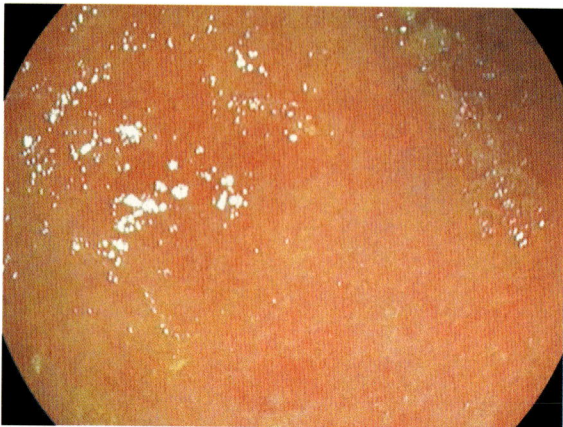

Fig. 1.6: Biliary gastritis. Bile reflux into the stomach can be readily seen at endoscopy and the accompanying mucosal inflammation makes it an easy diagnosis.

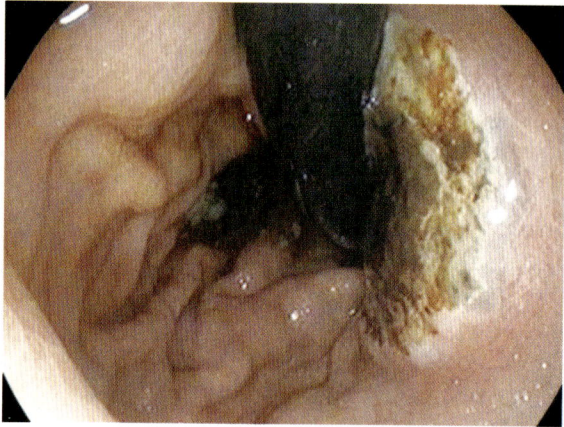

Fig. 1.7: Retroflexing the scope reveals a raised lesion with altered blood. This is an adenocarcinoma.

Helicobacter eradication. Investigations for Zollinger–Ellison syndrome include a fasting gastrin level. Sometimes calcium levels may also be elevated in MEN1 (Multiple Endocrine Neoplasia Type 1) syndrome. These patients have tumors in the 3 Ps—pituitary (e.g. prolactinoma), pancreas (gastrinoma), and parathyroid. The gastrinomas tend to be multiple. Imaging with computed tomography (CT) scanning is often sufficient to locate the lesions but other modalities like magnetic resonance imaging (MRI) can also be very useful. Transabdominal ultrasound may even be sufficient in some cases of locating a lesion. Pancreatic gastrinomas can also be localized using endoscopic ultrasonography, which has a higher sensitivity and specificity for pancreatic and duodenal gastrinomas.

Duodenitis

Duodenitis is usually an endoscopic or histological diagnosis rather than a clinical one. Many patients with duodenitis have little or no symptoms or symptoms that are indistinguishable from duodenal ulceration. Treatment is purely symptomatic.

Is it a Gallbladder Disease?

Gallstones are extremely common and are frequently completely asymptomatic. A common error is to attribute nebula symptoms of abdominal discomfort, bloating and fat intolerance to the gallstones. This may lead to unnecessary cholecystectomy. Patients would then still complain of the same functional symptoms despite the cholecystectomy. It is therefore important to make the firm diagnosis that the symptoms are attributable to the presence of gallstones.

Gallstones can cause two varieties of pain. This may be due to inflammation or it could be due to stones or tumor that is obstructing the outflow of the gallbladder. Forcible contractions against such an obstruction would result in pain. Pain also occurs if the gallstones are impacted infundibulum or the neck of the gallbladder or if they are extruded into the common bile duct and can obstruct the common bile duct.

A typical feature of biliary pain is epigastric or right upper quadrant pain that often radiates to the back or to the right shoulder blade associated with nausea or flatulence. These symptoms mimic the pain of IBS or peptic ulcer disease or even cardiac ischemia. If examinations carried out at a time when the patient has symptoms, tenderness in the right upper quadrant may be a useful sign.

The pain of biliary colic can be quite characteristic. It is often very memorable, very severe, and it rises to a crescendo and plateaus for about 30 minutes or so before diminishing again. Patients may have episodes of these pains and may be able to recall the episodes quite succinctly. These characteristic symptoms would point to a biliary cause for the patient's pain. If the patient just complains of a vague, generalized pain in the right upper quadrant this is usually not caused by biliary colic and removal of the gallbladder with or without stones usually is unproductive.

When stones dislodge into the common bile duct, then abnormal liver function tests (LFTs) may result with or without a rise in serum bilirubin; but when obstruction gets complete, then jaundice is inevitable. Sometimes stones impacted in the neck of the gallbladder can cause local edema, which can compress on the common bile duct and cause a degree of jaundice or abnormal LFTs. This is sometimes referred to as Mirizzi's syndrome.

Pain of an inflamed gallbladder is usually a constant right upper quadrant pain and can be exquisitely tender on palpation.

Radiology

The best way of imaging a gallbladder is to perform an ultrasound scan. A well-performed ultrasound scan is usually very instructive. A well-fasted patient will have a distended gallbladder and gallstones usually cast an acoustic shadow giving characteristic pictures. The size of the common bile duct may also be measured and it should be no more than a few millimeters. Anything in excess of 6 mm usually suggests some ongoing pathology although the size of the duct will be dilated after cholecystectomy and becomes increasingly dilated with advancing age.

If other lesions are suspected, then a computed tomography (CT) scan would be a very useful investigation as it would likely image the pancreas rather better than an ultrasound scan. If stones in the common bile duct are suspected either from raised LFTs or if there is a dilated common bile duct without obvious stones, then it is reasonable to proceed to magnetic resonance cholangiopancreatography (MRCP), which is valuable in assessing the presence of common bile duct stones. The presence of common bile duct stones will require therapy with endoscopic retrograde cholangiography (ERCP) (Figs. 1.8 to 1.10).

Adenomyomatosis of the Gallbladder

Ultrasound scan can often pick up cholesterol accumulation in the gallbladder known as cholesterolosis and may also be associated with adenomyomatosis. This is a benign condition characterized by hyperplastic changes of the gallbladder wall, causing overgrowth of mucosa, thickening of muscle wall and formation of intramural diverticula or sinus track sometimes known as Rokitansky–Aschoff sinuses. It may be seen on ultrasound scan as a tumor-like lesion but these are completely benign. Occasionally, ultrasound scan

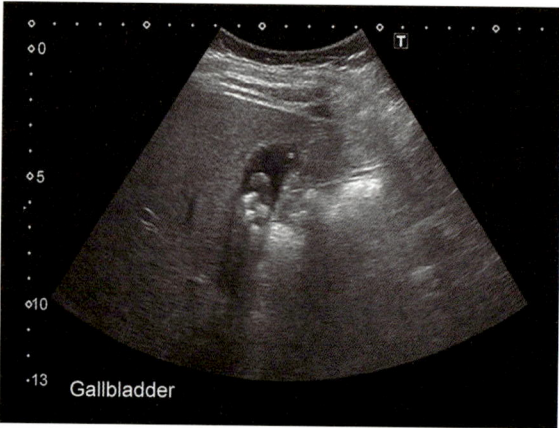

Fig. 1.8: Ultrasound showing gallstones: note the acoustic shadows cast by the stones.

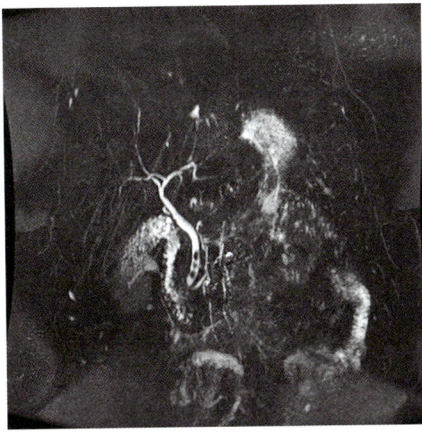

Fig. 1.9: Magnetic resonance cholangiopancreatogram (MRCP) showing three stones in the common bile duct as well as stones in the gallbladder.

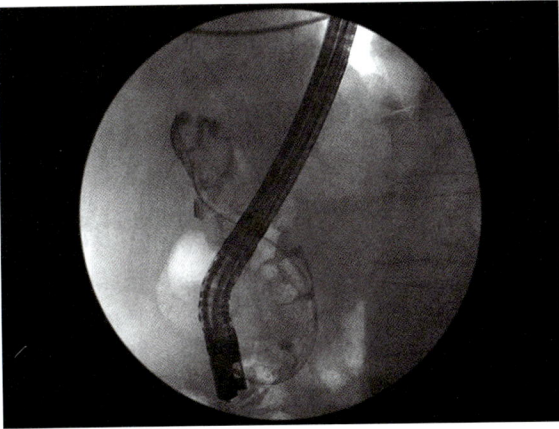

Fig. 1.10: Endoscopic retrograde cholangiopancreatography showing biliary duct stones.

cannot differentiate between adenomyomatosis and gallbladder cancer and further imaging may be considered including MRI or CT scanning.

Gallstones

About 15% of the British adult population have gallstones. Hence, it is not uncommon to have patients presenting with right upper quadrant pain and found to have incidental gallstones, but the presence of gallstones does not necessarily mean that they are the cause of the patient's symptoms. If the patient has a definite acute cholecystitis, then there would be evidence on ultrasound scan of a thickening gallbladder. Then it is almost certain that the pain experienced would be related to the gallbladder and cholecystectomy would be the correct treatment option. Often patients present with more diffuse symptoms and therefore endoscopy is often required to make sure that there are no other upper GI causes of the pain and symptoms before considering cholecystectomy on the patient. Because the symptoms may not be related to the gallbladder and may really reflect underlying functional problems in many patients, as many as 40% still continue to have symptoms despite a cholecystectomy. Hence, it is important to get an accurate reliable history before proceeding to cholecystectomy. Additionally, it must be noted that the absence of a gallbladder carries with it its own problems. This is sometimes referred to as postcholecystectomy syndrome and includes biliary gastritis, reflux symptoms and diarrhea. Diarrhea is caused by unbuffered bile reaching the colon and irritating the colon.

Is it a Pancreatic Disease?

The pancreas is a difficult organ to investigate. It lies behind the duodenum and the stomach and therefore ultrasound scans can be unreliable because of overlying gas. Upper GI endoscopy only reveals gastric and duodenal mucosa and unlikely to pick up evidence of pancreatic disease. The vast majority of patients with epigastric pain will have functional bowel pain and not necessarily underlying pancreatic disease. A high index of suspicion of neoplastic disease is necessary if one is to avoid the common mistake of missing early and therefore treatable pancreatic lesions. Pain from the pancreas can be quite diverse. Pain arising from the head of the pancreas may cause a right upper quadrant type pain and sometimes radiating to the back. Lesions in the body are frequently epigastric and more likely to radiate to the back and lesions in the tail may present as left upper quadrant pain. Initially, pain may be provoked by meals, particularly meals high in fat content but gradually it will be more severe, constant and patients are often more comfortable sitting forward rather than lying on the back.

Biochemical Tests for Pancreatic Disease

Serological markers such as CA19-9 detect carbohydrate antigens expressed by mucus glycoproteins. When ducts of the pancreas are blocked, these mucus glycoproteins spill into the blood circulation and can be detected in very high levels in the blood. Hence, the very high levels of CA19-9 may indicate pancreatic tumor. However, the test is nonspecific and there are many other causes of elevated CA19-9. Any other mucus-secreting tumor or ascites may also cause a raised CA19-9. However, presence of raised CA19-9 would trigger the need for more radiological imaging of the pancreas.

Radiology

An ultrasound scan performed by a good operator in a non-gaseous abdomen can pick up pancreatic lesions. However, CT scans are more reliable. CT scans would show a pancreatic lesion and also help stage the lesion. Size of the lesion is perhaps less important than the invasion of the lesion into neighboring vascular structures like the superior mesenteric artery and portal vein, which would severely compromise the ability for the surgeon to do a curative resection.

When the pancreatic lesion is in the head of the pancreas, the patient often presents with jaundice as a result of obstruction of the common bile duct. Once again a CT scan is helpful in staging the disease and making a diagnosis. An endoscopic ultrasound is also very helpful in further staging of disease, especially when it is in the head or the neck of the pancreas. Lesions in the tail of the pancreas are less accessible to endoscopic ultrasound (Figs. 1.11 to 1.17).

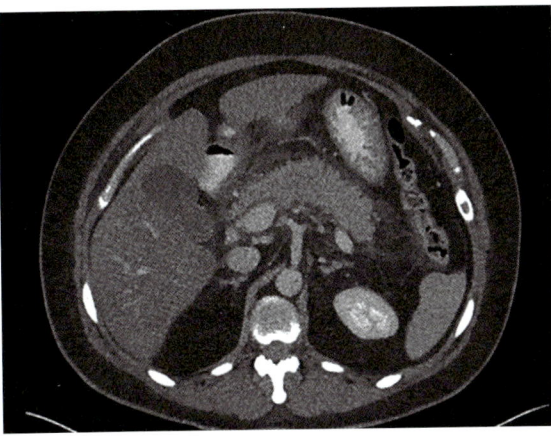

Fig. 1.11: Computed tomography of an inflamed swollen pancreas: This patient had azathioprine-induced pancreatitis.

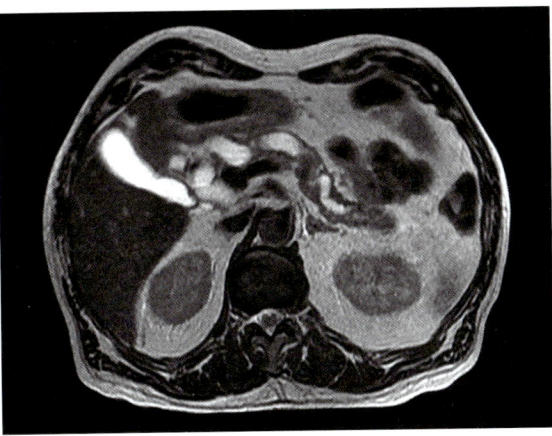

Fig. 1.12: Intraductal papillary mucinous neoplasm (IPMN) of the pancreas are potentially malignant intraductal epithelial neoplasms that are composed of mucin-producing columnar cells often present as incidental findings on scanning. The MRI shows a grossly dilated pancreatic duct.

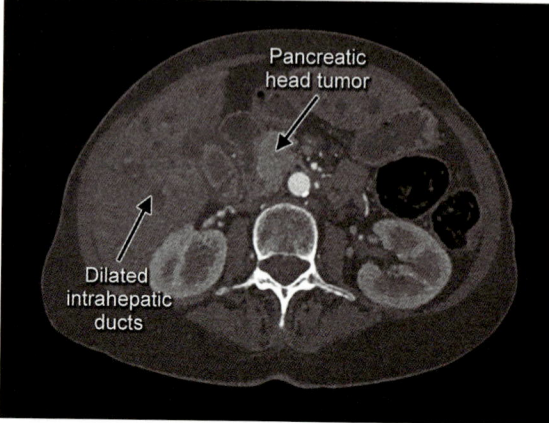

Fig. 1.13: Computed tomography scan showing dilated intrahepatic ducts and a pancreatic head tumor.

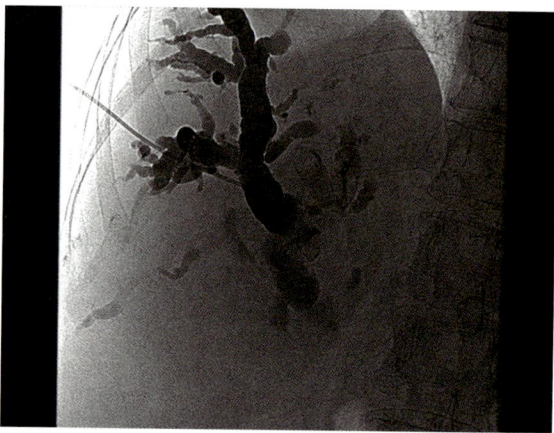

Fig. 1.14: Percutaneous transhepatic cholangiogram (PTC) showing dilated intrahepatic ducts and a tumor obstructing the lower end of common bile duct.

Is there an Intestinal Disease?

Pain arises from intestinal disease usually arises either from contractions of the intestine (colic) or due to distention of the bowel. Colicky-type abdominal pain can arise spontaneously as in IBS or as a result of an obstruction caused by a stricture. Because IBS is so common, in the absence of any "red flag" symptoms, it is wise to make a firm diagnosis of IBS rather than embark on expensive and sometimes unpleasant investigations. In patients without any of these alarming symptoms, a negative CRP, blood count and fecal calprotectin would exclude the majority of organic diseases and enables the physician to confidently make a diagnosis of IBS. A simple algorithm is found in Figure 1.2.

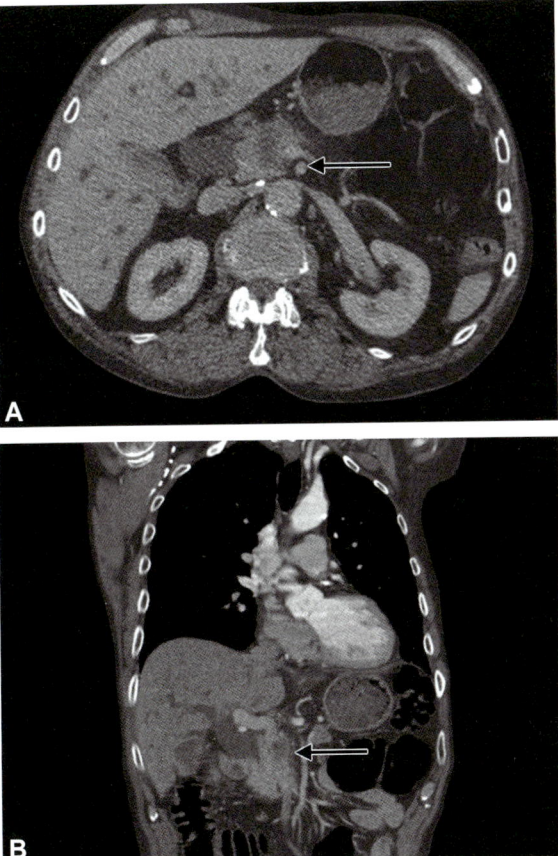

Figs. 1.15A and B: Pancreatic tumor with dilated intrahepatic ducts. (A) Transverse and (B) Coronal images of tumor.

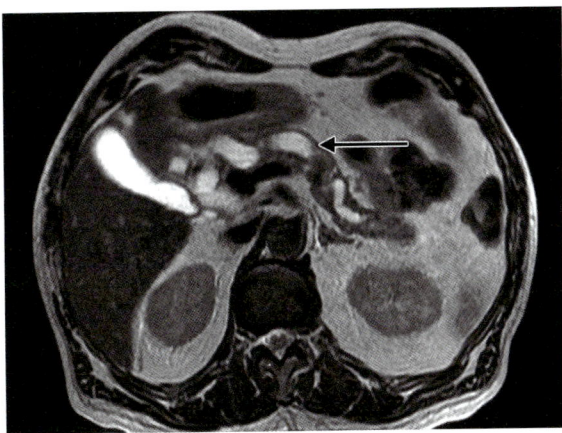

Fig. 1.16: Magnetic resonance imaging showing chronic pancreatitis with dilated pancreatic duct.

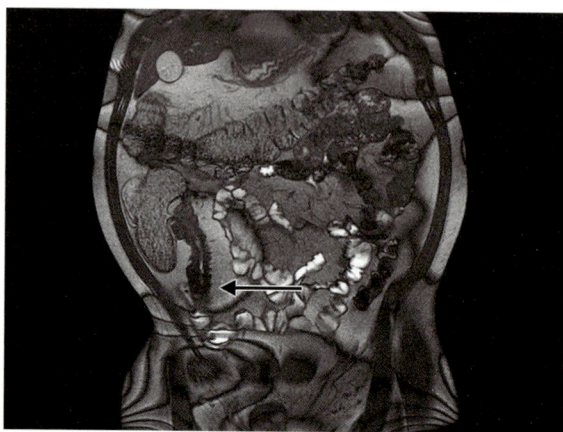

Fig. 1.17: Magnetic resonance imaging showing marked thickening of the terminal ileum with surrounding inflammation: This is typical of terminal ileal Crohn's disease.

Imaging

In a younger patient with symptoms of abdominal pain with weight loss, mild anemia or positive fecal calprotectin, always suspect inflammatory disease of the bowel like Crohn's disease. If there is associated rectal bleeding or diarrhea, it could suggest colonic involvement with inflammatory bowel disease, either ulcerative colitis or Crohn's disease. In general, ulcerative colitis, being a mucosal disease, does not result in abdominal pain except when there is a complication like perforation or megacolon. Crohn's disease being a transmural disease can cause irritation of the parietal peritoneum and therefore pain is often a predominant feature.

In the older patient presenting with any of these symptoms, the principal condition to exclude is colonic neoplasia. Some form of imaging is therefore necessary in both groups of patients.

Colonoscopy is by far the best imaging modality as it would pick up any colonic neoplasia and the majority of patients with colonic or ileocolonic inflammatory bowel disease. A skillful colonoscopist should be able to enter the terminal ileum and assess the terminal ileum in over 90% of patients. Inflammatory changes in the colon are very common in patients with Crohn's disease, even in those with predominant ileal disease. If the patient is unable to have a colonoscopy for whatever reason, then the alternative is CT colography or MRI scanning. In patients where colon cancer is being suspected, particularly the older age group, CT colography can be a useful alternative to colonoscopy. It may be an alternative in individuals for whom colonoscopy is deemed too invasive, especially in the frail elderly patient. There are limitations to CT colography. Polypoidal lesions can be difficult to differentiate from particulate feces and it is clearly not possible to carry out biopsies and histological examination of any lesions seen. Often when a lesion is suspected or found the individual will need a colonoscopy eventually. There is also an issue of radiation exposure and therefore colonoscopy is still regarded as the investigation of choice. MRI scanning is also valuable. It is particularly useful in detecting small bowel Crohn's disease, especially in parts where the colonoscope is unable to reach. A modified way of performing an MRI with the ingestion of a polyethylene glycol drink allows imaging of the small bowel with contrast (magnetic resonance enterography; MRE). This will pick up areas of intestinal stenosis caused by inflammation and also fissures and ulcerations of the mucosa. MRE also gives a good impression of the thickness of the bowel, another indication of infiltrative or inflammatory condition. A standard CT of the abdomen is also a valuable investigation. It has the advantage of being somewhat cheaper than MRI and it can show quite a lot of detail. It will also show the presence of abscess formation or diverticular disease of the colon. Finally, if lymphoma is suspected, a CT scan of the abdomen would pick up associated lymphadenopathy, which usually is generalized and may be associated with splenic enlargement (Figs. 1.17 to 1.21).

Is it Volvulus or Intussusception?

Occasionally, patients may have intermittent severe pain due to intermittent volvulus. If volvulus is suspected, a plain X-ray is often very helpful (Fig. 1.22). Gastric volvuluses can be picked up and are often associated with a large diaphragmatic defect and a chest/upper abdominal film would be quite revealing. A volvulus affecting the sigmoid would present with constipation and abdominal distention and often a large "coffee bean" shadow on

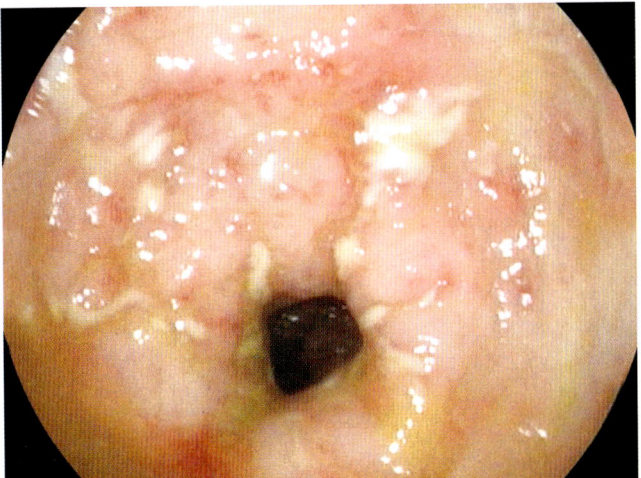

Fig. 1.18: Colonoscopic findings of deep fissuring ulcers with skip lesions favor a diagnosis of Crohn's disease.

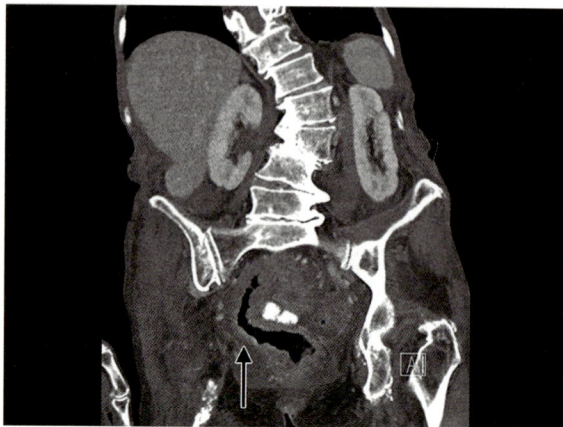

Fig. 1.19: Sigmoid inflammation. Thickened sigmoid colon clearly demonstrated by CT.

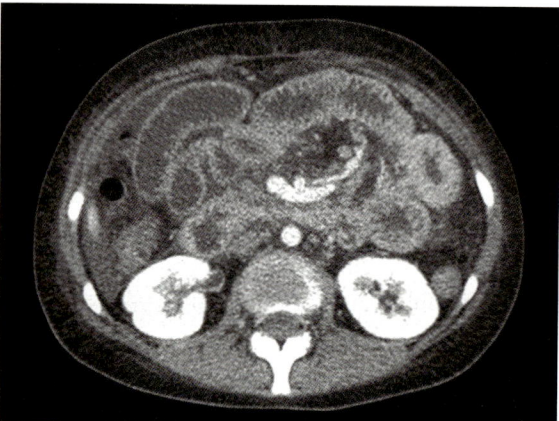

Fig. 1.20: Extensive mucosal inflammation and edema: This patient has raised peripheral eosinophil count and should alert the clinician to possible eosinophilic enteritis.

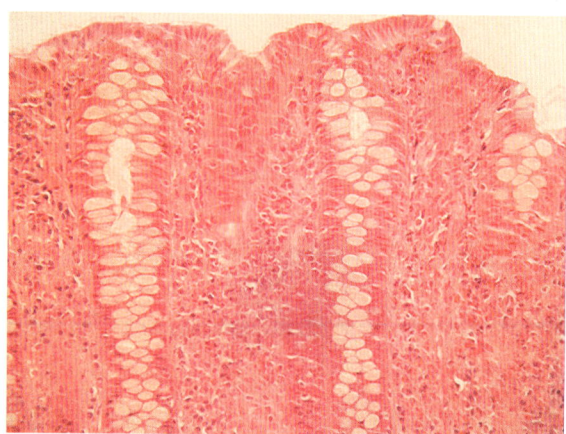

Fig. 1.21: Eosinophilic infiltration of colon suggests a diagnosis of eosinophilic enterocolitis.

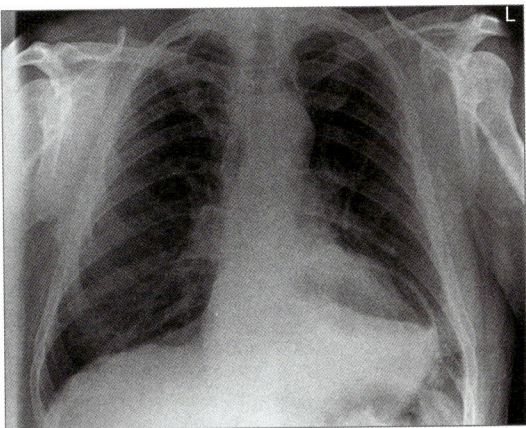

Fig. 1.22: Large hiatus hernia. Much of the stomach is in the chest.

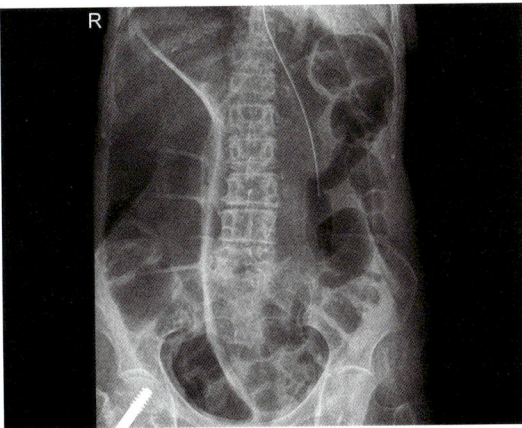

Fig. 1.23: Sigmoid volvulus. Massively dilated sigmoid colon giving the "coffee bean" sign.

the abdominal film is seen (Fig. 1.23). Both problems may be intermittent and may present acutely as a surgical emergency but sometimes may be chronic and persistent or even be asymptomatic (Figs. 1.24A and B).

Is it Mesenteric Ischemia?

Mesenteric Ischemia should be considered in an older patient. It can present acutely as an area of bowel infarction. This can occur after an episode of hypotension when areas of vascular watershed like the splenic flexure of the colon can become ischemic. Patients may present with pain, rectal bleeding with or without diarrhea. Acute intestinal infarction can also occur in patients with embolic disease like atrial fibrillation. Atheromatous diseases tend to present with chronic intestinal ischemia with a chronic pain often

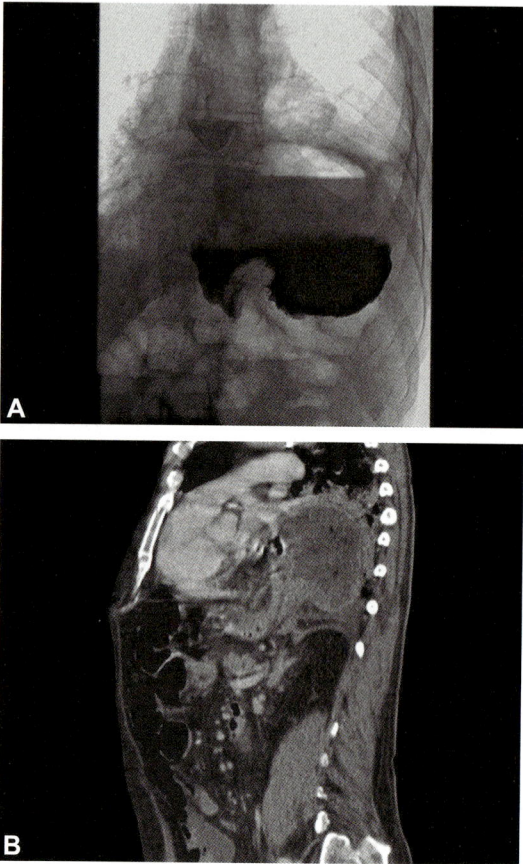

Figs. 1.24A and B: Gastric volvulus. (A) The gastrografin meal shows a gastric volvulus flipped along its axis (organo-axial volvulus); (B) CT image shows the same.

associated with food and eating, sometimes referred to as intestinal angina. These patients therefore reduce their food intake and can lose weight quite dramatically. A good history is the key. It is strongly associated with smoking and diabetes and they often have evidence of arteriopathy elsewhere, like peripheral vascular disease or ischemic heart disease. It can be extremely difficult to diagnose, CT may show calcified vascular atheroma. MRI angiography can be helpful in this situation, confirmation and treatment requires direct angiography and angioplasty can be attempted.

Is it Diverticular Disease?

Diverticulosis of the colon is extremely common. Like gallstones, it is easy to attribute symptoms to diverticular disease but they may not necessarily be the cause of the patient's complaint. Diverticular disease is easily picked up on barium enemas, abdominal CTs or colonoscopy. Typically, diverticulosis causes few symptoms. However, when they get inflamed (diverticulitis) they can cause discomfort, pain and altered bowel habit. The pain is usually in the left iliac fossa as the commonest site of diverticular disease is in the sigmoid colon.

Is there an Underlying Metabolic Disease?

Metabolic diseases are rare. However, physicians should always be alert to a possibility in unusual presentation of organic diseases suspected and none found. Hypercalcemia and porphyria are metabolic diseases that can present as abdominal pain. In the case of hypercalcemia, serum calcium is easily checked by chemical profile. Hence, it is important to cast an eye on the calcium level when attending to a patient with abdominal pain. In hypercalcemia, pain can be caused by acute as attacks of acute pancreatitis or chronic pain due to dyspepsia or ulcer disease caused by hypersecretion of acid. This is due to the raised serum gastrin found in patients with hypercalcemia. The helpful *aide memoire*: "stones, bones and abdominal groans" summarizes hypercalcemia with renal stones, bone lesions and abdominal pain. Hyperlipidemia syndromes may also present with acute abdominal pain because it can cause attacks of acute pancreatitis.

Porphyria can cause abdominal pain. Acute intermittent porphyria, porphyria variegata but not porphyria cutanea tarda, can cause acute intermittent episodes of severe abdominal pain rather than chronic pain. There may be neurological complications such as behavioral disturbances, epilepsy, coma or peripheral neuropathy. During an acute attack of hyponatremia; hypertension and uremia are common. Other rare causes of abdominal pain include lead poisoning, C1 esterase inhibitor insufficiency, familial Mediterranean fever and neurological conditions like multiple sclerosis and peripheral neuropathy. Abdominal pain is also a common problem in patients with longstanding diabetes. They are at increased risk of gallstones, duodenal ulcer disease, intestinal vascular insufficiency and pancreatitis.

A high index of suspicion and the specific diagnostic test is required to make the correct diagnosis.

Is there an Occult Malignant Disease?

If the patient remains unwell with persistent pain, there is always a lingering worry that malignant disease may have been missed. The next step would be a review of all the investigations carried out to date making sure that there are no gaps left unplugged. Abdominal CT scan is probably the best investigation to exclude intra-abdominal malignancies and if in doubt should be reviewed by an experienced radiologist. Colonoscopy remains the best investigation for colonic neoplasia but occasionally it may be missed because of a bad prep or incomplete examination. Hence, a review of the colonoscopy and a repeat procedure by an experienced endoscopist should be considered if there is a high degree of clinical suspicion. If there is still some doubt, then a "wait and

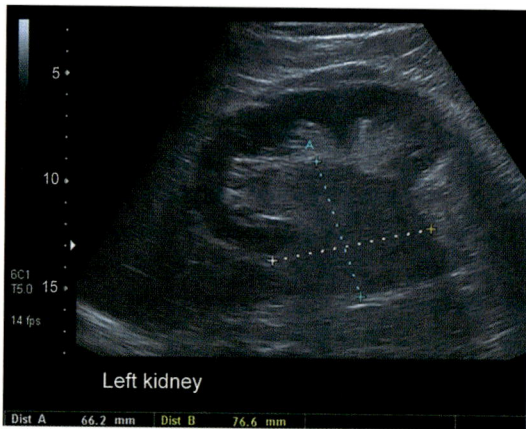

Fig. 1.25: Renal cancer: This is most often picked up incidentally by ultrasound.

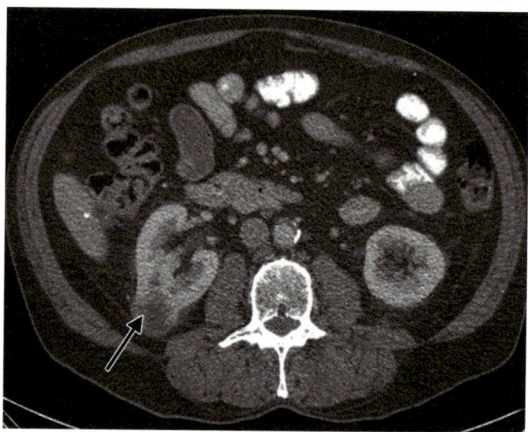

Fig. 1.26: Renal cell cancer on CT scanning.

see policy" or an interval CT scan, perhaps 2 or 3 months down the line would be helpful, but with modern imaging it is rare to miss lesions unless they are extremely small or elusive. Finally, in patients where the diagnosis remains elusive and the suspicion is still high, a laparoscopy may be considered, but it would be unusual to resort to such invasive measures (Figs. 1.25 and 1.26).

Is it Endometriosis?

Lower abdominal and pelvic pain associated with hemorrhagic phase of the menstrual cycle is suggestive of endometriosis. Up to 25% of these patients may have bowel involvement and that often results in abdominal pain. The endometriosis tends to occur on the serosal surface and bleeding into the gut is really quite rare. Endometriosis can cause stricture and adhesions and sometimes mistaken for neoplastic disease or Crohn's disease.

Laparoscopy usually is diagnostic and treatment with cauterization is possible laparoscopically.

CONDITIONS CAUSING CHRONIC OR RECURRENT ABDOMINAL PAIN: NATURAL HISTORY AND MANAGEMENT

Irritable Bowel Syndrome

Natural History

Irritable bowel syndrome should be considered as one of a group of functional GI conditions that occur throughout the elementary tract. It is by far the commonest of the functional GI diseases. It can be very varied in presentation and can mimic serious organic diseases. It is very troublesome to the sufferer and can be challenging to manage.

Symptoms: The cardinal symptom that most patients complain of being abdominal pain. There may be continuous dull ache but most frequently it is a colicky-type abdominal pain that comes as spasms lasting only a few minutes or several hours. The site of the pain can be very variable, often flitting, but sometimes predominantly in an area typically the left iliac fossa or the right iliac fossa. When asked to point where the pain is, patients often move their hands in a circular fashion over the abdomen suggesting a varied or diffuse site. Along with the pain, the two other principal symptoms are abdominal bloating/distention and a change in the bowel habit. This can vary from predominant constipation to predominant diarrhea or a mixture of constipation alternating with diarrhea. Definitions of IBS have been proffered and it can be quite difficult to pin down precisely. For the purposes of clinical trials, strict definitions are required and several have been devised. The Rome III criteria (Rome Foundation for Functional GI Diseases) included recurrent abdominal pain or discomfort for 3 days out of a month in the past 3 months associated with two or more symptoms which include:

- Improvement with defecation
- Onset associated with change in stool frequency
- Onset associated with change in stool form.

This definition is rather loose and all-encompassing and has since been replaced by Rome IV in 2017. NICE (National Institute of Clinical Excellence) offered an alternative, simpler definition that is more suitable for everyday clinical use and the definition is:

Abdominal pain/discomfort relieved by defecation or associated with altered stool frequency/form plus 2 or more of:

- Altered stool passage
- Abdominal bloating/distention
- Symptoms made worse by eating
- Passage of mucus.

From a clinical point of view, the patients presenting with the classic pattern of abdominal pain associated with bloating and a change in bowel habit are usually easy to pick out and patients with predominant constipation or alternating constipation and diarrhea probably require no further investigation. However, patient with persistent diarrhea would probably benefit further investigation to detect cases of small intestinal bacterial overgrowth, bile salt diarrhea and microcytic/collagenous colitis.

Psychology: Anxious obsessional patients are certainly more likely to consult a doctor if they develop IBS, but the psychological aspects of this condition are probably over emphasized. Many patients who are psychologically normal to have this syndrome. It is true that patients will often bring out stress as a major trigger for their symptoms. However, it would be a mistake if the physician overemphasized that aspect and deprive the patient of simple treatments that might improve their symptoms and overly focus on the psychological aspects. Suggesting that the condition is all in the mind is likely to upset the patient and create barriers between physician and patient.

Epidemiology: A survey has shown that over 14% of apparently healthy British subjects have IBS by the ROME 1 criteria. Furthermore, over half the patients attending British gastroenterology clinics have a predominant functional bowel problem. Although 65% are women, an increasing number of young men also suffer from this condition. In many of these patients, the problems are longstanding and when questioned, these patients would often have a very long history starting from early adulthood or childhood.

Etiology and Pathogenesis: This syndrome has many complex and contributory factors. Looking at the predominant symptoms in turn.

Abdominal Pain: The mechanism of abdominal pain is complex. There is good evidence that patients with IBS have increased visceral sensitivity. Inflating a balloon in the rectum of a patient showed that they experienced discomfort at lower volumes than normal subjects. There is also evidence that patients with IBS handle pain abnormally. This probably occurs at the modulation level in the spinal cord. In patients with postinfective IBS, there is also microinflammation and inflammatory cells may release pain causing chemicals at the nerve endings.

Bloating: Bloating is a very common symptom of IBS. Its etiology is also quite complex. There is evidence for abnormal gas handling. The tone of the bowel may be altered causing gas to be trapped in parts of the bowel and there may be altered gas production as well. Altered gas production may be due to bacterial fermentation processes. In patients where there is small bowel bacterial overgrowth, there is increased gas production in the small bowel. Patients who are intolerant of carbohydrates and also with celiac disease may also have abnormal gas production due to poorly digested sugars fueling colonic bacterial fermentation. Furthermore, ingestion of fermentable carbohydrates is also a possible source of gas. Patients with slow gut transit found in those with predominant constipation will also get abdominal distention from fecal loading. Finally, some hormones, particularly estrogens, can cause abdominal bloating. However, all the causes of gas production above does not account for the degree of distention that many patients display. It also does not account for how quickly the distention can occur and regress in the course of a day. It is now known that the most important contributor to bloating is phrenic dyssynergia. This occur when the diaphragm is contracted unconsciously, and simultaneously the abdominal wall muscles to relax. The cause for this is still unknown (Fig. 1.27).

Change in Bowel Habit: A change in bowel habit is characteristic of IBS. Thus, IBS may be classified as being IBS-D when there is predominant diarrhea, IBS-C when there is predominant constipation and IBS-M when there is an alternating or mixed picture. The etiology is complex and probably multifactorial. The change in motility of the gut may be a result of delayed gastric emptying, small bowel or colonic transit changes. This is often triggered by food or emotion. In a number of patients, there is also evidence of small bowel bacterial overgrowth.

The stool type correlates very well with gut motility and the Bristol Stool Chart has become a very useful visual aid in clinics for patients to point out which type of stools they have. Stool types 1 and 2 (Fig. 1.28) are associated with constipation and the gut transit is slow, whereas patients with Bristol types 6 and 7 have rapid gut transit and diarrhea.

Postinfective Irritable Bowel Syndrome: In a number of patients presenting with IBS, there is a clear history of an infective episode prior to the onset of IBS symptoms. There will be a history of some kind of infectious diarrhea whether or not a pathogen becomes cultivated. During the acute episode, there is usually diarrhea plus vomiting, rather than diarrhea alone. The patients then

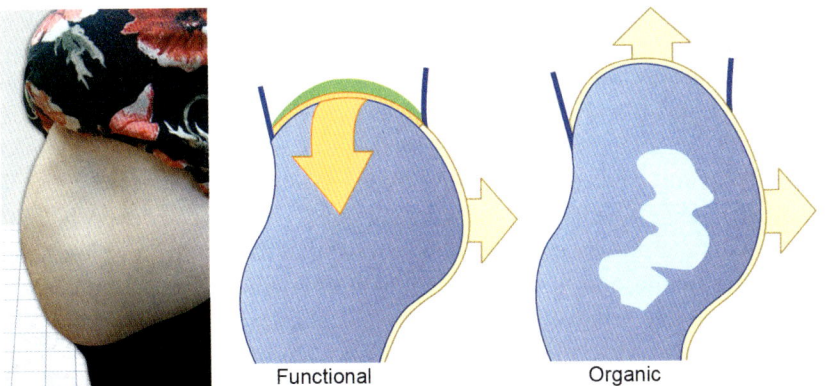

Fig. 1.27: Bloating: It is a combination of gas as diaphragmatic contraction and relaxation of abdominal wall muscles.

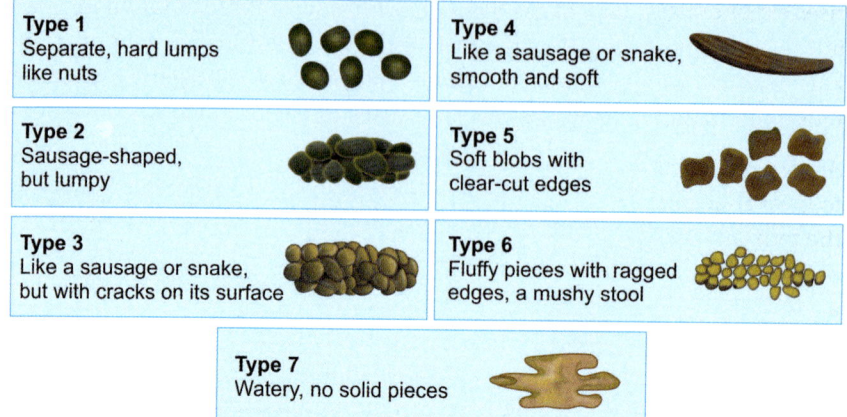

Fig. 1.28: Change in bowel habit.

start having episodes of the typical IBS that lasts long after the acute episode. There is a predominance of diarrhea (IBS-D) as opposed to the constipation or alternating type. There is often a higher anxiety score prior or during the infection. Patients often acquire the infection while travelling, often on holiday or away from home.

Algorithm for Diagnosing Irritable Bowel Syndrome: It is important to make a firm diagnosis of IBS early without recourse to complex and unpleasant investigations. NICE has issued a set of guidelines that are quite helpful. If the patients do not have alarm symptoms and have the typical symptoms outlined above, then a firm diagnosis of IBS can be made. The alarm symptoms include:
- Age (>40)
- Strong family history of colorectal cancer/IBD
- Rectal bleeding
- Anemia
- Weight loss
- Abdominal mass.

In this group, only a simple noninvasive test is required. Blood tests including a full blood count, biochemistry, CRP and thyroid function test along with celiac antibodies can be carried out. Stool tests, including fecal calprotectin and culture if there is the reason to suspect an infective cause. If diarrhea is predominant, a hydrogen or methane breath test can be very helpful. This detects the presence of small bowel bacterial overgrowth that ferments glucose or lactulose and releases hydrogen or methane in the breath. The test is simple and relatively cost-effective. Fecal calprotectin or lactoferrin is emerging as a very helpful test in this situation. Calprotectin and lactoferrin are released by inflammatory cells into the GI tract and this is excreted in the feces and easily detected. When there is inflammation, the level of fecal calprotectin rises exponentially. Laboratory standards vary, but any fecal calprotectin over 50 μg/g of feces is usually indicative of possible inflammatory bowel disease. However, a negative calprotectin does not exclude other organic diseases or indeed Crohn's disease in remission. A simple algorithm is shown in Figure 1.2.

Abnormal Bile Salt Handling: Nearly 30% of patients with IBS have been found to have abnormal bile salt handling. When bowel salts are not reabsorbed in the terminal ileum then some gets into the colon and that irritates the colon and can cause diarrhea-predominant symptoms. It is possible to carry out a SeHCAT scan. This, however, can be quite expensive. Empirical treatment with cholestyramine is safe and cheap and should be tried in patients with diarrhea-predominant IBS.

Often doubt still exists as to whether or not the patient has inflammatory bowel disease and probably the single most useful investigation in this situation is to perform a colonoscopy. For patients with diarrhea-predominant symptoms, inflammatory bowel disease can be difficult to exclude. Patients with microcytic and collagenous colitis can be very difficult to diagnose without endoscopic examination and may have negative fecal calprotectin and ultimately can only be diagnosed with biopsies, particularly of the right colon.

Management

Reassurance: The most important part of management of IBS is reassurance. Make a firm diagnosis and explain that it is a benign condition. The mechanisms of pain and altered bowel habit in a healthy intestine should be explained simply and clearly to the patient. It should be made clear that the doctor understands the severity and genuine nature of the patient's symptoms and that the patient can be reassured that the condition is not harmful and the frequency and severity of symptoms would diminish with time. Treating the patient dismissively as a neurotic will lead the patient to assume that symptoms have not been taken sufficiently seriously. This will increase any cancer phobia and the patient will almost certainly seek a second opinion.

Having established a rapport, the physician should look at exploring some of the triggers. If there is evidence of an infective trigger, then probiotics may be proffered although clinical trial evidence for its use is sketchy. If there is a degree of stress or anxiety involved, that should be addressed at a suitable time. Other psychological treatments like hypnotherapy and counseling have a place if available.

Dietary Advice: Dietary advice or dietetic referral may be helpful. It is directed at specific symptoms.

Constipation: Patients with predominant constipation should be encouraged to eat more foods containing soluble fibers. This is found in many foods like fruit and cereals.

Diarrhea: Diarrhea can be more difficult to treat with dietary measures. Avoidance of certain foods like dairy and gluten may be important. Even patients without celiac disease may have poor carbohydrate handling and gluten intolerance and it is well worth trialing them on a gluten avoidance diet.

Bloating: Foods that produce a lot of gas are the ones that are fermentable. A group of foods known as FODMAP (Fermentable Oligo-Di-Mono-saccharides and Polyols) are shown to produce more gas and therefore abdominal distention. Avoidance of these foods can be difficult as they are very varied but a session with a dietitian can be very helpful.

Pharmacological Treatments: Once a patient is reassured that the condition is benign, it is important then to explain that you have means of treating the specific symptoms. Abdominal pain can be treated with antispasmodics like mebeverine, hyoscine and alverine. If the pains are spasmodic and episodic then patients can have these drugs on demand rather than on a maintenance fashion. If the pain is more constant then treatment with a small dose of a tricyclic like amitriptyline has been shown to be effective although tricyclics tend to cause constipation and therefore best avoided in patients with constipation-predominant irritable bowel. Conversely, tricyclics can be very helpful in patients with diarrhea-predominant IBS. An alternative to tricyclics are the selective serotonin reuptake inhibitors (SSRIs). They tend to cause diarrhea probably a better drug to try on patients with constipation-predominant IBS. It is important to emphasize that you are using the drugs to control the symptom not because you think they are depressed as such.

Newer drugs have been recently evaluated for use in IBS with constipation. For IBS-C linaclotide have recently been introduced. A longer discussion of these drugs on constipation is in the Chapter 4. For IBS-D, symptomatic treatment with loperamide is helpful and new agents like eluxadoline have been recently approved for this indication. Rifaximin, a poorly absorbed antibiotic, has also been approved for IBS-D (*see* Chapter 3).

Patients with evidence or suspicion of bile salt malabsorption could be given a trial with cholestyramine. Bile excretion is maximal in mornings, so this is best given first thing in the morning, 30 minutes before breakfast. If there is evidence of small intestinal bacterial overgrowth, antibiotic therapy, notably with rifaximin, could be given.

Duodenal Ulcer

Natural History

Diagnosis: The principal means of diagnosing duodenal ulcer disease is endoscopy. However, if patients present with dyspeptic symptoms it is not unreasonable to perform a test for *H. pylori* on the onset. The noninvasive methods of testing for *H. pylori* are cheap and that could be serology, breath testing or fecal antigen testing. The latter has increasingly gained acceptance as being both sensitive and specific. The presence of *H. pylori* in a symptomatic patient would justify *H. pylori* eradication. This "test and treat" method has gained general acceptance in recent years.

Symptoms: The symptoms of duodenal ulcer disease can be rather nonspecific. Duodenal ulcers may be completely asymptomatic and it is not uncommon for patients to be admitted to hospital with a bleeding ulcer and give no history of previous dyspepsia. The most common symptom is epigastric pain that wakes the patient at night and periodic pain. Periodic pain refers to relapses of pain lasting several days or weeks interspersed with pain-free periods for weeks or months. Less reliable association is relief of pain with antacids or food. Major complications of duodenal ulcers are perforation and bleeding and in the elderly and patients with multiple comorbidities like cardiac, renal failure and malignancy, it carries a significant mortality rate.

Epidemiology: Previous epidemiological studies have shown that as many as 9% of women and 12% of men have been told they have a diagnosis of duodenal ulcer disease at some point. However, the discovery that *H. pylori* is a major cause of duodenal ulcer disease has led to eradication of the bacteria. This has completely altered the natural history of the disease from a recurrent condition to permanent cure. Furthermore, as the prevalence of *H. pylori* infection decreased in many Western nations, so has the prevalence of duodenal ulcer disease. However, there is an increase in incidence of nonsteroidal-induced peptic ulcer disease particularly in elderly patients. Smoking is strongly associated with duodenal ulcer disease as is alcohol.

Etiology and Pathogenesis: *H. pylori* infection and NSAIDs are the main etiological causes for duodenal ulcer disease. The mucosa of the stomach and duodenum need to defend itself against the effects of pepsin and acid. Mechanisms in which there is increased acid and pepsin action and reduced defenses by the duodenal mucosa would result in mucosal ulceration and breakdown. Defects in the healing and repair mechanisms are also contributory factors. Smoking and stress can elevate basal acid output, reduce mucus synthesis and inhibit healing.

Drugs like the anti-inflammatory drugs and aspirin cause ulceration either by direct toxic effects or inhibit prostaglandin synthesis by binding on cyclo-oxygenase (COX) active site (specifically COX-1). Aspirin even in low doses can cause ulceration by direct toxic chemical effects on the mucosa itself. Nonsteroidals drugs, however, tend to act by inhibiting prostaglandin synthesis. Prostaglandin depletion causes an increase in acid secretion,

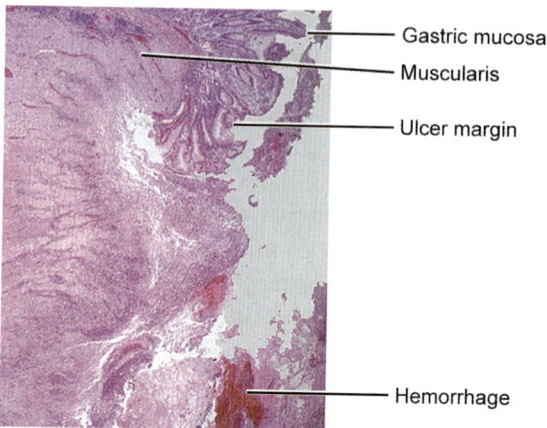

Fig. 1.29: Histology of gastric ulcer margin.

decreased mucin production and a decrease in bicarbonate secretions, all factors vital in promoting ulcer formation. Prostaglandin is also important in epithelial cell healing and therefore nonsteroidal drugs also reduce the ability of the mucosa to repair itself. Additionally, the analgesic effects of nonsteroidal drugs may account for the fact that many nonsteroidal-induced duodenal ulcer disease remain silent and may not present until bleeding or perforation occurs (Fig. 1.29).

Helicobacter pylori: *H. pylori* remains the major cause for duodenal ulcer disease and worldwide it is a massive health problem. It is strongly associated with duodenal ulcer disease but the most convincing evidence is the fact that when eradication of the bacteria is successfully achieved a cure results. However, the bacterium is very common and the majority of people harboring this bacteria in the stomach do not have duodenal ulcer disease or come to any apparent harm. The bacterium is a gram-negative rod and resides in the deep portions of the mucus, generally in the gastric mucosa. It is uniquely adapted to this hostile environment. It has multiple flagella that helps in motility and adhesion and produces very strong urea enzyme. This produces ammonia from urea which is alkaline and helps to neutralize any acid diffusing into the mucus layer.

The infection is probably acquired during childhood and spreads in areas and times of overcrowding. Initially, the bacterium tends to inhabit the antrum of the stomach and over time tend to migrate proximally. Apart from duodenal ulcer disease, *H. pylori* infection is credited to cause gastric ulcers, MALT lymphomas and gastric cancer. It is still not understood as to how the bacterium can cause the diverse pathology and yet, in a large number of individuals, it causes no symptoms or pathology at all. It is likely to be a combination of bacterial and host factors. The bacteria may have genetic determinants that result in increased pathogenicity. This includes

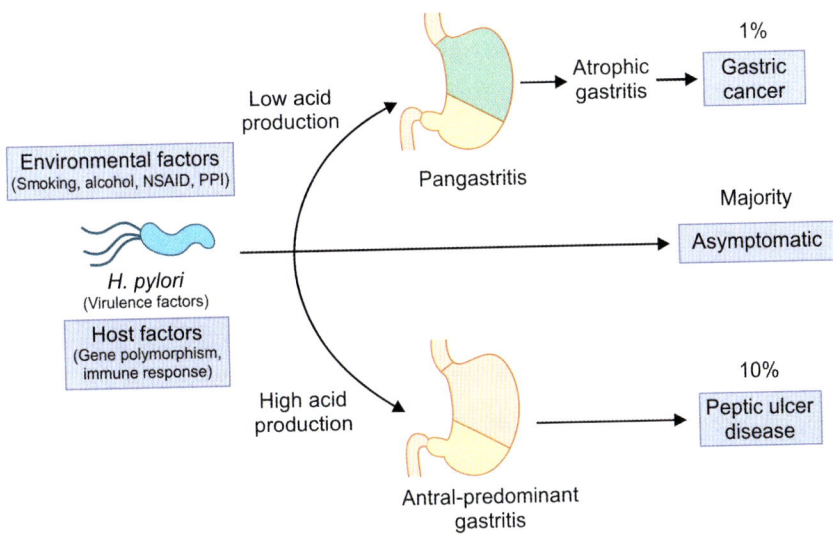

Fig. 1.30: Putative pathogenesis of *H. pylori* diseases.

its ability to produce certain enzymes like VacA and CagA or may have adhesins which facilitate attachment of the bacteria to the gastric epithelial cells. Amongst host factors may be the subject's ability to mount an inflammatory response and the specific site of the stomach where the bacteria tend to colonize.

Patients who predominantly have antral inflammation would lead the antral G cells to produce high levels of gastrin via the loss of negative inhibition from the D cells in the antrum. The result is an elevated gastrin level that stimulates the acid secreting parietal cell to secrete more acid. Patients who have predominantly body and fundus infection with *H. pylori* may find that the parietal cells themselves get affected and acid level output may actually be reduced. This may lead, in the long term, to chronic atrophic gastritis eventually leading to intestinal metaplasia, dysplasia and leading to gastric cancer. In the majority of patients with pangastritis, the infection tends to be non-pathogenic and therefore the bacterium inhabits the individual without producing any symptoms or disease (Fig. 1.30).

Management of Duodenal Ulceration

The management of duodenal ulcers has altered dramatically over the last 30 or 40 years. Operations frequently performed for duodenal ulcers in the past have given way to highly effective acid suppressing drugs like H2 antagonists and then followed rapidly by even more powerful acid suppressants like PPIs. *H. pylori* eradication has changed the natural history of the disease. However, increased bacterial resistances to antibiotics have hindered effective *H. pylori* eradication in many parts of the world.

H2 Antagonists and Proton Pump Inhibitors: H2 antagonists like cimetidine and ranitidine are safe and effective drugs for reducing gastric acid secretion and are now found in many over-the-counter medications for dyspepsia. They do heal duodenal ulcers by suppressing acid by inhibiting the H2 receptors, one of the three receptors that cause the parietal cell to secrete acid. The other two receptors are acetylcholine receptor and gastrin receptor. Hence, it only partially inhibits the excretion of acid. The final pathway is the migration of the "proton pump" which is ATPase. This migrates to the canaliculus membrane and the pumping of a hydrogen ion (Proton) accompanied by potassium chloride that leads to the production of hydrochloric acid. This is pumping against a huge concentration gradient and acquires energy that is supplied in the form of the breakdown of ATP into ADP.

Inhibitors of the proton pump include omeprazole, esomeprazole, lansoprazole, pantoprazole and rabeprazole. Thus, almost complete blockage of acid secretion is the result. These drugs also have a long biological life as the inhibition is irreversible and parietal cells have to manufacture new proton pumps to replace those blocked. Ranitidine in clinical trials has shown to heal up to 70% of duodenal ulcers at 8 weeks whereas PPIs would heal duodenal ulcers at > 90% at 8 weeks. However, unless the underlying cause for the ulcers (e.g. *H. pylori* and nonsteroidal drugs) is removed then the ulcers would tend to recur (Fig. 1.31).

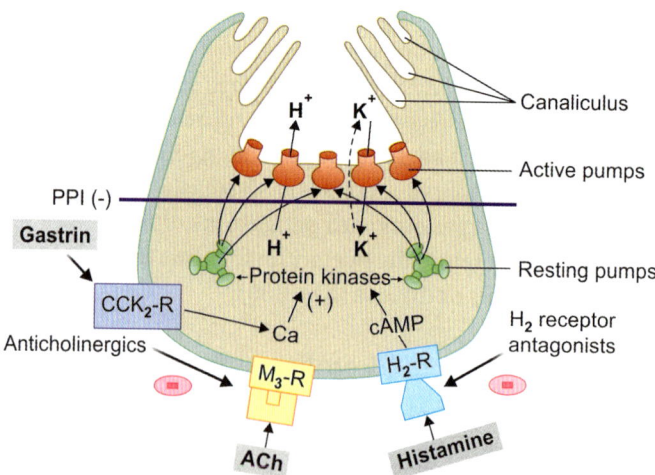

Fig. 1.31: Parietal cell function: The gastric parietal cells are the producers of acid in the stomach. Gastrin acetylcholine and histamine receptors are present in the inner membrane where hormonal (gastrin), neural (vagus nerve releasing acetylcholine) and inflammatory (histamine) stimuli activate the proton pump ATPase. Inhibition of this enzyme stops parietal cell acid production.

Anti-Helicobacter Therapy: Eradication of *H. pylori* will result in curing of *H. pylori*-associated duodenal ulcer disease. As this accounts worldwide for the majority of duodenal ulcer cases effective *H. pylori* eradication is much sought after. The typical regime would be a "triple therapy," which comprises of a PPI like omeprazole or lansoprazole with two antibiotics typically a combination of either clarithromycin or amoxicillin or metronidazole or tinidazole. The treatment is usually carried out for 14 days. Shorter regimes tend to be less effective and promote bacterial resistance. Even with 14-day triple therapy eradication may not exceed 70% and may be even lower in parts of the world where antibiotic resistance is common. Hence, in refractory cases other treatment strategies have been sought. One strategy is quadruple therapy with the addition of bismuth in the form of tripotassium dicitratobismuthate. Other regimes have also been recently trialed. One particular promising regime is "sequential therapy" that usually takes the form of 5 days of lansoprazole and amoxicillin followed by 5 days of lansoprazole, clarithromycin and metronidazole.

Failure to Heal: A repeat endoscopy to check for healing is not usually necessary. Effective *H. pylori* eradication can be checked either by using urea breath tests or fecal antigen tests, both of which are equally reliable. However, if the patient remains symptomatic it may be necessary to re-endoscope such patients. If patients are compliant with treatment and *H. pylori* eradication is confirmed then one would also have to question whether patients have been taking aspirin or nonsteroidal agents. Rare conditions such as Zollinger–Ellison syndrome should also be considered. Effective treatment with *H. pylori* eradication should result with an effective cure. However, in some patients the *H. pylori* may be resistant to therapy. In a few patients, it would be necessary to be placed on maintenance therapy with PPIs.

Surgery: Surgery for duodenal ulcer disease thankfully is extremely rare nowadays. Operations are usually now reserved for complications such as bleeding and perforation. The operations performed are mainly of historic interest but there remain some patients from the "pre-*Helicobacter* discovery era" who may have had such procedures carried out on them (Fig. 1.32).

Duodenitis

Duodenitis is often reported in endoscopy reports for endoscopies carried out for dyspeptic symptoms. However, there is a very poor correlation between symptoms and endoscopic appearances. Even endoscopic and histological appearances are poorly correlated. Many asymptomatic patients may have duodenitis as incidental endoscopic findings. However, it is clear that *H. pylori* infection in the duodenum often leads to gastric metaplasia. This occurs when gastric type mucosa starts proliferating in the duodenum.

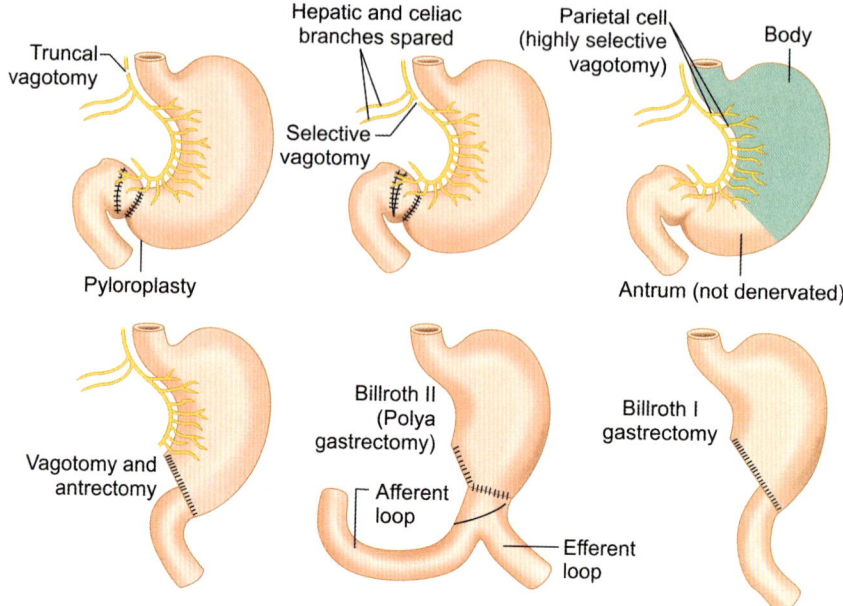

Fig. 1.32: Surgical procedures for ulcer diseases.

Gastric metaplasia may also be caused by increased acid secretion. Non-steroidal drugs and aspirin are also implicated in causing duodenitis. Duodenitis is also strongly correlated with smoking and patients with poor nutritional intake.

When widespread duodenal inflammation occurs, it is also important to consider Crohn's disease; celiac disease; Whipple's disease and small bowel lymphoma. Biopsies would be indicated if the endoscopist is unsure of the exact pathology or if these conditions are suspected. Usually, however, the inflammation is mild, confined to the first part of duodenum and is usually of little consequence to patients.

Non-ulcer Dyspepsia/Functional Dyspepsia

Natural History

The term "non-ulcer dyspepsia" is unsatisfactory with different meanings to different clinicians. The term is now largely replaced by the more useful term of "functional dyspepsia". Fundamentally, it is presence of symptoms, such as:
- Epigastric pain
- Nausea
- Bloating
- Belching
- Fat intolerance

Chronic or Recurrent Abdominal Pain

- Heartburn
- Early satiety.

When endoscopy is carried out it is usually normal and is thus regarded as a functional condition. There is evidence of poor pyloric relaxation and gastric emptying and there is also evidence of visceral hypersensitivity with pain or intolerance when the stomach is distended with fluid.

Management

Due to variety of symptoms and the benign nature of the condition treatment is largely symptomatic. However, it is important to exclude *H. pylori* infection and if *H. pylori* is found then it is reasonable to give a trial of *H. pylori* eradication as previously discussed.

The management of functional dyspepsia includes the following:
- If a patient has endoscopy negative upper abdominal pain and no other organic causes found either through history or by ultrasound then a diagnosis of functional abdominal pain should be made and treatment is more in line with IBS with efforts directed to control of pain and bloating. Apart from tricyclics, prokinetic agents like prochlorperazine and metoclopramide can also be helpful in this situation. The latter two drugs carry a risk of extrapyramidal side effects. Due to risks of cardiac complications domperidone use in this condition is not encouraged.
- If heartburn is a predominant symptom, then the use of antacids and other antireflux treatments is perfectly reasonable. Use of PPI has also been shown to marginally improve symptoms in this group of patients. Even in the absence of endoscopic appearance of esophagitis, reflux can occur.
- Diet would also play a role. Diets containing high levels of fat tend to inhibit gastric emptying and can encourage symptoms like bloating.

Zollinger–Ellison Syndrome

Natural History

In Zollinger–Ellison syndrome, there is duodenal ulceration due to increased acid production. The ulcers are multiple and usually in the distal duodenum and even in the jejunum. This syndrome is rare and probably accounts for <1 in 10,000 of all patients with duodenal ulceration but it is often left undiagnosed.

Gastrin is produced by the G cells of the gastric antrum. In Zollinger–Ellison syndrome, excessive gastrin is produced by non-beta islet cell tumors of the pancreas or duodenum. This is not under the natural feedback mechanism and leads to constant over stimulation of the parietal cells that leads to overproduction of acid. This results in hypertrophy of the gastric body and a high basal acid output. The acid is dumped into the duodenum and upper duodenum and causes ulceration.

The tumor is malignant in about 65% of patients and about 25% of tumors are sited in duodenal wall and may be very tiny and difficult to diagnose.

However, the majority of the tumors will be found in the duodenum or the neck of the pancreas or even the porta hepatis.

Acid also inactivates pancreatic lipases and results in fat malabsorption. Diarrhea is therefore a very common symptom along with the classic symptoms of duodenal ulceration.

Diagnosis of Zollinger–Ellison Syndrome

Fasting gastrin levels is the best screening test for Zollinger-Ellison syndrome. It is also important to check the calcium levels as it may be part of a multiple endocrine neoplasia Type 1 syndrome (MEN1). Gastric acid secretion tests are rarely performed these days. In doubtful cases, a provocation test using secretin and a measurement of serum gastrin can also be helpful to make the diagnosis.

Imaging with CT scan would be necessary to locate the tumor but it is only possible to locate the tumor in 50% of the patients. Endoscopic ultrasound can also be very useful. Frequently tumors are <1 cm and easily missed on scanning. Somatostatin receptor scintigraphy (octreotide scan) is the best imaging modality. It uses radiolabeled somatostatin analog that binds to the receptors found on these tumors (Fig. 1.33). Finally, endoscopy which shows unusually severe ulceration of duodenum should alert the clinician to consider this diagnosis.

Management of Zollinger–Ellison Syndrome

The management depends on the operability of the primary secreting tumor. If it is operable then it would be considered curative. Medical therapy for controlling gastric acid output is achieved using PPIs often at higher than usual doses. In patients where surgical resection is not possible, palliative therapy with chemotherapy, interferon, and octreotide may be helpful but the response to these agents in most studies has been poor.

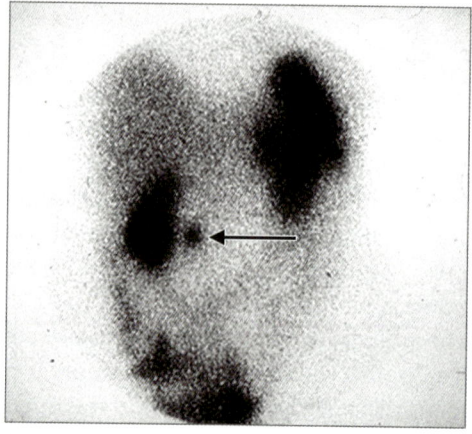

Fig. 1.33: Octreotide scan. This shows a hot spot in the pancreas from a neuroendocrine tumor. Similar hot spot may be be seen in Zollinger–Ellison syndrome.

Benign Gastric Ulcer

Natural History

Symptoms: The symptoms of benign gastric ulceration are highly variable and can often be vague. Pain is usually but not always present in the upper abdomen. Usually the pain is less prominent in benign gastric ulceration than in the duodenal ulcers. Response to food is also variable, while half of the patients may get relief from eating another third may actually have pain exacerbated by food. Other symptoms include epigastric discomfort, belching, nausea and water-brash (a sudden outpouring of saliva). Patients may present with complications of gastric ulcers like bleeding and weight loss is not an uncommon symptom making it difficult to distinguish between malignant and benign conditions from symptoms alone.

Epidemiology: Gastric ulcers are less common than duodenal ulcers. In the United Kingdom as in most of Western Europe and North America, the overall incidence is decreasing but with an increasingly elderly population and a high use of nonsteroidal drugs and aspirin the incidence of complicated gastric ulcers have remained fairly constant.

Etiology and Pathogenesis: Gastric ulcers like peptic ulcer may be associated with *Helicobacter* infection. This is particularly true for ulcers in the prepyloric area and antrum. In the elderly population in particular, nonsteroidal agents are a major cause for gastric ulcers. Typically, they cause ulcers in the lesser curve of stomach and antrum at the junction between the antral and body-type mucosa. The inhibition of prostaglandins is likely to be the major contributory factor to these ulcers. Other contributory factors include smoking, genetic factors and poor diet. Steroid therapies are often blamed for ulcers but there is no evidence that it increases the risks of gastric ulcers but it may certainly delay healing. Ulcers associated with stress tend to be the superficial variety and can occur in severe trauma, burns (Curling's ulcers) and acute sepsis. Prophylactic use of acid suppression with PPIs may prevent these ulcers from forming.

Management

Establish that the Ulcer is Benign: The first priority is always to establish that the ulcer is truly benign. This will require endoscopy with biopsy and possibly brush cytology if available. Biopsy should be performed even if it looks benign and after treatment at an interval of about 6–8 weeks endoscopy should be repeated to ensure complete healing. Ulcer that fails to heal adequately should be treated with suspicion.

Drug Therapy: H. pylori is implicated in about two-thirds of gastric ulcers and if it is detected eradication therapy is indicated. Details of eradication therapy have been discussed earlier. Gastric ulcers can take longer to heal than duodenal ulcers particularly if they are very large. Treatment with PPIs is effective and the ulcers should be reviewed with further endoscopy after 6–8 weeks of treatment to ensure complete healing. If in doubt further biopsies should be performed.

Avoidance of nonsteroidal agents would be important in patients who have nonsteroidal-induced gastric ulcers. Aspirin and antiplatelet drugs like clopidogrel should be reviewed. However, these are often prescribed for major cerebrovascular and cardiovascular indications like stroke and ischemic heart disease. The morbidity and mortality from these conditions may outweigh the risks of the gastric ulcers and therefore coprescription with PPI and aspirin together is acceptable and often results in lower overall morbidity and mortality.

Gastritis

Strictly speaking, gastritis should refer to histological evidence of inflammation of the stomach. Different classification exists. It can be a clinical classification based on whether it is acute gastritis or chronic gastritis, or one based on histological or endoscopic appearances, or one based on its etiology. As a result, there is no universally accepted classification system despite attempts like the Sydney Classification. Gastritis is also often reported by endoscopist based on endoscopic appearance of inflammation or redness. However, there is often no correlation between an endoscopic appearance and underlying histology or etiology of the gastric mucosal inflammation. Additionally, inexperienced endoscopists may report vascular abnormalities such as gastric antral vascular ectasia (GAVE) as "gastritis" (Fig. 1.34).

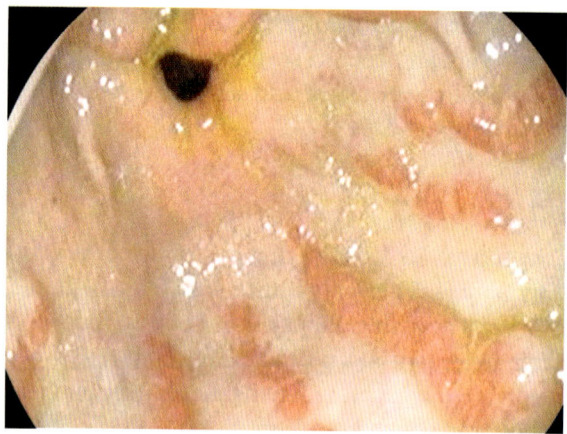

Fig. 1.34: Gastric antral vascular ectasia (GAVE) gives an appearance not unlike a watermelon and sometimes referred to as watermelon stomach. It is often misdiagnosed as "gastritis" by inexperienced endoscopists.

Probably the best way of classifying gastritis is probably by its etiological origin.

Acute Erosive Gastritis

Acute erosive gastritis usually affects the antrum but sometimes the corpus of the stomach and occurs after major trauma, burns, sepsis, renal failure and also ingestion of alcohol, aspirin or ingestion of toxic substances. It is often asymptomatic but can cause acute upper GI bleeding. Its cause is unknown but probably related to high acid and poor cytoprotection in such patients. Management of the underlying pathology is obviously the key to prevention of acute erosive gastritis along with prophylactic use of PPIs.

Chronic Gastritis

Chronic gastritis can be broadly divided into two forms, either infectious origins or noninfectious conditions (Table 1.2).

Helicobacter-associated Chronic Gastritis

Helicobacter pylori is the principal cause of chronic gastritis, peptic ulcer disease, gastric adenocarcinoma and primary gastric lymphoma. It has a worldwide distribution and rates of infection vary between countries. The effects of *H. pylori* infections vary according to the site of colonization of the bacterium. There are both bacterial factors and host factors that would also decide on the final outcome of the *H. pylori* infection. Gastritis is almost universal. It may affect the whole stomach (pangastritis), predominant antral infection (antral gastritis) or a body type infection (corpus gastritis). When gastritis affects predominantly the antrum of the stomach then gastrin secretions are abnormally high especially with meal stimulated release of gastrin. These patients would tend to develop peptic ulcer disease.

Table 1.2: Gastritis.	
Acute gastritis	Acute hemorrhagic and erosive gastropathy Acute *Helicobacter pylori* gastritis
Chronic gastritis: Common forms	*Helicobacter pylori* gastritis Chemical gastropathy Aspirin and NSAIDs Bile reflux Alcohol Atrophic gastritis Autoimmune
Chronic gastritis: Uncommon forms	Eosinophilic gastritis Other infectious gastritis like *Mycobacterium avium-intracellulare* (MAI), tuberculosis (TB), viral, etc. Crohn's disease—associated sarcoidosis Lymphocytic gastritis Ménétrier's disease

Helicobacter pylori pathogenicity is decided by certain inherent virulence factors in the bacterium. Strains that produce a protein CagA associated with greater risk of developing gastric cancers and peptic ulcers.

Some patients develop a multifocal atrophic gastritis pattern where the infection of the corpus of the stomach eventually leads to a pattern of gastric atrophy with loss of gastric glands and eventually replacement of gastric glands by intestinal-type mucosa (intestinal metaplasia). This will eventually develop into dysplasia and gastric cancer. Because of gastric atrophy, the acid levels tend to fall and carcinogenic agents such as nitrosamine are not neutralized by acid.

The majority of patients with *H. pylori*-associated chronic gastritis, however, remain asymptomatic. Only a small number will develop duodenal ulcer disease and gastric cancer (Figs. 1.35 and 1.36).

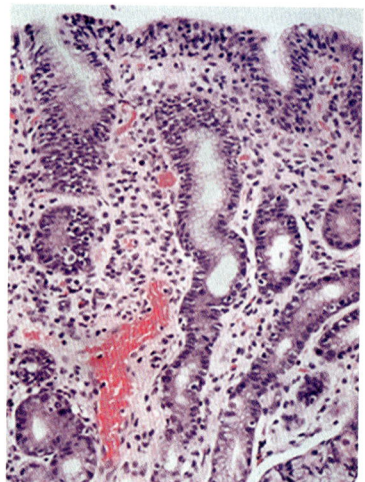

Fig. 1.35: Gastritis. Histologically, this is a severe gastritis.

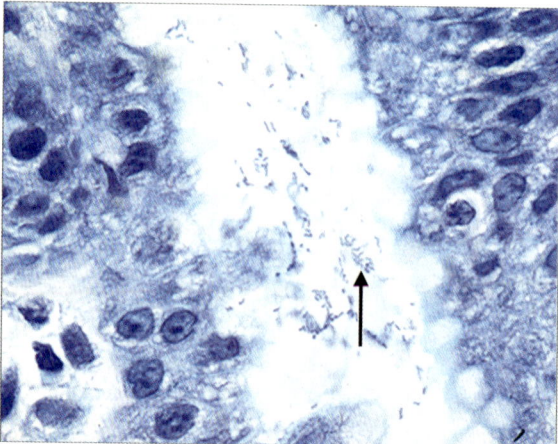

Fig. 1.36: *Helicobacter pylori* is easily identified on the biopsy of the stomach.

Other Infectious Gastritis

Granulomatous gastritis is a rare condition that may be caused by tuberculosis or *Cryptococcus*. Immunocompromised patients may occasionally acquire cytomegalovirus or mycobacterial infections involving *Mycobacterium avium-intracellulare* (MAI) species.

Gastritis Caused by Autoimmune Causes

Patients with autoimmune gastritis may have elevated antibodies such as an intrinsic factor and parietal cell antibodies. Two types of atrophic gastritis have been identified:
1. In type A gastritis, the fundus is primarily affected resulting in reduced acid secretion. This causes the hyperplasia of gastrin-producing G cells and results in hypergastrinemia.
2. In type B gastritis, the antrum is primarily affected and patients have normal serum gastrin.

Atrophic gastritis can be as a result of *H. pylori* infection when the *H. pylori* causes a pangastritis or a corpus gastritis. Thus, infection must be excluded by fecal antigen testing or any other readily available tests.

Atrophic gastritis may result in lower gastric acid production and may result in increased risk of gastric cancer. Atrophy of parietal cells also results in reduced production of B12 and development of B12 deficiency and pernicious anemia.

In terms of diagnosis, the endoscopic appearance of an atrophic stomach can be quite obvious with lack of rugal folds and biopsies would also be helpful in making the diagnosis.

Eosinophilic infiltration of gastric mucosa would result in eosinophilic gastritis. This condition is rare although it is increasingly being diagnosed. There may be a peripheral blood eosinophilia and they are sometimes associated with asthma and other allergic conditions. Patients may present with abdominal pain, fever, diarrhea or even ascites. Large antral folds may simulate other infiltrative processes like lymphoma and therefore biopsies are usually required to make a diagnosis. Patients may present with gastric outlet obstruction due to edema of the pylorus and infiltration of the antrum of the stomach (Fig. 1.37).

Biliary or Alkaline Reflux Gastritis (See Fig. 1.6)

Bile reflux causes a reddening appearance of the stomach on endoscopy. It is almost invariable as a consequence to partial gastrectomy and is termed biliary gastritis. It has a specific histological appearance characterized by foveolar hyperplasia.

Other Rare Gastritis

Hypertrophic gastritis or Ménétrier's disease is a very rare condition in which the fundic glands are replaced by a hypertrophic epithelium and forming massively enlarged mucosal folds. There is variable degree of inflammation.

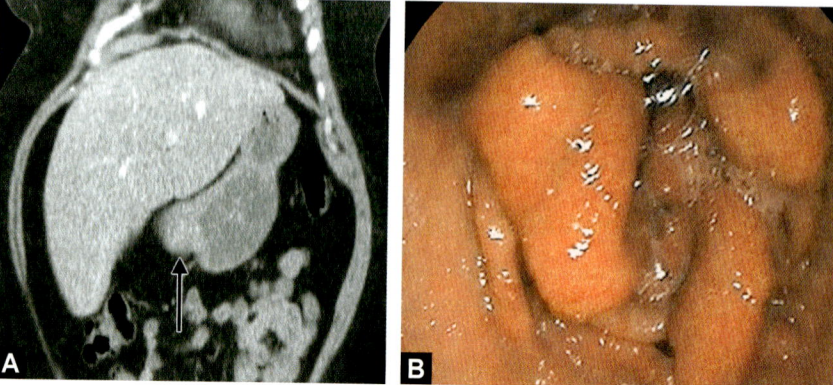

Figs. 1.37A and B: Eosinophilic gastritis. CT image (A) shows thickened gastric antrum correlating with the endoscopic image (B) of the same patient.

Patients may present with pain, vomiting, bleeding or signs of hypoalbuminemia, which results from excessive protein loss as mucous is shed from the gastric mucosa. Other rare causes of gastritis include sarcoidosis, granulomatous gastritis and lymphocytic gastritis.

Management

Acute Erosive Gastritis: Acute erosive gastritis may cause bleeding, requiring resuscitation and even emergency surgery. More usually, the bleeding can be controlled endoscopically and if nonsteroidal drugs are used, then they should be stopped and PPIs initially intravenously followed by oral PPI may be indicated. Very ill patients with septicemia shock, renal failure or hepatic failure may also develop acute ulcers, which may require PPI prophylactically.

Atrophic Gastritis: Atrophic gastritis may result in B12 deficiency so parenteral B12 replacement is required. If the atrophic gastritis is a result of *H. pylori* infection eradication of *H. pylori* would be wise.

Eosinophilic Gastritis: Eosinophilic gastritis usually responds very rapidly to corticosteroids, which may initially be necessary to give intravenously but that can easily be followed by a short course of oral prednisolone, usually starting with a dose of 30 mg and reducing over a week or so. Elimination of specific food allergies, use of leukotriene inhibitors montelukast or zafirlukast may also be helpful. Patients may have recurrence of this condition and may require a steroid sparing agent like azathioprine if they have repeated recurrence of this condition (*See* Figs. 1.20, 1.21 and 1.37).

Helicobacter-associated Gastritis: Treatment for *Helicobacter*-associated gastritis is *H. pylori* eradication, which has been discussed earlier. However, in asymptomatic individuals with *H. pylori*-associated gastritis, controversy exists as to whether they should have eradication or not. On balance with the hope of reducing the patients' risk of developing gastric cancer, then *H. pylori* eradication is justified if found.

Biliary Reflux Gastritis: Biliary reflux gastritis responds well to bile chelating agents like cholestyramine. Aluminum hydroxide is also worth trying because it also has a bile acid–binding effect.

Carcinoma of the Stomach

Natural History

Symptoms and Signs: Gastric cancers are usually asymptomatic until invasion occurs through the submucosa and beyond. Hence, they often present late. The principal clinical features that they present with are weight loss, abdominal pain and vomiting. Weight loss is often the result of anorexia and pain on eating and early satiety (Table 1.3). Pain is often indistinguishable from those of peptic ulceration and may be relieved by PPIs and antacids or H2 antagonists. It usually takes the form of a vague upper abdominal discomfort often associated with a feeling of fullness. When the tumor is proximal to stomach there may be dysphagia as well. This may be from direct tumor obstruction or invasion of the nerve cells of the Auerbach plexus. The latter would cause pseudoachalasia syndrome with grossly dilated esophagus. Early satiety may be due to a diffuse form of gastric cancer (linitis plastica) where the stomach distends poorly because of the cancer. Distal tumors that block the pylorus or antrum will cause a gastric obstruction presenting with nausea and vomiting and sometimes hematemesis (Figs. 1.38 to 1.42).

A palpable mass may be found on examination. Signs of tumor spread may also be presenting features. Prominent left supraclavicular lymph node (Virchow's node) may be a sign of metastatic spread of gastric cancer and is also the most common sign of metastatic disease. When there are hepatic metastases then the liver may be often palpable and ascites may also be detected when there is peritoneal carcinomatosis.

Epidemiology: The incidence of gastric cancer in the United Kingdom and other developed countries is declining. Prevalence in the Far East and some Latin American countries remain very high. The increased risk in these areas is probably related to high rates of *H. pylori* infection. There is an encouraging decline in mortality from gastric cancer in the European centers (Fig. 1.43).

Table 1.3: Alarming symptoms.
Age >40
Strong FH CRC/IBD
Rectal bleeding
Anemia
Weight loss
Abdominal mass

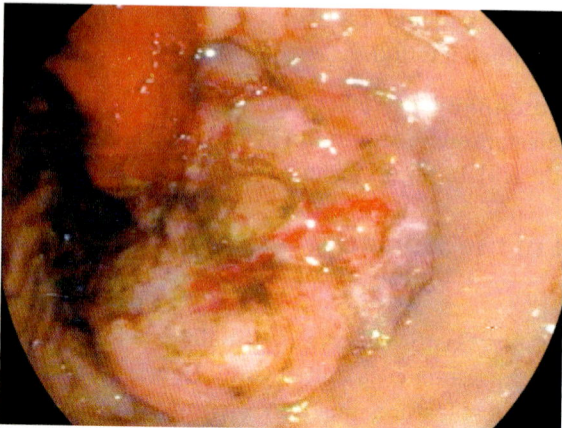

Fig. 1.38: Endoscopy showing a large gastric cancer.

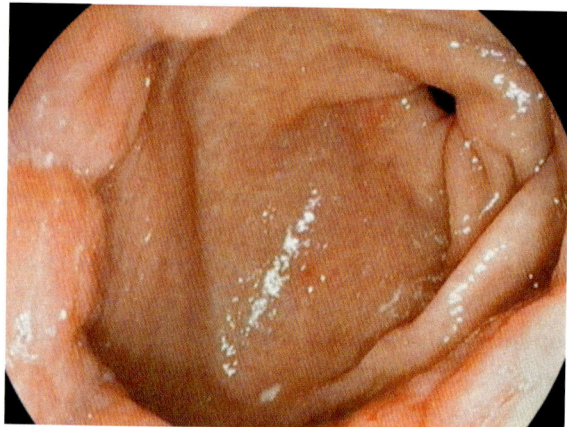

Fig. 1.39: Endoscopy: It appears unremarkable but the stomach was not distending with insufflation. This proved to be linitis plastica.

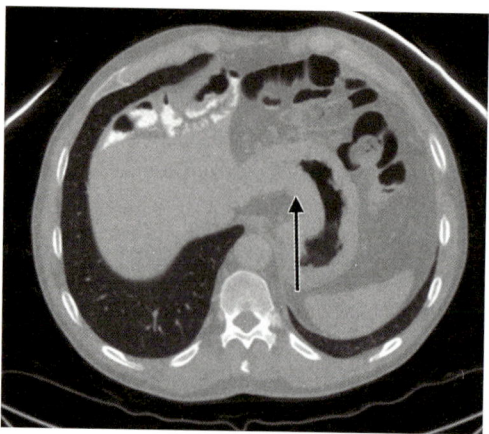

Fig. 1.40: CT scan of the above showed linitis plastica: a thickened stomach infiltrated with malignant cells.

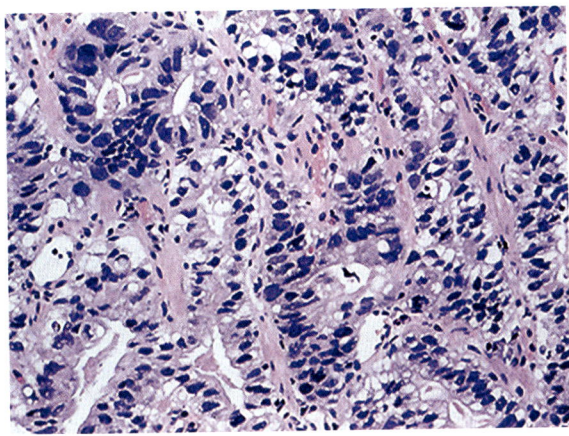

Fig. 1.41: Gastric adenocarcinoma. Moderately well-differentiated carcinoma.

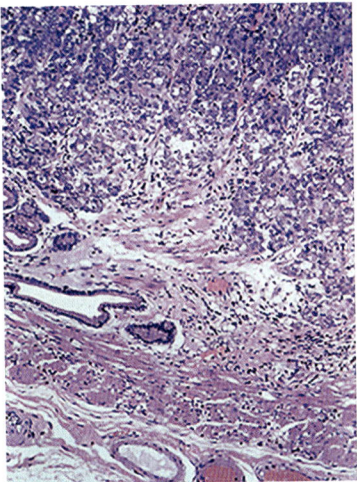

Fig. 1.42: Gastric adenocarcinoma. Poorly differentiated carcinoma.

Management of Gastric Cancer

When gastric, etc. cancer is suspected a prompt endoscopy should be made. When cancer is found, multiple biopsies and brush cytology should be carried out and the patient then fully staged. The commonest staging system used is the TNM criteria. It is based on the tumor (T) nodal (N) metastases (M). This is being revised at present moment and the physician should consult the American Joint Committee on Cancer website for details.

The imaging modalities required to adequately stage patients include:

Abdominal and Pelvic CT Scan: CT scan of the abdomen and pelvis is very helpful in staging a disease. It will adequately pick up affected lymph nodes, liver metastases or ascites. However, lesions <5 mm may be missed by

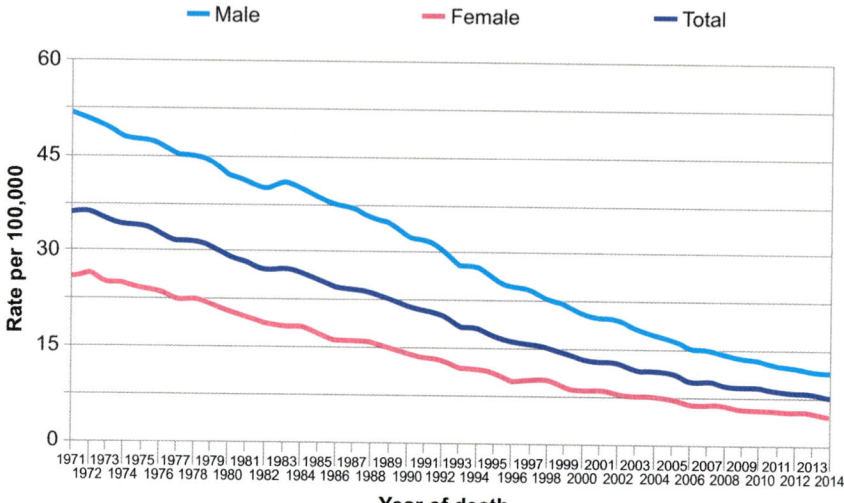

Fig. 1.43: Stomach cancer: 1971–2014. European age-standardized mortality rates per 100,000 population, UK.
Source: cruk.org/cancerstats.

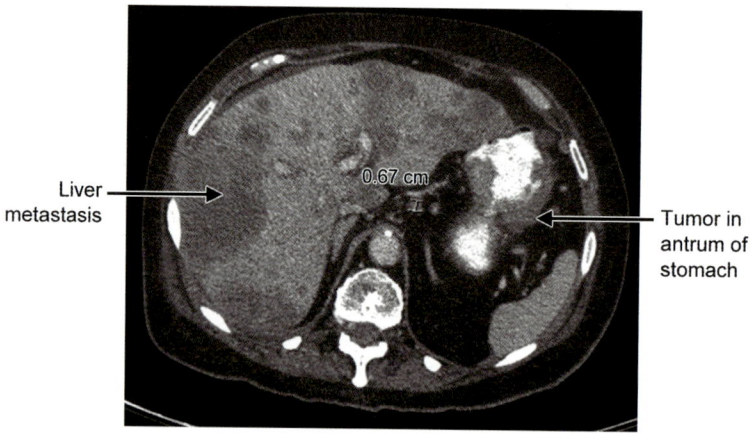

Fig. 1.44: Gastric cancer with liver metastasis.

CT scanning. Patients with proximal gastric cancer should have a CT scan of the thorax as well (Fig. 1.44).

Endoscopic Ultrasound: Endoscopic ultrasound (EUS) is helpful in gastric cancer staging. It is the most accurate method of staging the depth of tumor invasion. If the depth of invasion as evaluated at EUS shows that it is very superficial and not invaded submucosa then endoscopic resection may be possible. However, it is more useful as a tool for picking up tumors that have invaded the muscularis and also detects any local nodal involvement. In this situation patients may be offered neoadjuvant chemotherapy or chemoradiotherapy prior to surgery.

Positron-emission Tomography Scan: Positron-emission tomography (PET) using a radio labeled (positron emitting) isotope of glucose (FDG). The FDG is taken up by tumor cells and is therefore valuable in detecting any distant metastases. However, patients with peritoneal carcinomatosis may be missed on PET scanning.

Staging Laparoscopy: If there is any doubt as to whether the tumor is operable or not then a staging laparoscopy is usually recommended. This is especially true if CT or EUS show more advanced tumors, particularly stage T3/T4 tumors but no metastases. Laparoscopy may be needed to establish operability.

Treatment of Gastric Cancer

If it is possible, surgical resection of the tumor is still the primary treatment. However, the treatment of gastric cancer is based on the staging of the tumor. A combination of neoadjuvant chemotherapy; adjuvant chemotherapy and chemotherapy and surgery is available to the patient.

Neoadjuvant chemotherapy refers to chemotherapy given before surgery to downstage the tumor. This is given in patients with bowel T3 or T4 tumors or patients with perigastric nodes.

Adjuvant chemotherapy refers to chemotherapy given along with surgery. The aim of adjuvant chemotherapy is to improve survival by eliminating any residual tumor after surgery.

The exact treatment protocol for each individual patient is usually discussed at the multidisciplinary team meeting where the imaging, histology and overall patient fitness are discussed. If the patient is fit for surgery, then every attempt is made to improve surgical outcome. Best treatments are still a subject for research and patients should be considered for entering many of the clinical trials that are currently running.

Prognosis and Screening

Successful surgical resection of an early gastric cancer carries a 90% 5-year survival rate. Invasive gastric cancers, however, have a very poor prognosis. In countries where there is high incidence of gastric cancer such as Japan, screening may be a viable option and pick up cases of early gastric cancer. This remains the best way of improving outlook of the disease. However, in countries where gastric cancer incidence is low risk, like in the United Kingdom, screening is not viable or a cost-effective option.

Gastric Lymphomas (Figs. 1.45 to 1.50)

Gastric lymphomas account for about 5% of gastric malignancies and for about 60% of all GI lymphomas. Symptoms and endoscopic features may be indistinguishable from those of gastric cancers. The endoscopic appearance may be that of a polypoidal lesion, ulcerating lesion or an infiltrating lesion.

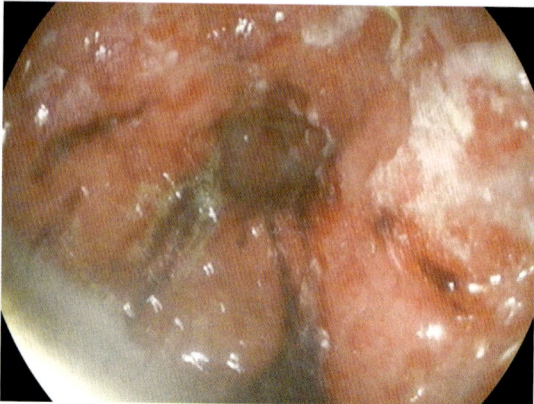

Fig. 1.45: Gastric lymphoma. On endoscopy, the appearances can vary from discrete ulcers to diffuse infiltrative picture.

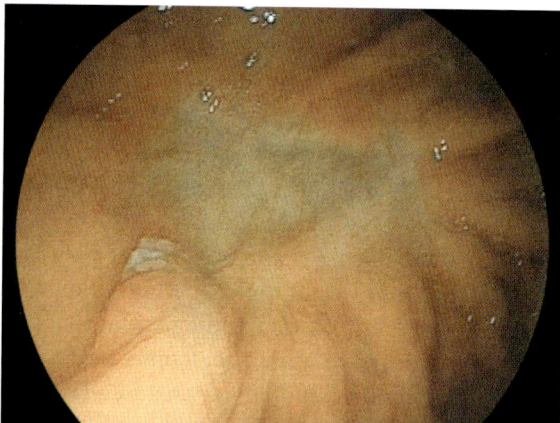

Fig. 1.46: Gastric lymphoma. Appearance after chemotherapy shows scarring.

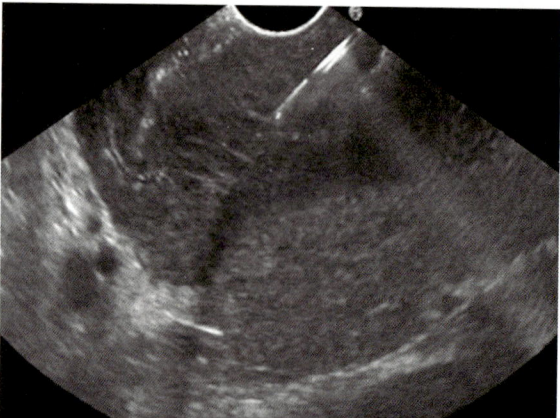

Fig. 1.47: Gastric lymphoma. Sampling of the deeper tissue may be necessary to make a diagnosis. Here a fine needle aspirate was taken using endoscopic ultrasound.

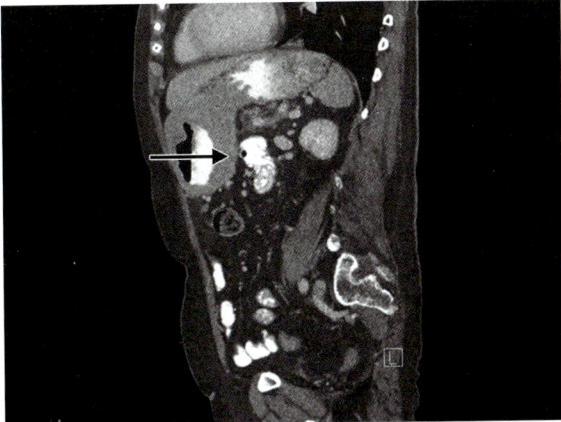

Fig. 1.48: Gastric lymphoma. Grossly thickened stomach is clearly demonstrated.

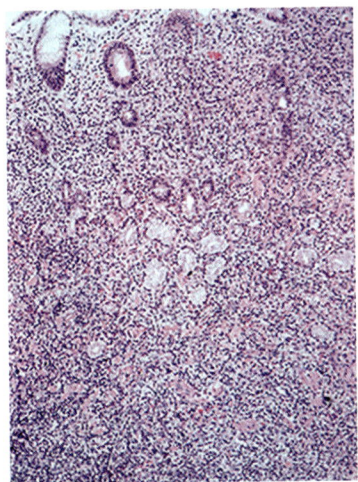

Fig. 1.49: Gastric lymphoma. Proliferation of infiltrative lymphoma cells.

However, clues that the lesion is a lymphoma rather than gastric carcinoma may be the younger age group or patients who had previous organ transplantation receiving immune suppressive therapy. Almost all the gastric cancers are the B-cell variety and are divided into two types: (1) those with mucosa-associated lymphoid tissue (MALT lymphomas) that account for about half of the gastric lymphomas encountered, and (2) those with diffuse, large B-cell lymphoma that account for the other half. MALT lymphomas (also referred to as extranodal marginal zone B-cell lymphoma) is often associated with *H. pylori* infection. Eradication of *H. pylori* infection may result in involution of these tumors.

Management

Proper staging evaluation includes CT scanning and PET scanning. Discussions at the multidisciplinary meeting as to best management will

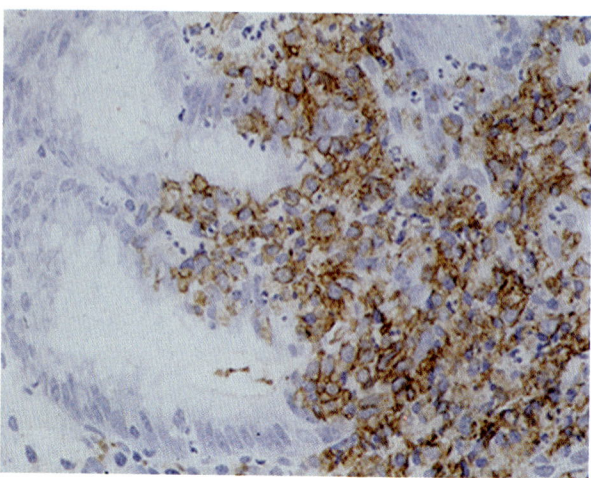

Fig. 1.50: Gastric lymphoma. Immunohistochemical staining helps identify the cell type. The vast majority are B-cell lymphomas and about 40% are mucosa-associated lymphoid tissue (MALT) lymphomas which are associated with *H. pylori* infection.

depend upon tissue type, grade of malignancy and extent of disease. A combination of *H. pylori* eradication if indicated, radiotherapy, chemotherapy and immunotherapy is available depending upon the specific stage and type of lymphoma. Prognosis is usually good.

Gastric Polyps

Natural History

Gastric polyps are frequently encountered on endoscopy. The commonest type of polyps found is fundic gland polyps (Fig. 1.51) (also known as cystic fundic polyps). They account for over 90% of gastric polyps. They pose no significant overall risk to the patient. They have no malignant potential. These polyps as their name implies are found mainly in the fundus of the stomach although they do occur in the body of stomach and occasionally in antrum as well. They are cystic in nature. They are also commonly seen in patients who have been on long-term PPIs. Patients with familial adenomatous polyposis (FAP) may also have proliferation of these fundic gland polyps and if there is a family history then investigation of colon would be advised.

True adenomas of the stomach are relatively rare, occurring in about 5% of gastric polyps. They have a similar premalignant potential as colonic adenomas. Hence, they are best removed endoscopically if possible. It may be difficult endoscopically to decide the nature of the polyps then biopsies are best performed to establish diagnosis.

Other polyps that may be encountered in the stomach include hamartomatous polyps found in polyposis syndromes such as Peutz–Jeghers. Also, quite rare are gastric carcinoids. Four types of gastric carcinoids have

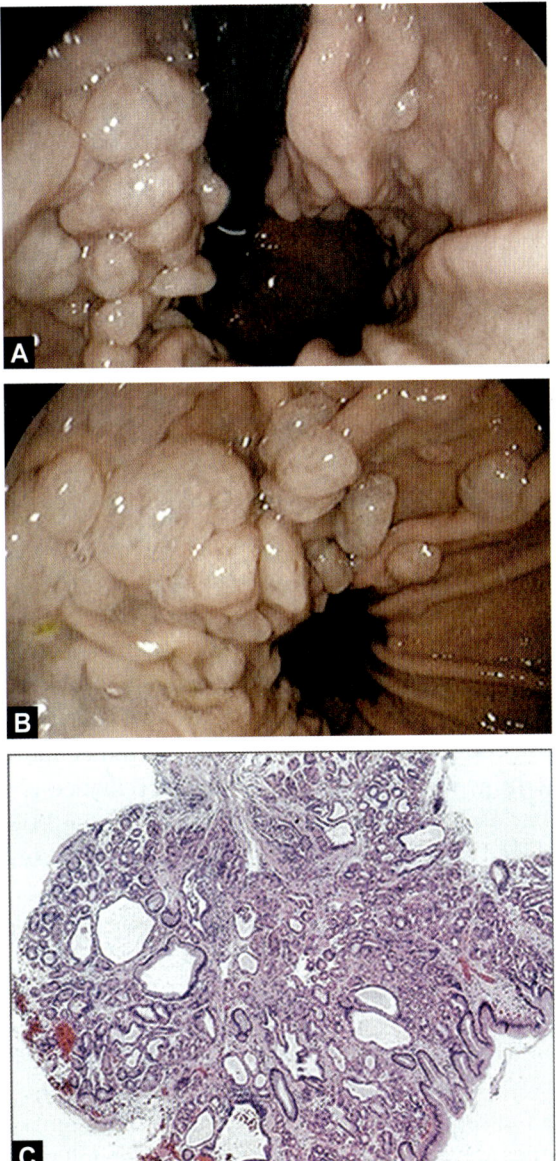

Figs. 1.51A to C: Fundic gland polyps are a common finding on endoscopy and are usually associated with acid suppression (PPI use). It may rarely be associated with polyposis syndromes.

been identified. The most common is Type I which is well differentiated and associated with atrophic gastritis usually in the elderly and of relatively good prognosis, whereas Type II is multifocal and associated with multiple endocrine neoplasia and Zollinger–Ellison syndrome. Type III is solitary, well differentiated but in the absence of gastric atrophy and Type IV is the poorly

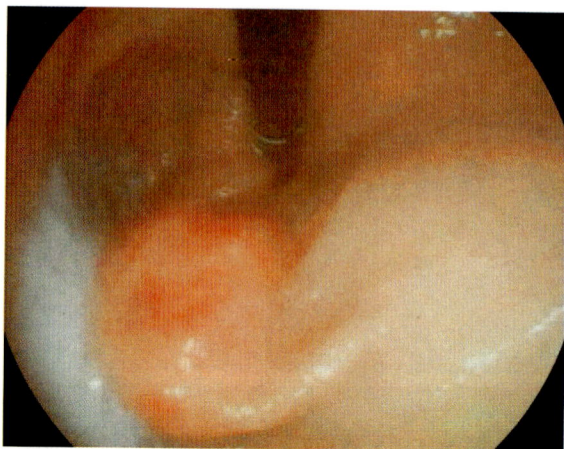

Fig. 1.52: Gastrointestinal stromal tumor (GIST) lesion. A polypoid lesion sometimes with an umbilicated center. This proved to be a GIST.

differentiated variety. Types III and IV are more aggressive and would require resection.

Other lesions that look like polyps include gastrointestinal stromal tumors (GIST) (Fig. 1.52). These may be asymptomatic and may look like an elevated umbilical lesion in the stomach and are usually solitary. Occasionally, they might cause complications like bleeding and may undergo malignant transformation. In general, if they are <2 cm surveillance is probably not necessary. If they are >2 cm then it is worth considering EUS followed by surgery if it is judged to have malignant features. If in doubt, surgical excision should be considered.

Gallstones

Natural History

Cross-sectional studies have shown that in European studies more than 75% of patients with gallstones are asymptomatic. In a large cohort study with a median follow-up of over 17 years, <20% of patients with asymptomatic gallstones develop symptoms. Also in their follow up, their initial symptoms are typically not severe. It is therefore widely accepted that cholecystectomy for patients with asymptomatic gallstones is not advised. However, of the patients who do develop symptoms, a significant number develop complications. Once symptoms develop, probably about one-third will continue to have symptoms in the subsequent 2 years. Finally of the patients who do have symptoms, up to 10% develop serious complications after a median follow-up of 10 years. These complications include, acute cholecystitis, choledocholithiasis with or without acute cholangitis and gallstone pancreatitis. Hence, patients with symptomatic gallstones should be offered therapy.

Epidemiology

About 8% of white populations in the United Kingdom have gallstones and the incidence is increasing. The prevalence increases with age and 80% are female. The incident varies considerably with population groups. Western Caucasian, Hispanic and Native American populations have the highest incidence whereas African, Eastern European and Japanese populations have a relatively low incidence. Large ultrasound-based studies in Europe suggest that in individuals between the ages of 30 and 70 years, 18% of women and 9% of men have gallstones.

Etiology and Pathogenesis

The majority of gallstones found among European Caucasian populations are cholesterol-based gallstones. Here, there are several risk factors that increase the tendency to produce gallstones. Obviously, the older the patient, the more time they have to produce gallstones. Women are twice as likely to produce stones as men presumably due to the presence of sex hormones. Pregnancy itself is a major risk factor. This may be caused by estrogen stimulating increasing cholesterol secretion in the bile. Similarly, oral contraceptives may affect gallstone production presumably by the same mechanism.

Family history and genetics play an important part as does obesity itself. Curiously, rapid weight loss is a risk factor of gallstone formation and one of the complications of bariatric surgical operations. Other risk factors include diabetes, liver disease and Crohn's disease. Pigment stones are more likely in patients with hemolytic anemia from any cause. Drugs such as octreotide are also known to promote formation of gallstones. This may be due to its effects on gallbladder motility and increasing the chance of gallbladder stasis. Gallstone formation may be also a complication of total parenteral nutrition. This is probably due to its effects of causing biliary stasis. Surgical removal of terminal ileum will also affect enterohepatic circulation of bile acids and promote the formation of gallstones.

Management

In the absence of any symptoms, there is no justification in carrying out any specific treatment of gallstones. Furthermore, many patients have nonspecific abdominal symptoms and the finding of gallstones by ultrasound may be quite incidental. It is therefore important to ascertain that the symptoms are directly caused by the presence of gallstones. This may be very difficult and ultimately is a clinical decision.

The mainstay of treatment is laparoscopic cholecystectomy. In expert hands, conversion rate to open cholecystectomy is usually <2% and duct injuries <0.1%. The main complications are bile leak, hemorrhage and retained stones.

For patients with previous cholecystitis, cholangitis or pancreatitis, risk of recurrence is high and therefore cholecystectomy is recommended.

If the LFTs are abnormal or there is dilatation of the common bile duct on ultrasound, then an MRCP is recommended before embarking on surgery to ensure that there are no stones in the common bile duct (Fig. 1.9). Stones in the common bile duct can be removed by ERCP and that should be performed prior to surgery (Fig. 1.10).

Medical Management of Gallstones: The medical management of gallstones have proved very disappointing. The mainstay of treatment uses hydrophilic bile acids such as chenodeoxycholic acid or ursodeoxycholic acid. For dissolution to be successful, the stones must be predominantly of cholesterol origin and not to be calcified. CT scanning is a good method to see if there is significant calcification of the stones. The stones must also be of small size, preferably <10 mm and the gallbladder must be functioning adequately. Even with all the above criteria met, the drug has to be given for a minimum of a year to achieve adequate dissolution. Hence, it is only in very exceptional circumstances that medical therapy for gallstones is appropriate.

Management of Polypoidal Lesions in the Gallbladder: Polypoidal lesions of the gallbladder are frequently found on ultrasound. The commonest polypoidal lesion is adenomyomatosis. This is characterized by mucosal thickening and localized muscle wall thickening and sometimes with a prominent diverticula formation. It is thought to be predominantly asymptomatic. If the patient exhibits symptoms that sound biliary, then it may be worth considering cholecystectomy in limited cases. The association between adenomyomatosis and gallbladder cancer is a controversial one and there is no direct evidence to suggest that the two are causally linked.

Chronic Mesenteric Ischemia

Natural History, Symptoms and Signs

Clinically, significant obstruction of one of the main mesenteric vessels (celiac axis of the superior/inferior mesenteric arteries) usually present with acute infarction of the bowel. However, intermittent bowel ischemia resulting in abdominal angina can occasionally occur. Typically, the patient experiences a pain in the central abdomen usually 15–30 minutes after meals and it may last for several hours. This pain results in fear of eating and with bowel ischemia there is also poor absorption of nutrients and the two factors result in marked weight loss. Typically patients are elderly, have evidence of atheromatous disease elsewhere like cardiac disease and peripheral vascular disease and smoking is a major risk factor.

Computed tomography scanning is helpful in its diagnosis in identifying stenosis of the mesenteric vessels. The presence of high-grade vascular stenosis in at least two of the major vessels (celiac, superior/inferior mesenteric) are clues that the symptoms are due to mesenteric ischemia. MR angiography is also a valuable modality.

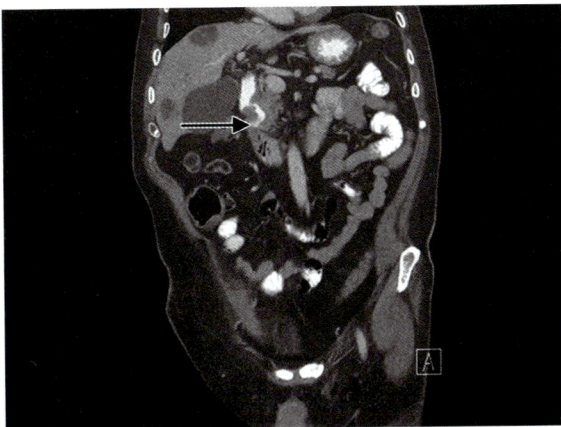

Fig. 1.53: Duodenal tumor obstructing the gastric outlet.

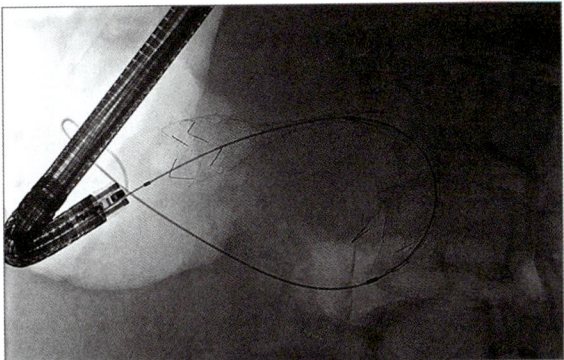

Fig. 1.54: Obstruction in duodenum can be stented.

Management

True intestinal ischemia carries a poor prognosis. Some form of revascularization would be necessary. The treatment of choice is angioplasty and stenting carried out by interventional radiologists. Open surgery may be required if endovascular treatment is not successful.

Miscellaneous Conditions: True duodenal cancers are rare and may be associated with familial adenomatous polyposis syndromes (FAP) (*see* Chapter 5) (Figs. 1.53 and 1.54).

■ FURTHER READING

Irritable Bowel Syndrome
1. Collins S. A role for the gut microbiota in IBS. Nat Rev Gastroenterol Hepatol. 2014;11(8):497-505.
2. Ford AC, Talley NJ, Spiegel BM, et al. Effect of fibre, antispasmodics, and peppermint oil in the treatment of irritable bowel syndrome: systematic review and meta-analysis. BMJ. 2008;337:a2313.

3. Ford AC, Quigley EM, Lacy BE, et al. Effect of antidepressants and psychological therapies, including hypnotherapy, in irritable bowel syndrome: systematic review and meta-analysis. Am J Gastroenterol. 2014;109(9):1350-65.
4. Talley NJ. Irritable bowel syndrome. Intern Med J. 2006;36(11):724-8.
5. Wedlake L, A'Hern R, Russell D, et al. Systematic review: the prevalence of idiopathic bile acid malabsorption as diagnosed by SeHCAT scanning in patients with diarrhoea-predominant irritable bowel syndrome. Aliment Pharmacol Ther. 2009;30(7):707-17.

Helicobacter pylori and Peptic Ulcer Disease

6. Lanas A, Chan FK. Peptic ulcer disease. Lancet. 2017;390(10094):613-24.
7. Malfertheiner P, Megraud F, O'Morain CA, et al. European Helicobacter Study Group. Management of *Helicobacter pylori* infection—the Maastricht IV/Florence Consensus Report. Gut. 2012;61(5): 646-64.
8. Tsai HH. *Helicobacter pylori* for the general physician. J R Coll Physicians Lond. 1997;31(5):478-82.

Functional Dyspepsia

9. Brun R, Kuo B. Functional dyspepsia. Ther Adv Gastroenterol. 2010;3(3):145-64.

Gastric Cancer

10. Fuchs CS, Mayer RJ. Gastric carcinoma. N Engl J Med. 1995;333(1):32-41.
11. Macdonald JS, Smalley SR, Benedetti J, et al. Chemoradiotherapy after surgery compared with surgery alone for adenocarcinoma of the stomach or gastroesophageal junction. N Engl J Med. 2001;345(10):725-30.
12. Neugut AI, Hayek M, Howe G. Epidemiology of gastric cancer. Semin Oncol. 1996;23(3):281-91.

Gallstones

13. Heuman DM. Gallstones (Cholelithiasis) Clinical Presentation: History, Physical Examination. http://emedicine.medscape.com/article/175667-clinical#b3.
14. Portincasa P, Moschetta A, Palasciano G. Cholesterol gallstone disease. Lancet. 2006; 368(9531):230-9.

CHAPTER 2

Acute Abdomen

Benjamin Chan, Barry Taylor

■ REACHING A DIAGNOSIS

The patient with acute abdominal pain has always presented a diagnostic challenge to clinicians, as there is a little time for sophisticated investigations other than computed tomography (CT) scans, and the preliminary diagnosis remains largely reached on clinical grounds. The three crucial questions are:
- What is the diagnosis?
- Does the patient need further imaging?
- Does the patient need an emergency operation?

The answer to the first question is derived using a combination of clinical, laboratory and imaging criteria as discussed later. The answers to the second and third questions depend almost exclusively on the answer to the first.

Like many disciplines of medicine, after a full history has been obtained, a diagnosis should become apparent for approximately 75% of patients. The examination, biochemical markers and radiological imaging are directed at confirming this diagnosis.

History

The characteristics of the pain should be elicited, along with any associated features such as gastrointestinal disturbance or systemic upset. Visceral pain is poorly localized, but once peritoneal irritation is established, the site of the pain and maximal tenderness becomes good indicators of the site of pathology.

Associated features may include shortness of breath or chest pain if there is a medical cause for the acute abdominal pain, such as basal pneumonia or myocardial infarction. Other features, such as jaundice or an alteration in bowel habit, or previously documented gastrointestinal disease, are obviously crucial. The nature of any previous surgical intervention needs to be clarified, ideally by inspecting operation notes.

- Previous abdominal surgery is particularly relevant to small bowel obstruction.
- Mesenteric ischemia or infarction needs to be considered in any patient with vascular disease or atrial fibrillation.
- A patient with an obstructed kidney or bladder may have previous genitourinary problems.

A complete drug history is essential. Most patients with a perforated peptic ulcer are elderly and are taking non-steroidal anti-inflammatory agents (NSAIDs), while a variety of drugs, including furosemide and azathioprine, have been implicated in acute pancreatitis. Anticoagulants are important to be aware of if surgical intervention is a possibility. Other drugs, including non-prescription drugs, tobacco and alcohol, should also be noted.

A careful family history should always be taken. Many causes of an acute abdomen (e.g. ulcers, gallstones, vascular and inflammatory bowel disease) show a familial tendency, and sometimes the family history may suggest the diagnosis (e.g. acute pancreatitis or intermittent porphyria).

Examination

The physical examination of a patient with an acute abdomen aims to provide:
- A diagnosis
- An assessment of the patient's general condition, particularly peritoneal irritation, so the need for and urgency of an operation can be decided upon

If these are not satisfactorily met after the initial examination, it must be repeated at regular intervals until they are.

Powerful analgesia should be used sparingly until a diagnosis has been made and it has been decided whether or not a laparotomy is necessary.

It is essential to make an initial assessment of the patient's general observations, including pulse rate, respiratory rate blood pressure and temperature, with these measurements repeated regularly. It must be stressed that an inexorably rising pulse rate is often the first sign of an impending intra-abdominal catastrophe, particularly in the young fit patient, and usually occurs before any apparent changes in blood pressure. Of course, the patient with a rupture of abdominal aneurysm may be significantly hypotensive from the outset, but such patients are in the minority, and tend to be relatively elderly.

The patient's hydration status should also be assessed, as any pathological process leading to unrelieved intestinal obstruction and/or peritonitis will be accompanied by significant dehydration. The extracellular fluid volume should be considered to be depleted by at least 3 L if dehydration is clinically apparent in an otherwise healthy, normal-sized adult. If there is proximal intestinal obstruction, dehydration is likely to be severe, since fluid is sequestered in the gut proximal to the obstructing lesion and may also be lost as vomitus. Acute pancreatitis is another cause of rapid dehydration, since large fluid shifts occur as fluid is sequestered in the peritoneal cavity and third space.

The general physical examination should include:
- Inspection of the hands for signs of anemia and liver disease
- Palpation of all lymph node groups throughout the body
- A thorough inspection of the face, mouth and tongue, noting any jaundice, conjunctival pallor, anemia, cyanosis and dehydration, and rare signs such as the circumoral pigmentation of Peutz–Jeghers' syndrome.

It is well known that acute chest conditions and myocardial infarction may be confused with acute upper abdominal conditions, and may occasionally be accompanied by guarding and even rigidity in the upper abdomen. The next logical step is therefore a thorough examination of the cardiorespiratory system in an attempt to exclude conditions such as basal pneumonia, pulmonary embolism and infarction, pneumothorax, pleurisy and acute myocardial infarction. It is usually possible to exclude these conditions after the examination, but various confirmatory tests will be discussed later. The other notable intrathoracic catastrophe that may cause epigastric guarding and rigidity is Boerhaave's syndrome, or ruptured esophagus, which is usually caused by forced vomiting against a closed glottis. This diagnosis is sometimes considered only after a negative laparotomy has been carried out, and the importance of the physical sign of subcutaneous crepitus in the neck cannot be overstated in this situation.

Abdominal Examination

Finally, attention needs to be directed to the abdomen. As initial inspection should include the following:
- An assessment of the patient's ability to move the abdominal wall with or without pain. This can be reliably obtained by watching the patient's abdominal wall during normal breathing and coughing, and by asking the patient to sit up unaided. The general size and shape of the abdomen and any obvious mass, visible peristalsis and distension, should be noted.
- An inspection of the groins (inguinal and femoral regions) for the presence of hernias, which may have escaped the patient's notice. The external genitalia should also be examined, especially in children.
- An inspection for signs of retroperitoneal bleeding. Although in general a rather later manifestation, Cullen's/Grey Turner's sign (bruising periumbilically or the flanks) may provide useful confirmatory evidence of hemorrhagic pancreatitis in the absence of other abnormal investigations.

The abdomen should then be gently palpated in all quadrants to assess for the presence of guarding or rigidity. Palpating a rigid abdomen (a feature of an acutely perforated peptic ulcer) is rather like palpating a table-top (board-like rigidity). If there is guarding, the patient's abdominal wall will only move a small amount before the abdominal wall muscles contract, rendering an informative palpation impossible. Palpable masses should be sought and assessed to decide on their likely organ of origin. Patients with acute urinary retention occasionally present with severe abdominal pain and a lower abdominal mass (the bladder), with surprisingly little in the way of pre-existing genitourinary symptoms. Moving masses will only be appreciated if the palpating hand remains still, and failure to keep the hand still is the commonest reason why aortic aneurysms, however large, are missed by relatively inexperienced examiners.

The site of maximum tenderness then needs to be defined. In generalized peritonitis with rigidity any attempt at localization is futile, but otherwise the location of maximum tenderness will often give useful clues to the underlying diagnosis, for example appendicitis, biliary pain and pelvic colon diverticulitis.

Persistent and well-localized pain with local guarding (as occurs over an ischemic loop of bowel in small bowel obstruction) implies peritoneal irritation for whatever reason, and is usually a good indication for urgent surgical intervention.

Auscultation of the abdomen in general is not very helpful although very high-pitched "tinkling" bowel sounds often accompany small bowel obstruction. The presence of normal bowel sounds does not exclude generalized peritonitis, since the ileus that develops is often a rather late effect of peritoneal inflammation. Occasionally, a vascular bruit will be heard in patients with mesenteric vascular stenosis or aortic disease.

Finally, the importance of a digital examination of the anorectum performed by an experienced clinician cannot be overstated. To fail to carry out this part of the assessment, particularly in an adult patient, risks missing a diagnosis such as a pelvic abscess or a rectal or prostatic carcinoma.

> **Assessment of the patient with an acute abdomen**
> - Repeated examination is essential when the diagnosis is in doubt.
> - If dehydration is clinically apparent in an adult, the extracellular fluid volume is probably depleted by at least 3 L.
> - Beware of the battle-scarred abdomen, consider Munchausen's syndrome.
> - An inexorably rising pulse is often the first indication of impending intra-abdominal catastrophe.

A STEP-BY-STEP APPROACH TO ACUTE ABDOMINAL PAIN

Should the Patient be Referred to a Hospital?

If, on the basis of the clinical examination, the general practitioner feels that the diagnosis is probably a surgical condition such as acute appendicitis or cholecystitis, the patient should clearly be referred to hospital. It is difficult to set rigid rules if the diagnosis is not clear, but it is wise to refer to hospital any patient with:

- Tachycardia >90 beats per minute
- Pyrexia >37.5°C
- Hypotension, with systolic <100 mm Hg
- Persisting pain >4 h
- Pain uncontrolled with simple analgesia such as paracetamol.

The threshold for referral should be lower for children <16 years of age and for adults >65 years of age.

Should the Patient be Admitted to the Hospital?

Over 90% of patients referred to hospital with acute abdominal pain will be admitted for observations overnight or longer. A small number of patients with mild pain or who have symptoms that resolve during their visit to the hospital are discharged after an assessment in the emergency department by an experienced surgeon. It should be remembered, however, that no test is 100% sensitive for any cause of an acute abdomen: a normal full blood count does not exclude appendicitis, and a normal serum amylase on admission does not exclude pancreatitis. If there is any doubt, an admission with regularly repeated observation is the sensible approach.

Should the Patient have a CT Scan?

Computed tomography is now a well-recognized imaging modality to complement clinical assessment in the acute abdomen. This should particularly be considered in patients with recent surgery, complex comorbidities and atypical presentations. Raised biochemical markers (such as white blood count (WBC), C-reactive protein (CRP) and lactate) are helpful adjuncts and should raise the clinician's index of suspicion. While these markers are non-specific, one study has shown that a CRP >130 mg/L has a high specificity in determining positive findings on CT, and should be undertaken especially if there is diagnostic uncertainty.

Magnetic resonance imaging (MRI) is an establishing modality that has also been validated, and may be particularly helpful in pregnant patients and others where exposure to X-rays may be contraindicated.

Is it Appendicitis?

Patients with appendicitis typically present with central abdominal colic associated with vomiting, which is followed by right iliac fossa pain as peritoneal irritation progresses. There may be urinary symptoms and an alteration in bowel habit in pelvic appendicitis. A fever is common, as is a fetor.

Well-localized tenderness in the right iliac fossa (McBurney's point) and guarding are the cardinal signs, although the site may vary in pelvic

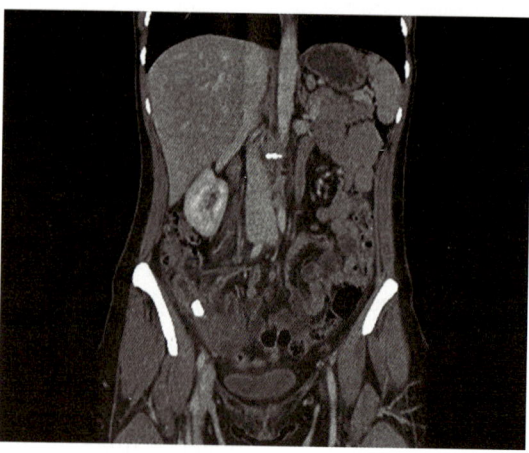

Fig. 2.1: Coronal reformat of a CT in the portal venous phase. In the RIF, we can see the appendix contains a calcified fecolith and the appendix itself is dilated, with surrounding fat stranding due to inflammation. (CT: Computed tomography; RIF: Right iliac fossa)
Courtesy: Keegan C.

appendicitis or pregnancy. When the appendix is retrocecal or retroileal, there may be surprisingly little to find on palpating the anterior abdominal wall, and a high index of suspicion is important.

There are no confirmatory biochemical markers. A rise in inflammatory markers such as WBC and CRP is common but not diagnostic. While various scoring systems such as the Alvarado score have been proposed, the diagnosis remains largely clinical.

Imaging in the form of ultrasound may visualize an abnormal appendix or exclude gynecological causes, but cannot reliably exclude appendicitis. CT should be considered early, and is particularly useful in atypical presentations or when there is a suspicion of alternative pathology, while MRI as mentioned earlier may be particularly helpful in pregnant patients (Fig. 2.1).

When the diagnosis is in doubt, repeated examination is important, since the signs will usually either improve or worsen. In young women, a diagnostic/therapeutic laparoscopy may have a role to exclude gynecological causes and, possibly, to remove the appendix without a conventional incision.

Is it Acute Cholecystitis?

The patient with acute cholecystitis, who is commonly a woman in her 40s or 50s, presents with epigastric and right upper quadrant pain, which often radiates to the back and may by associated with vomiting. There may be a history of biliary colic, and usually low-grade pyrexia.

Clinical examination reveals marked tenderness with guarding in the right upper quadrant. A marked increase in discomfort caused by inspiration while the examining hand is in the right upper quadrant (Murphy's sign) may also be

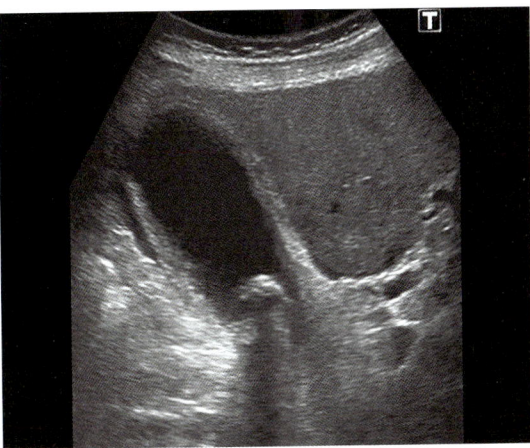

Fig. 2.2: Ultrasound scan of the gallbladder showing wall thickening, pericolic fluid and an obstructing stone in the gallbladder neck casting an acoustic shadow. These findings are keeping with acute cholecystitis.
Courtesy: Keegan C.

evident, and the patient may be mildly jaundiced, depending on the position of the stones. A swinging pyrexia and severe tenderness suggest an empyema, while a sudden deterioration in the patient's condition with spreading peritonitis suggests that the gallbladder has ruptured. A combination of pain, jaundice and pyrexia (Charcot's triad) suggests ascending cholangitis, usually due to ductal calculi and demands urgent treatment. However, in a patient with painless jaundice and a palpable gallbladder, the cause is unlikely to be gallstones, but more often a malignant obstruction of the common bile duct (Courvoisier's law).

Biochemically, inflammatory markers WBC and CRP are often raised, while bilirubin and liver enzymes may be deranged, and a serum amylase is crucial to help exclude acute pancreatitis.

Plain radiography is of little use. Gallstones are radiopaque in only approximately 10% of patients, and their presence does not necessarily implicate them as the cause of pain, since many stones are asymptomatic. Ultrasound (ideally within 48 h of admission) is the simplest method for confirming the presence of gallstones, and will also provide valuable information about the thickness of the gallbladder wall, the size of the common bile duct, the appearance of the liver (especially the presence or absence of intrahepatic bile duct dilation) and possibly also the pancreas (Fig. 2.2).

Is it Acute Pancreatitis?

Most patients with acute pancreatitis presents with a relatively sudden onset of severe epigastric pain, which usually radiates to the back and is often associated with vomiting. There may be a pre-existing history suggesting biliary tract disease or a history of alcohol abuse. Easing the pain by sitting forward is a classical feature.

There are no specific signs in the acute phase except extensive tenderness and guarding in the epigastrium, usually with diminished bowel sounds. Grey Turner's sign (bruising in the flanks) or Cullen's sign (periumbilical bruising) indicates retroperitoneal pancreatic necrosis and hemorrhage, and is usually associated with a poor outcome, but often does not appear until the disease is well established.

To establish a diagnosis of acute pancreatitis, two of the following three criteria should be met:

- Clinical history and examination consistent with acute pancreatitis
- Biochemically, a raised serum lipase or amylase (80% sensitivity, limited specificity) three times greater than the upper limit of normal. In total, 1–2% of the population has persistently high level of serum amylase due to the presence of an abnormal protein, which is not readily excreted (macroamylasemia). A urinary amylase >5,000 units/24 h may be helpful in diagnosing a delayed presentation and distinguishing macroamylasemia, as it will not be freely filtered by the glomerulus.
- Radiological findings of acute pancreatitis, commonly on CT, or alternatively on ultrasound or MRI (Fig. 2.3).

Plain erect chest radiographs are helpful in excluding visceral perforation, while abdominal films may identify a sentinel loop of small bowel reflecting a localized ileus produced by the inflammatory process. Ultrasound or MRI may be useful in establishing the etiology, and assessing the biliary anatomy.

Diagnosis of acute pancreatitis

- Clinically: Vomiting is common, pain may be eased by sitting forward.
- Biochemically: Serum amylase (80% sensitivity, limited specificity) is the most commonly used in the United Kingdom.
- Radiologically: CT will aid confirmation.

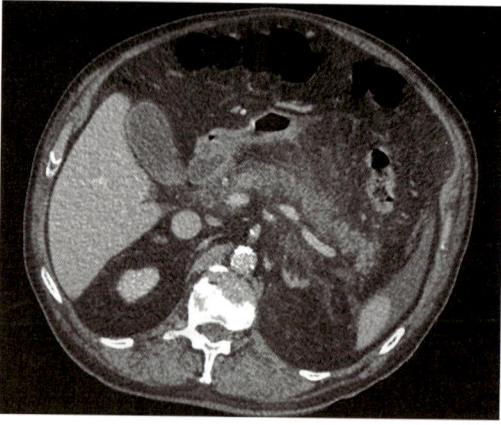

Fig. 2.3: Axial CT in the portal venous phase demonstrating acute pancreatitis as characterized by the adjacent inflammatory fat stranding. (CT: Computed tomography.) *Courtesy:* Keegan C.

Is it Acute Diverticulitis?

A typical patient with acute diverticulitis is over 60 years of age, although it seems to be becoming more common in younger age groups as well. They complain of acute left iliac fossa pain, a low-grade fever and marked tenderness to deep palpation in the left iliac fossa. Other features are variable: a mass may be palpable either in the left iliac fossa or pelvis. Surprisingly, a previous history of altered bowel habit is often absent, but there is usually some degree of abdominal distension and constipation during the attack. Commonly, there is a history of previous similar attacks and the patient may have already been investigated for the symptoms.

Biochemically, inflammatory markers such as WBC and CRP are often raised, and there may be white cells in the urine.

Plain chest radiographs are usually normal, but may demonstrate a diverticular perforation, while abdominal films may show distension of the proximal colon with the suggestion of a left iliac mass. CT is now the gold standard for confirming diverticulitis in the acute phase, assessment of complications such as perforation and corresponding degree of contamination (Hinchey classification) (Fig. 2.4).

Once a clinical diagnosis of acute diverticular disease without perforation has been made, treatment is commenced with broad-spectrum antibiotics and further endoscopic investigation may be delayed for 6–8 weeks to allow for inflammation to subside. While there is only low quality evidence for colonoscopy after acute diverticulitis has been confirmed on CT scan, it has been shown to detect a small number of cancers and advanced adenomas.

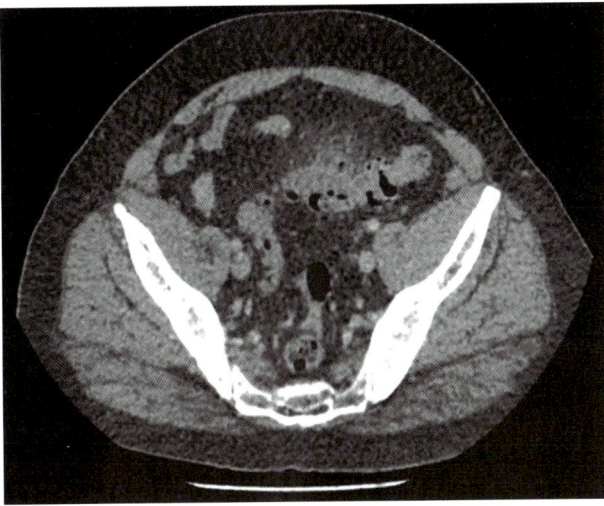

Fig. 2.4: Axial CT showing uncomplicated acute sigmoid diverticulitis. The bowel wall is thickened with adjacent inflammatory fat stranding focused around the diverticulum. No perforation or collection. (CT: Computed tomography.) *Courtesy:* Keegan C.

Is there a Perforated Viscus?

Most patients with a perforated viscus have severe abdominal pain and guarding or rigidity, but occasional patients, particularly frail elderly patients receiving NSAIDs or immunosuppressants, will have minimal or no signs. Conversely, severe abdominal pain with guarding may occur in the absence of intra-abdominal pathology in conditions such as esophageal rupture and pulmonary embolism. The diagnosis is further complicated by the fact that few patients with a perforated peptic ulcer or diverticular disease give a previous history suggesting the diagnosis.

The systemic disturbance in patients with a perforated viscus varies enormously, from the fit young patients with little systemic effect, but severe abdominal pain, to the patients with gross septicemia and shock on admission. The effect obviously depends on a variety of factors, including the patient's age and underlying comorbidities, duration of perforation, extent of contamination and nature of contaminating enteric content. A low-grade pyrexia is common.

Biochemically, inflammatory markers WBC and CRP are usually raised, as is the serum amylase (though not usually over 100 IU/L). Hemoglobin may be low if there has been blood loss, but is more likely to be relatively high, along with a raised hematocrit and urea, reflecting hypovolemia.

A plain erect posteroanterior chest film demonstrates free gas in approximately 70% of patients with perforated viscus, with a left lateral decubitus abdominal X-ray (AXR) an alternative in those not able to stand upright (Fig. 2.5). A plain abdominal film is likely to be normal but an ileus is common, with gas-filled loops of normal-sized small bowel centrally. In a hemodynamically stable patient with the absence of peritonitis, imaging in the form of CT offers higher sensitivity for detecting small amounts of free intraperitoneal air, as well as assessing the possible site of perforation and any other intra-abdominal pathology (Fig. 2.6).

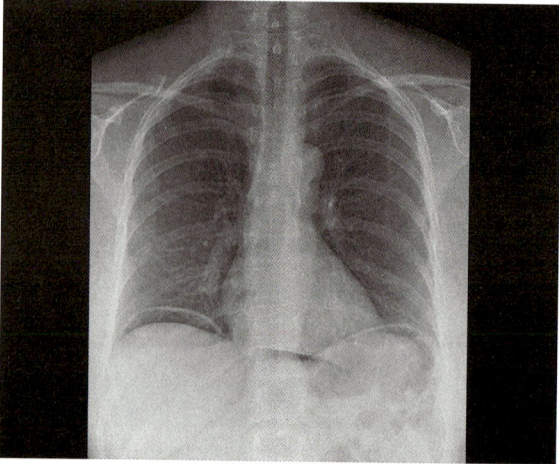

Fig. 2.5: An erect PA chest radiograph demonstrating pneumoperitoneum. Extensive subdiaphragmatic free air is seen. (PA: Posteroanterior.) *Courtesy:* Keegan C.

Acute Abdomen

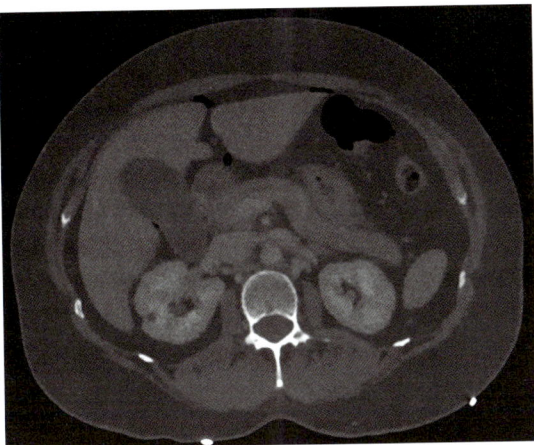

Fig. 2.6: Axial CT demonstrating pneumoperitoneum. Locules of air can be seen anterior to the liver edge and within the gallbladder fossa. This is viewed using bone windows but lung windows are also useful for identifying free intra-abdominal air. (CT: Computed tomography.)
Courtesy: Keegan C.

Is there Evidence of Peritonitis?

The clinical condition here will be very similar to that described with intestinal perforation, but causes also extend to mesenteric infarction and rupture of the gallbladder.

The patient with peritonitis becomes rapidly unwell over 4–6 h, and shows increasing signs of endotoxemia with tachycardia, hypotension, oliguria and prostration, movement of any kind worsens the abdominal pain, so the patient tends to remain very still. Involuntary guarding and rigidity of the abdominal wall on palpation are the hallmarks of the condition, and these signs alone may be an adequate reason for recommending laparotomy.

If there remains some uncertainty about the underlying cause of the problem after the initial assessment, a diagnostic laparoscopy may be considered.

Is there Intestinal Obstruction?

A diagnosis of intestinal obstruction is based on the combination of a suggestive history and typical radiographic changes, and confirmed by CT (Figs. 2.7 to 2.9).

Features in the history include colicky abdominal pain, abdominal distension, nausea and vomiting, and an alteration in bowel habit. The relative importance of each of these features depends on the level of the obstruction:
- Proximal obstruction may have early vomiting and a scaphoid abdomen.
- Distal obstruction may have constipation and a distended abdomen.

Previous abdominal surgery or the presence of a painful irreducible hernia in the groin may point to an underlying cause. Other features to look for during the clinical assessment include visible peristalsis, signs of hypovolemia, hyperactive bowels sounds and abdominal masses.

Computed tomography is the gold standard in confirming the diagnosis, dilation of small bowel loops >2.5 cm or large bowel >7 cm together with a paucity of intestinal gas distally is the hallmark of intestinal obstruction. It is also useful for identifying the site and potential etiology such as cancer, adhesions, hernia or volvulus. Equally CT is an excellent modality to differentiate ileus (e.g. in the postoperative period) from a mechanical small bowel obstruction, or pseudo-obstruction (Ogilvie's syndrome) from mechanical large bowel obstruction.

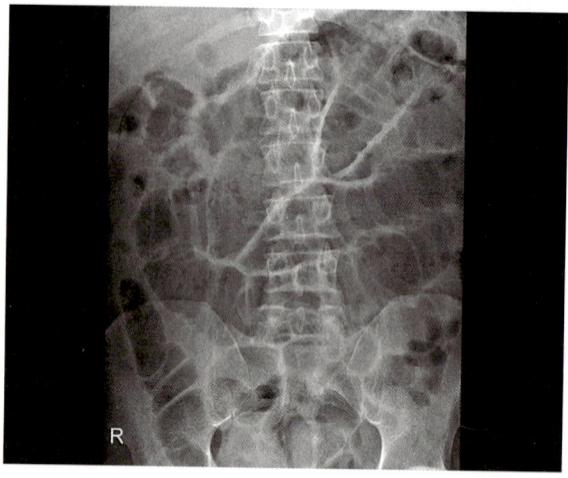

Fig. 2.7: Supine abdominal radiograph demonstrating incomplete small bowel obstruction, as there is some gas in the large bowel, its central positioning and valvulae conniventes passing across the full width of the lumen. *Courtesy:* Keegan C.

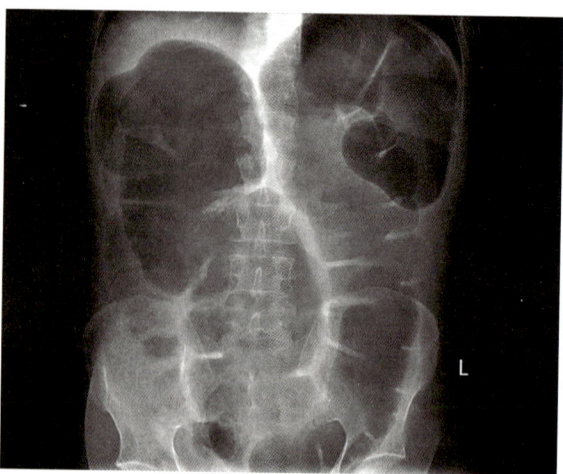

Fig. 2.8: Abdominal radiograph demonstrating large bowel obstruction, demonstrated by its peripheral positioning and haustral markings not completely traversing the bowel. *Courtesy:* Keegan C.

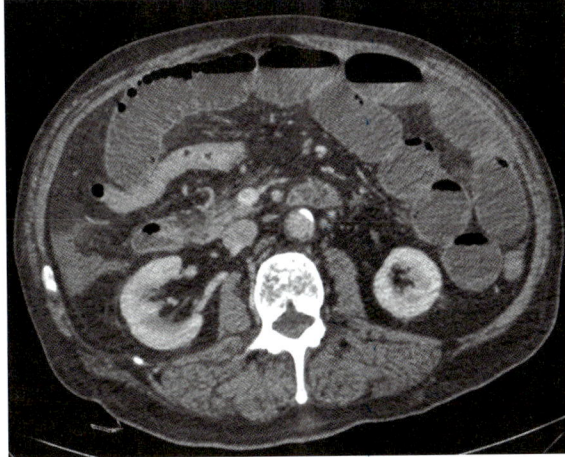

Fig. 2.9: Axial CT in the portal venous phase demonstrating dilated loops of small bowel. These can contain fluid as in this case, which may make identification on a plain radiograph difficult. There is also free fluid in the right paracolic gutter. (CT: Computed tomography.) *Courtesy:* Keegan C.

Is there an Evidence of Ischemia?

Having decided that a patient has an obstructed intestine, the possibility of ischemia secondary to adhesive obstruction should be considered. There are no clinical features or tests that are 100% accurate in the early stages. There may be clinical signs of a systemic inflammatory response syndrome and elevated inflammatory markers WBC and CRP, but both are nonspecific. Severe, persistent and well-localized tenderness on abdominal palpation is the most useful sign since it suggests significant peritoneal irritation and implies ischemia of an adjacent bowel loop.

The adage "never let the sun set on an obstructed abdomen" has much to recommend it because it reduces the risk of an ischemic segment becoming frankly necrotic and perforating with potentially severe consequences.

Is there an Intestinal Infarction?

A diagnosis of intestinal infarction should be near to or at the top of a list of differential diagnoses in a patient with known arteriopathy or who is in atrial fibrillation and has severe abdominal signs or symptoms. Initially, there is often a discrepancy between the symptoms (which are severe, with agonizing pain) and signs (which may be relatively unimpressive until the intestine infarcts and perforates). Vomiting and diarrhea are often prominent in early stages.

There are no reliable diagnostic tests in the early stages, but neutrophilia and lactic acidosis are common, while amylase may be marginally elevated. Radiographs are often normal, though there may be an ileus. Portal venous gas is usually a grave prognostic sign. A high index of suspicion is needed for patients at risk, with early laparotomy if there is any doubt. CT is often helpful in confirming the diagnosis (Figs. 2.10 and 2.11).

Infarction due to venous thrombosis presents in a similar way, but there is often a more prolonged prodromal illness lasting a few days in which nonspecific symptoms such as vomiting and diarrhea predominate. Hemoconcentration is common and there may be splenomegaly. Once the acute problem has been dealt with, the underling hypercoagulable state, which is usually present, will need investigation. This will include measuring antithrombin III, protein S and C levels, and anticoagulation following surgery is mandatory if further venous infarction is to be avoided.

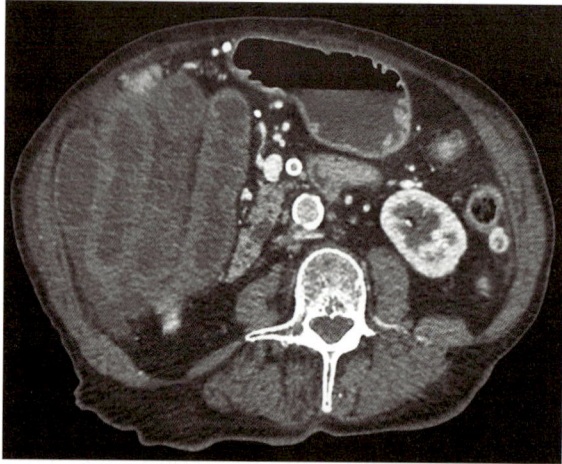

Fig. 2.10: Axial CT in the portal venous phase demonstrating thickened, dilated distal ileum with no enhancement of its walls and surrounding free fluid, confirming small bowel infarction. (CT: Computed tomography.) *Courtesy:* Keegan C.

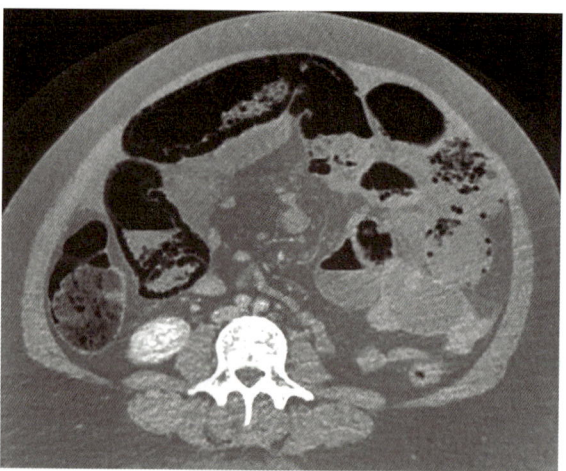

Fig. 2.11: Axial CT (lung window) demonstrating dilated loops of small bowel and circumferential pneumatosis intestinalis, indicating infarction of bowel wall. (CT: Computed tomography.) *Courtesy:* Keegan C.

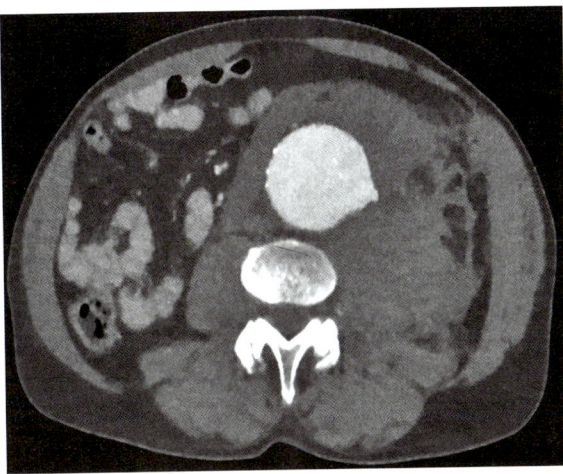

Fig. 2.12: Computed tomography aortic angiogram demonstrating a large abdominal aortic aneurysm that has ruptured with extensive surrounding hematoma.
Courtesy: Keegan C.

Is there a Leaking Aortic Aneurysm?

The emergency presentation of an abdominal aortic aneurysm can vary from sudden collapse and death to a patient with vague abdominal and/or back pain in whom an aneurysm is detected during a routine physical examination. More commonly, the patient, usually a man who is over 60 years of age, has a previous history of backache for a few weeks and presents with a sudden severe pain in his back and abdomen, which is followed by collapse and prostration.

The diagnosis can be missed easily unless the clinician palpates the abdomen with this in mind because:
- Pulsation may be weak if there is marked hypotension.
- If back pain predominates, renal colic may be mistakenly diagnosed instead.

An emergency bedside ultrasound scan will confirm the presence of an abdominal aortic aneurysm, and should be followed by a prompt CT in a stable patient. CT is the gold standard for diagnosis, but also allows for potential preoperative endovascular planning. More commonly, immediate surgical intervention will be required especially in the critically unstable (Fig. 2.12).

Is there a Gynecological Problem?

Several gynecological conditions can cause an acute abdomen, typically in relatively young women.

Rupture of Ectopic Pregnancy

The most important gynecological condition causing an acute abdomen is a ruptured ectopic pregnancy, which can be rapidly fatal if not dealt with urgently and effectively. An entirely normal menstrual history does not exclude a ruptured ectopic pregnancy, and this diagnosis must be considered in any women of childbearing age with sudden, severe, lower abdominal pain and collapse. Shoulder tip pain suggests diaphragmatic irritation from intraperitoneal blood. A history of relative infertility is common.

The most common site for the ectopic pregnancy is in the ampulla of the fallopian tube, so when the rupture occurs, the tube is badly damaged and has to be removed. If the condition is diagnosed before it ruptures, the tube can usually be reconstructed, but the primary concern of the surgeon in the emergency situation must be to control hemorrhage and prevent an avoidable death.

Acute Salpingitis

Acute salpingitis can be caused by a variety of infecting organisms. The patient typically presents with pelvic peritonitis, which is often associated with vomiting and a high fever. There is usually marked tenderness in both iliac fossae, and pain when the cervix is moved during vaginal examination.

The most important differential is acute appendicitis, and diagnostic laparoscopy can be extremely useful in this situation.

Acute salpingitis can progress to pyosalpinx, which is usually bilateral and characterized by the presence of a tender, boggy swelling the pouch of Douglas. A sudden severe deterioration with spreading peritonitis suggests an intraperitoneal rupture of a pyosalpinx. Complications from scarring include chronic pelvic pain, infertility, ectopic pregnancy or spread to external surface of the liver (Fitz–Hugh–Curtis' syndrome).

Torsion of an Ovarian Cyst

Torsion of an ovarian cyst typically causes acute, severe pain and vomiting, but little systemic disturbance. A tender mass in the pelvis can usually be felt on bimanual examination. As the condition progresses and pelvic peritonitis ensues, it may become impossible to palpate the mass without a general anesthetic due to guarding in the lower abdomen.

Occasionally, massive ovarian cysts give rise to an acute abdominal presentation, usually because of torsion or simple infarction.

Spontaneous Rupture of an Endometriotic Cyst

Spontaneous rupture of an endometriotic cyst, usually of the ovary, gives rise to a clinical picture that can resemble both ruptured ectopic pregnancy and acute salpingitis. In this condition, irregular nodularity palpable on bimanual examination in the pouch of Douglas and in the broad ligament will suggest the etiology.

Investigating Possible Gynecological Causes of Acute Pelvic Peritonitis

If there is a possible gynecological cause for an acute pelvic peritonitis, useful investigations include pelvic ultrasound, transvaginal ultrasound and laparoscopy. Diagnostic laparoscopy offers the benefit of being a possible therapeutic tool without resorting to a laparotomy.

A gynecological opinion should always be sought prior to any radical excisional surgery.

> **Initial management of the patient with acute abdomen**
> - A completely normal menstrual history does not exclude an ectopic pregnancy.
> - Check the serum amylase before carrying out a laparotomy for abdominal pain.
> - Surgical intervention should be early in intestinal obstruction and when ischemia is a possibility.

Is Emergency Laparotomy Indicated?

The decision to perform an emergency laparotomy is usually based largely on clinical grounds and should not be particularly difficult to make.

- For patients with probable appendicitis, an appendicectomy should be carried out without delay, except in women of childbearing age, for whom preliminary laparoscopy may be preferable. If, however, an appendix mass has developed, surgery may be safely delayed to allow conservative management with antibiotics.
- Emergency intervention is indicated for a probably ruptured abdominal aortic aneurysm unless there is evidence of some other life-threatening condition or terminal disease.
- A diagnosis of peritonitis, of whatever cause, based on the findings of abdominal rigidity and involuntary guarding, and usually accompanied by systemic signs such as a tachycardia and fever, is a clear indication for laparotomy.
- Impressive local signs that render adequate palpation of the whole abdomen impossible (e.g. those that might develop over an empyema of the gallbladder or ischemic bowel loop) should generally precipitate a laparotomy to prevent the peritonitis that may well develop otherwise.
- Patients with intestinal obstruction should generally have a laparotomy within 24 h of presentation, but only after the diagnosis has been adequately confirmed radiologically, unless adhesions are thought to be the most likely cause and the patient's condition improves rapidly with conservative measures. It is not acceptable to wait for several days for an episode of presumed adhesive obstruction to settle.

- If there is concern about a patient's progress following a laparotomy, either because of protracted ileus or anxiety about an anastomosis, CT or occasionally a diagnostic laparoscopy are options prior to a second laparotomy.
- Finally, if there is any question of ischemic intestine, for example in a patient with small bowel obstruction or in a patient with known arteriopathy with abdominal pain, a laparotomy should be considered earlier rather than later.

> **Common medical causes of an acute abdomen**
> - Diabetic ketoacidosis
> - Inferior myocardial infarction
> - Basal pulmonary emboli
> - Basal pneumonia.

Common Misdiagnoses

Several medical conditions can present with abdominal symptoms and signs that are severe enough to precipitate an emergency laparotomy. Any acute cardiopulmonary condition may present with predominantly epigastric or upper abdominal pain. Epigastric pain, usually without tenderness, is a common feature of inferior myocardial infarction, while in basal pneumonia or basal infarction due to pulmonary emboli there may be severe tenderness and guarding. Chest radiography and electrocardiography will usually resolve the dilemma. However, linear atelectasis on the radiograph may be due to either pulmonary infarction or a reaction to problems below the diaphragm. Any further uncertainty can be resolved with CT.

A young patient with diabetes presenting with ketoacidosis may have impressive abdominal signs and if there is any suggestion of acidosis in such a patient, blood and urine glucose and arterial blood gases must be checked urgently.

Less common medical conditions that occasionally present as emergencies with abdominal pain include sickle cell disease, acute intermittent porphyria, systemic vasculitis, complement C1-esterase inhibitor deficiency and familial Mediterranean fever. Of these, porphyria is arguably the most important to consider since mismanagement, particularly the administration of inappropriate drugs, is likely to be fatal.

Other Pitfalls

- The removal of a normal appendix is hardly a catastrophe, but the normal appendicectomy rate should be about 10%, except in young females, among whom it should be possible to reduce this figure by introducing a policy of preliminary laparoscopy.
- Misdiagnosis of a leaking abdominal aortic aneurysm for left renal colic is not uncommon, and the abdomen of any patient with acute back pain

must be palpated carefully for an aneurysm. A finding of aneurysmal femoral arteries on palpating the groins should alert the clinician to the possibility of an aortic aneurysm.
- A lengthy delay before carrying out a laparotomy in a patient with intestinal obstruction and/or ischemia is potentially disastrous.
- Carrying out a laparotomy in a patient with colonic pseudo-obstruction in the belief that the instruction is mechanical is not acceptable. A CT scan will differentiate the two.
- Carrying out a laparotomy in a patient who has Munchausen's syndrome is a mistake that often cannot be avoided. However, if the syndrome is suspected, collateral history from the relatives, review of previous admissions/imaging and a CT scan should be helpful.
- Failing to diagnose a femoral hernia in a patient with small bowel obstruction is unfortunately very common, and usually delays appropriate surgical intervention.

> **Further points in the diagnosis of an acute abdomen**
> - Intrathoracic esophageal rupture may present as an acute abdomen.
> - If a ruptured aortic aneurysm is suspected, a CT scan must not be delayed.
> - In intestinal infarction, the signs are often unimpressive in the presence of severe symptoms, and an air in the portal vein is a grave prognostic sign.

CONDITIONS CAUSING ACUTE ABDOMINAL PAIN: NATURAL HISTORY AND MANAGEMENT

Acute Appendicitis, Appendix Abscess and Appendix Mass

Natural History

Acute appendicitis is a common condition affecting all ages, the current incidence being approximately 1 in a 100 per year. It is relatively uncommon at the extremes of life, and there is a peak incidence in the second decade.

Etiology and Pathogenesis

The etiology remains unknown, but it seems to be a condition of developed societies, and the pathological process in the organ is often related to luminal obstruction, either by a fecolith or by lymphoid hyperplasia. Occasionally, patients with cecal tumors present with appendicitis after the appendiceal lumen is obstructed by the tumor.

Management

Once acute appendicitis has been diagnosed, an emergency appendicectomy should be carried out without further delay. Appendicectomy is also indicated for those patients in whom there may be some doubt about the diagnosis, but whose right iliac fossa pain and tenderness fail to resolve or worsen with time. Prophylactic antibiotics should be used, and continued if the appendix appears abnormal.

The approach used depends partly on the clinical situation:
- A classical, muscle-splitting oblique incision in the right iliac fossa is used most frequently, offering excellent access, can be extended easily and heals well.
- A midline incision is probably wiser in the older patient in whom alternative, more sinister diagnoses are possible.
- In pregnancy, the incision must be sited over the position of maximum tenderness, which depends on the stage of pregnancy and may be in the right upper quadrant.
- A laparoscopic approach offers excellent visualization of intra-abdominal pathology and may be used as a diagnostic or as a therapeutic tool.

An appendix abscess should be drained at the time of appendicectomy, which may be very difficult if the appendix is partially necrotic.

An appendix mass, if diagnosed before the patient is anesthetized, can be treated conservatively with broad-spectrum antibiotics and close observation to ensure that it resolves. Signs of sepsis, such as swinging pyrexia, indicating the development of an abscess, would suggest a failure of conservative management. Persistence of a mass should suggest alternative diagnoses such as Crohn's disease or a cecal lesion. If the patient is already anesthetized when the mass is first felt, an appendicectomy should still be carried out, but in this situation, it is often wise to involve a more senior surgeon because a more extensive procedure might be necessary.

A normal appendix will be removed in approximately 10% of cases despite modern imaging. It is the authors' practice to remove a macroscopically normal looking appendix at laparoscopy if no other pathology is identified, to exclude endoluminal appendicitis and avoid future confusion as to whether the appendix has been removed. Alternative causes (Crohn's disease, *Yersinia* infection, perforated peptic ulcer, cholecystitis, Meckel's diverticulitis or gynecological problems, particularly on the right side) should be looked for. Some of these alternative causes can be managed conservatively or treated using the same access, but occasionally a conversion to midline laparotomy will be necessary. An uncomplicated Meckel's diverticulum should not be interfered with.

Prognosis

Timely surgical intervention has a very high success rate, and usually morbidity and very occasional mortality mainly occur when diagnosis is delayed (Figs. 2.13 and 2.14).

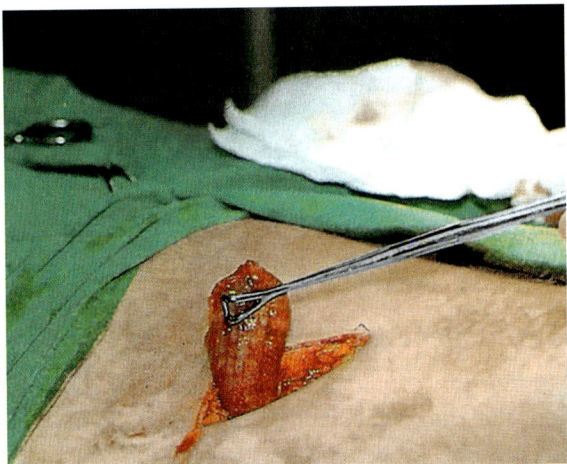

Fig. 2.13: An acutely inflamed appendix delivered via a conventional "Lanz" incision.

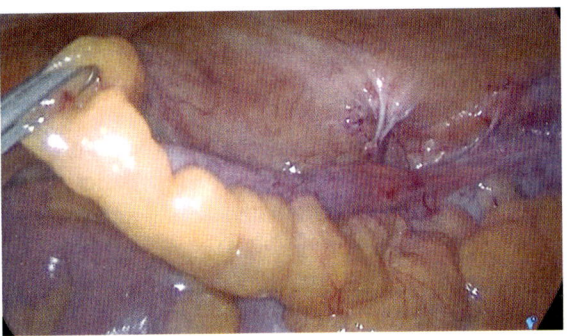

Fig. 2.14: An acutely inflamed appendix identified laparoscopically.

> **Important points in the diagnosis and management of appendicitis**
> - Raised inflammatory markers are not universal.
> - A diagnostic laparoscopy especially in women aged 15–45 years can be a helpful tool.
> - In pregnancy, the incision is placed at the site of maximal tenderness.
> - The diagnosis is most difficult if the patient is mentally impaired, very young or very old.
> - If ileal Crohn's disease is discovered, appendicectomy will not affect the risk of fistula formation.

Acute Cholecystitis, Empyema and Mucocele

Natural History

Most people with gallstones are asymptomatic. The most common presentations seem to be recurrent attacks of biliary colic (a clinical diagnosis) leading ultimately to chronic cholecystitis (a histological diagnosis). However, a small proportion of patients with gallstones present with an acute abdomen secondary to acute cholecystitis or, more often, empyema and possible perforation.

Epidemiology

Gallstones are common and are present in approximately 40% of women and 20% of men by 80 years of age.

Etiology and Pathogenesis

In the small proportion of patients with gallstones who present with an acute abdomen, the cause is usually sudden impaction of a gallstone in the cystic duct, leading to an obstructed gallbladder containing infected bile. Occasionally in acute cholecystitis, there are no gallstones (acalculous cholecystitis), and this often follows a traumatic episode such as an esophageal resection or major burns, but may also occur in systemic vasculitis.

Management

Conservative measures including intravenous fluids, and usually (intravenous) antibiotics, are commenced for most patients once acute cholecystitis or empyema has been diagnosed clinically. Opiate analgesia is given to control pain until the diagnosis is confirmed. Deranged liver function tests and a raised serum amylase may suggest ductal calculi. If the diagnosis is confirmed within 7 days of the onset of symptoms, there are two main courses of action:
- Immediate cholecystectomy
- Continuation of conservative management with a view to delayed cholecystectomy 6 weeks later.

A small proportion of patients have signs of peritoneal irritation at presentation and fail to settle with conservative measures. The majority of such patients will require emergency cholecystectomy. A simple cholecystectomy can usually be carried out in such patients because the cystic duct is blocked, but facilities for an on-table cholangiogram should be available. In the very acute phase, the surgery is often facilitated by edema, but it must be stressed that inexperienced surgeons should not undertake this type of procedure. In patients with complex comorbidities, a radiologically guided tube drain is an alternative. Once 7–10 days from onset has lapsed, urgent surgery becomes difficult and further delay is probably justified to allow the inflammatory process to settle.

In practice, it is often the availability of an operating theater and/or a suitably experienced surgeon that limits the role of urgent surgery in this situation, but reducing the number and length of admissions for an individual patient can have advantages, both for the patient and hospital.

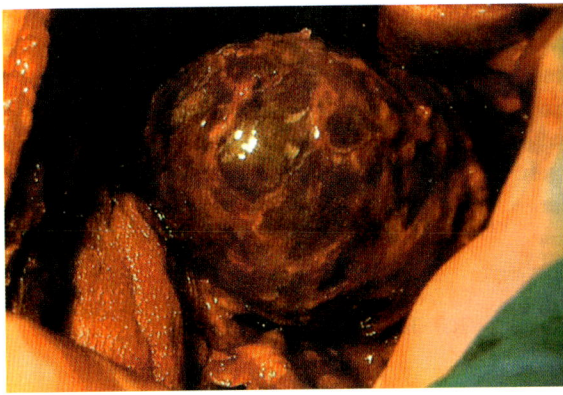

Fig. 2.15: Acute gangrenous cholecystitis.

A laparoscopic approach is the standard of care. One useful tip in the emergency situation is to aspirate the gallbladder at the start of the procedure, to facilitate traction and dissection. Again, the extent to which cholangiography or choledochoscopy is used will depend on the individual situation and the experience of the operating surgeon, but one or other facility should be available (Fig. 2.15).

Ascending Cholangitis

Parenteral fluids and antibiotics are commenced early for the patient with ascending cholangitis, but the single most important aspect is drainage of the common bile duct, commonly by emergency ERCP with sphincterotomy and extraction of stones. In the few patients where endoscopic drainage is not possible, a PTC drainage tube may be considered. The necessity for interval cholecystectomy is not universal, and generally the decision to recommend cholecystectomy in such patients can be taken on the basis of the presence or absence of ongoing biliary colic and/or cholecystitis.

> **Key points in biliary tract disease**
> - Suppurative cholangitis (a high fever, pain and usually accompanied by jaundice) is an emergency and requires decompression of the biliary system.
> - Cholangitis is not always accompanied by jaundice (although LFTs, particularly alkaline phosphatase, are nearly always abnormal).
> - If acute cholecystitis is diagnosed within 3–4 days of presentation, an urgent cholecystectomy should be considered.

Acute Pancreatitis

Natural History

Approximately 80% of patients with acute pancreatitis have a relatively mild and self-limiting illness. The remaining patients may follow a relatively stormy course with multiorgan dysfunction syndrome, peripancreatic fluid collection, pancreatic necrosis, or pseudocyst, and a significant eventual mortality, which may rise to 50% if infected pancreatic necrosis develops.

Gallstone-related disease may recur as acute attacks on an occasional basis, presumably as stones pass down the common bile duct, until the underlying biliary disease is corrected. Alcohol-related pancreatitis typically slips into a recurrent acute/chronic form, which tends to be exacerbated by alcoholic binges.

Etiology and Pathogenesis

- Gallstones are the most common etiological factor in the United Kingdom, accounting for approximately 60% of cases.
- Alcohol is the cause in approximately 30% of patients.
- A variety of conditions such as certain viral illnesses (notably mumps), some drugs (e.g. corticosteroids, azathioprine and diuretics), hypercalcemia, hypertriglyceridemia and some familial metabolic disorders are associated, usually with less severe forms of the disease.
- ERCP is complicated by a 3% risk of acute pancreatitis, particularly in young women with normal ducts. While usually mild, it may be severe, particularly if infection has been introduced.

It has been postulated that gallstone-related pancreatitis results from the reflux of infected bile into the pancreatic duct, but how the other forms of pancreatitis fit into this model is unclear.

Management

Management depends on the severity of the disease:
- A patient with mild acute pancreatitis may require almost no specific treatment.
- A patient with severe acute pancreatitis may require major ventilatory, circulatory and renal support.

Universal measures include intravenous fluid infusion and appropriate analgesia. This is followed by an assessment of severity; common assessment scores include APACHE II and Glasgow, while CRP has proved to be a reliable single predictive marker in clinical practice.

Blood gas estimation is also important because severe hypoxemia is not uncommon and may not be easy to recognize clinically. It presumably reflects physiological shunting as part of the syndrome of acute adult respiratory distress syndrome, which is a common consequence of severe pancreatitis.

Routine monitoring is commenced and may be extended to include regular assessments of central venous pressure and mean arterial pressures, depending on the severity of the attack. Plain films of the chest should be obtained early. Pleural effusion and pulmonary edema are features of severe pancreatitis.

The clinical progress of the patient will dictate the need for oxygen therapy and for the infusion of potentially large volumes of intravenous fluids to maintain central venous pressure and urine output. Hypovolemia may be severe and a common, but serious, error is an underestimation of fluid requirements, which may reach many liters in the first 24 h. Nutritional support may become necessary, preferentially by the enteral route, but possibly parenterally.

Deteriorating respiratory function may require intensive care nursing and possible intubation with mechanically assisted ventilation. A labile blood pressure, cardiac output and peripheral vascular resistance may require inotropic support, while a renal dose of dopamine may be required to maintain an adequate urine output. Ultimately, dialysis may be required.

Detecting Pancreatic Necrosis

Detecting pancreatic necrosis early during the course of a severe attack is not easy.

- An estimation of CRP provides a non-specific marker, a level higher than 150 mg/L at 48 h being a bad prognostic sign.
- The investigation of choice is a CT scan with intravenous contrast, since necrotic areas of the gland are not perfused and will not therefore enhance. There may also be evidence of infection such as gas formation.

Infected necrosis represents a significant worsening in prognosis, being associated with a mortality up to 50%, and should be managed in a specialized multidisciplinary unit with access to interventional radiology and endoscopy. Fine needle aspiration by either CT or USS guidance may help to differentiate between sterile and infected necrosis. However, many units now use organ dysfunction as the basis for surgical intervention.

Role of Surgery

The role, method and timing of surgery in the management of acute pancreatitis are controversial. The decision to abandon conservative measures in favor of an aggressive surgical approach in the patient with necrotizing pancreatitis is still made largely on clinical grounds, usually when and if the patient begins to show signs of sepsis. A practical approach is to defer surgery as long as possible in the absence of sepsis. Formal pancreatic resection in the emergency situation is extremely difficult and dangerous, whereas blunt necrosectomy can be relatively straightforward if sufficient time has elapsed since the start of the illness for viable and non-viable pancreas to be delineated adequately. When intervention is required, there is evidence to support a "step-up" approach with percutaneous drainage, followed by minimal access retroperitoneal pancreatic necrosectomy. Infected pseudocysts are managed along similar lines, with the addition of endoscopic approaches.

Gallstone-related Disease

For patients with more severe gallstone-related acute pancreatitis who fail to settle, there is much to commend an urgent ERCP with sphincterotomy to clear the distal common bile duct. This is especially true for patients with jaundice and exhibiting signs of sepsis. If an impacted stone is removed early in the course of an attack, the result can occasionally be dramatic, with a rapid resolution of symptoms. However, the majority of patients do not require this approach, in those who settle MRCP is almost always normal.

Definitive surgery in the form of cholecystectomy should be undertaken as soon as possible, ideally within 2 weeks of the attack.

Significant prognostic factors in acute pancreatitis within the first 48 h

Glasgow criteria: the presence of three or more of the following factors predicts a severe attack:
- P—PaO_2 <8 kPa
- A—age >55 years old
- N—neutrophilia: WCC >15 × 10^9/L
- C—calcium <2 mmol/L
- R—renal function: urea >16 mmol/L
- E—enzymes: LDH >600 IU/L; AST >200 IU/L
- A—albumin <32 g/L (serum)
- S—sugar: blood glucose >10 mmol/L

Perforated Viscus

Spontaneous perforation of the gastrointestinal tract is a surgical emergency that most often presents as an acute abdominal condition, though esophageal perforation may occasionally present with predominantly cardiorespiratory symptoms and signs, and perforation below the diaphragm is sometimes entirely silent. The natural history and management will obviously vary according to the site involved, and this section has therefore been divided along simple anatomical lines.

General Management

Once visceral perforation has been diagnosed or is considered to be the most likely underlying problem, initial management is similar irrespective of the suspected site of perforation. It is directed at correcting the constitutional disturbance before surgery, since surgical intervention is recommended for all except a few patients.

Having obtained the usual baseline blood tests (i.e. full blood count, urea and electrolytes, amylase, and group and save serum), nil by mouth, and an intravenous infusion being commenced, the rapidity of fluid replacement is dictated by the clinical situation. Broad-spectrum intravenous antibiotics according to hospital formulary are started immediately, and a urinary catheter is placed to monitor urine output. Routine observation is commenced and repeated frequently, depending on the clinical situation.

Critical care input may be required, and early involvement preoperatively may be beneficial. The endotoxemia and septic shock that can accompany fecal peritonitis may make it necessary for a hemodynamic monitoring such as PiCCO (Pulse Index Continuous Cardiac Output) device, particularly if there are any cardiorespiratory comorbidities. Pharmacological support in the form of pressor agents such as dopamine may be required to maintain urine output so that it exceeds 0.5 mL/kg/h or to sustain an adequate systolic blood pressure >100 mm Hg.

Esophageal Perforation

Natural History

Non-instrumental esophageal perforation (Boerhaave's syndrome) typically occurs in a patient who has over indulged in food and/or alcohol and results from vomiting against a closed glottis.

A sudden severe chest pain and shortness of breath after vomiting should alert the clinician about the possibility of an esophageal perforation, but the degree of prostration may confuse the issue and point toward alternative diagnoses such as acute myocardial infarction. Such patients may present with an acute abdomen and rigidity and the possibility of an esophageal perforation may only be considered after a negative laparotomy. If the diagnosis is in doubt, a CT chest and abdomen will confirm it.

The importance of the cardinal physical sign of subcutaneous emphysema, usually in the neck, but occasionally elsewhere, and also seen in the mediastinum on the chest X-rays, cannot be overstated.

Rapidly advancing respiratory embarrassment is typical, with the development of a hydropneumothorax, more often on the left side than on the right.

Management

Early recognition of esophageal perforation is vitally important. The general measures as mentioned earlier are important, but placement of an intercostal drainage tube may also be required with some urgency because a tension pneumothorax is an occasional problem. The chest drain will also remove some of the food debris contaminating the pleural cavity, and may be required bilaterally. At this stage, a decision will have to be made about the advisability of transferring the patient to a specialized thoracic unit, depending on the expertise of the local surgeons and the effectiveness of resuscitation.

The best surgical approach is to open the left chest to approach the distal esophagus because this is the most common site of perforation in Boerhaave's syndrome. If the perforation is recognized early and surgery is carried out within 24 h, a primary repair may be attempted. The muscular tear must be extended and the esophagus repaired in layers with non-absorbable material, the repair being buttressed with a patch of intercostal muscle or a 360° fundoplication. In most circumstances, the only realistic option is to resect the partially necrotic esophagus, carry out an extensive debridement and lavage the pleural cavity. Whether or not immediate reconstruction is attempted will depend on local surgical expertise and the condition of the patient in the knowledge that delayed secondary reconstruction is likely to be difficult. If reconstruction is attempted immediately, the intrathoracic stomach will probably be the organ of choice. If it is delayed, a colonic transposition in the anterior mediastinum may be considered. In either event, anastomosis placed in the neck is more likely to heal, and cause lesser problems if they do not heal, than those within the contaminated thoracic cavity.

A limited case can be made for aggressive conservative management using combined suction drainage of pleural cavities and the esophagus, but it tends to be reserved for patients whose prognosis is very poor from the outset. Furthermore, the pleural cavity obviously cannot be debrided if the chest is not opened, and such debridement constitutes a significant part of the conventional surgical approach.

Prognosis

The prognosis of esophageal perforation is relatively poor, with mortality up to 50%, largely due to gross contamination of the mediastinum and pleural cavities (Fig. 2.16).

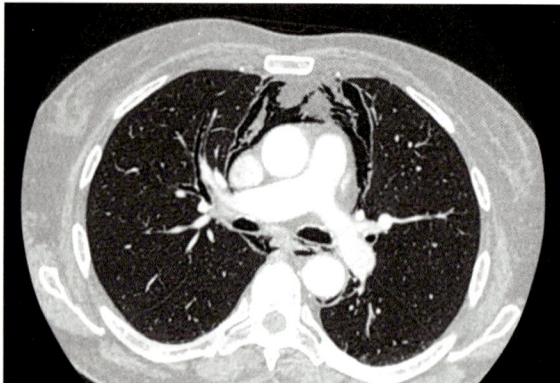

Fig. 2.16: Computed tomography thorax demonstrating pneumomediastinum, the anterior mediastinum is particularly affected here but there is also air tracking along the posterior mediastinum, which is more subtle on this image.

Gastric and Duodenal Perforation

Natural History

The patient with gastric or duodenal perforation presents with sudden severe epigastric pain with involuntary guarding. Shoulder tip pain represents subdiaphragmatic irritation, while appendicitis is sometimes simulated by the leakage of gastric contents into the right paracolic gutter. The constitutional disturbance can vary enormously, from no disturbance to severe prostration with dehydration, oliguria and hypotension. Occasionally, a patient has a silent perforation, and has no symptoms or signs.

Etiology and Pathogenesis

Most perforations of the stomach and duodenum are due to peptic ulceration, but occasionally a gastric neoplasm presents this way. Young dyspeptic men who smoke are still seen with an acute perforation of an anterior duodenal ulcer, but are now outnumbered by elderly women with an acute perforation of a gastric ulcer, almost all of whom give a history of taking NSAIDs.

Management and Prognosis

Having demonstrated a perforation of the stomach or duodenum, the main stream approach is surgical. The conservative (non-operative) approach risks missing alternative diagnosis such as perforated diverticular disease, and is probably best reserved for the following:
- Patients who refuse surgery
- Patients who are so compromised that any form of surgical intervention would be extremely hazardous
- Patients who are well and whose perforation can be well localized on imaging.

Operations for Perforated Gastric Ulcer

Patients at greatest risk should in general receive the simplest procedure, which is usually an oversew of the perforation with a wedge biopsy if there is a gastric ulcer. Since the availability of effective agents such as H_2 antagonists and proton pump inhibitors, many surgeons adopt a minimalist surgical approach for all patients with perforated ulcers. The elective operation of choice for gastric ulcer conventionally has been a Billroth I gastrectomy, but as most patients with a perforated gastric ulcer are relatively frail and elderly, biopsies from the ulcer or even ulcer excision, plus simple closure and postoperative proton pump inhibitors will be used almost universally. If malignant perforation is suspected, a Billroth II gastrectomy may be considered, but again most patients will not be suitable for such a radical approach in the emergency setting. Having said this, the prognosis for perforated gastric carcinoma is universally poor, because it has usually spread to the peritoneal surface and throughout the peritoneal cavity.

Operations for Perforated Duodenal Ulcer

The situation for a perforated duodenal ulcer is a little more complicated, partly because most patients are younger and reasonably fit. Ulcer-curing surgery obviously takes longer, and is therefore probably associated with an increased immediate morbidity, but simple ulcer closure itself is not without morbidity, and there is a risk to the patient from reperforation or bleeding after closure. A diagnostic laparoscopy with a view to closure or patch repair is commonplace with the benefit of faster recovery, and should especially be considered when there is diagnostic uncertainty.

A small portion of patients with a perforated chronic ulcer will need long-term medical management postoperatively or even further elective surgery at a later date after simple closure, and a small proportion of these patients may suffer a further life-threatening complication such as bleeding or gastric outlet obstruction.

Small Bowel Perforation

Natural History

The natural history of small bowel perforation depends entirely on the underlying diagnosis, which can be extremely varied. The patient usually presents with diffuse abdominal pain and generalized peritonitis, with a variable degree of systemic disturbance. It should be remembered that the condition found to be causing the perforation at the initial laparotomy may affect other parts of the gastrointestinal tract to a lesser degree, and this will obviously influence the long-term outlook.

Management

Small bowel perforation is managed by laparotomy and intestinal resection. The extent of the resection will be determined by the operative findings, the single most important consideration being the preservation of an adequate vascular supply to the bowel ends used for anastomosis. A conservative approach to the surgery for small bowel Crohn's disease is considered wise, with limited resection if possible.

Other technical points include:
- The use of defunctioning stomas as a temporary measure rather than an immediate anastomosis when there is excessive peritoneal contamination.
- The use of a "second-look" laparotomy at approximately 48 h postoperatively if the initial presentation has been caused by diffuse vasculitis or ischemia. A further resection can be undertaken if necessary before reperforation occurs.

Table 2.1: Conditions associated with small bowel perforation.	
Mechanical	Strangulating obstruction Foreign body Trauma
Idiopathic	Nonspecific ulceration
Drug-induced	Potassium supplements NSAIDs Corticosteroids Chemotherapeutic agents
Inflammatory	Jejuno-ileal diverticula Meckel's diverticulum Crohn's disease Zollinger–Ellison's syndrome Celiac disease
Neoplastic	Primary and secondary carcinomas Lymphomas Leukemias Carcinoid tumors Gastrointestinal stromal tumor Desmoids
Infective	Typhoid Tuberculosis
Parasitic	Ascariasis
Vascular	Mesenteric infarction
Connective tissue disorders	Polyarteritis nodosa Systemic lupus erythematosus Wegener's granulomatosis Scleroderma Rheumatoid arthritis
Metabolic	Amyloidosis
Iatrogenic	Operative injury Radiation damage

The prognosis will depend entirely on the underlying pathological diagnosis (Table 2.1).

Large Bowel Perforation

Natural History

Patients whose diverticular perforation is initially well-localized may present with an area of well-defined tenderness and a possible mass (acute diverticulitis); sudden deterioration with spreading peritonitis at a later stage suggests a communication of the peritoneal cavity. Patients with frank fecal contamination of the peritoneal cavity presents with lower abdominal peritonitis and commonly a severe constitutional upset, and the decision to recommend a surgical approach is not usually difficult.

Routine blood tests may reveal raised inflammatory markers in leukocytosis and CRP. There may also be free intraperitoneal gas on an erect chest radiograph. A CT will confirm the diagnosis and demonstrate the extent of contamination.

Etiology

In developed countries, large bowel perforation is usually secondary to diverticular disease, carcinoma or iatrogenic. There may, therefore, be a previous history of diverticular disease or carcinoma, or ongoing investigations of altered bowel habit or anemia suggesting the presence of an underlying problem.

Management and Prognosis

The success of the therapeutic approach to large bowel perforation depends almost entirely on the ability to control the gross sepsis that usually complicates the condition. The long-term prognosis of perforated diverticular disease should be excellent if sepsis is controlled and the patient survives any need for intervention, although all subsequent procedures will have their own inherent operative morbidity and mortality.

The risk of recurrent disease is high for patients with perforated carcinoma of the colon and higher than the risk for patients with non-perforated carcinoma of the colon at the same Dukes' stage. This is probably related to the spillage of tumor cells into the general peritoneal cavity through the perforation. However, not all colonic perforations associated with tumors occur at the site of the tumor. If there is large bowel obstruction, perforation may occur in the segment immediately proximal to the tumor (stercoral perforation); or in the cecum where the large bowel's diameter increases more rapidly in obstruction.

Perforated colonic carcinoma should be resected if at all possible. This may involve the in-continuity resection of adjacent organs such as small bowel or uterus, but the palliation achieved by resection is far superior to that achieved with lesser surgical procedures. Perforated proximal colonic neoplasms can almost always be resected with primary anastomosis, but a Hartmann's resection is more appropriate for tumors in the sigmoid colon and rectum with extensive contamination.

A second-look laparotomy at 48 h is occasionally indicated if there are any doubts about the viability of the remaining colon. A subtotal colectomy and ileostomy is usually the only safe option for colonic perforation secondary to acute inflammatory bowel disease, leaving the closed rectal stump in situ to preserve surgical options for a later procedure.

Other pathological processes that occasionally give rise to large bowel perforation include isolated cecal diverticulitis, which is usually indistinguishable from appendicitis, mesenteric vascular occlusion and unresolved sigmoid (or cecal) volvulus. Occasionally, patients with acute inflammatory bowel disease (Crohn's disease, ulcerative colitis or pseudomembranous colitis) present with large bowel perforation, but it is rare for there not to be some suggestive previous history.

Finally, infective causes such as amebiasis should not be forgotten if the patient is from a developing country or has recently returned from abroad.

> **Intestinal perforation**
>
> - 30% of patients with upper gastrointestinal perforation have no free gas on their admission chest radiograph.
> - An urgent CT would be required when in doubt.
> - Subcutaneous emphysema in the neck is the cardinal sign of esophageal perforation.
> - Warn patients with gastrointestinal perforations preoperatively about the possible need for an intestinal stoma.

Acute Diverticulitis

Patients presenting with an acute paracolic mass (acute diverticulitis) can usually be managed medically with intravenous broad-spectrum antibiotics, investigated with CT and occasionally percutaneous drainage. The decision to recommend surgery is made on the basis of the progression of the patient's general condition (worsening sepsis and/or peritonitis) and presumed severity of diverticulitis on CT (abscess formation and/or perforation), where a simple resection and primary anastomosis will suffice, but is often not necessary. Recent literature supports conservative management in complicated diverticulitis including Hinchey I (small confined pericolic or mesocolic abscess) and II (pelvic abscess) with the support of percutaneous drainage if suitable. The default management of "perforated" diverticulitis including Hinchey III (purulent peritonitis) and IV (feculent peritonitis) would be surgical resection, although there are several notable ongoing trials to determine whether a more minimalist approach such as diagnostic laparoscopy and washout may by suitable for Hinchey III patients. However, clear differentiation between Hinchey III and IV is often not possible from CT or even at laparoscopy.

Fistula formation will usually precipitate an earlier operation and when associated with frank sepsis, the formation of a temporary stoma might be considered safer than a primary anastomosis. If a larger inflammatory mass is found at laparotomy without evidence of free perforation, simple washout and drainage is an option, with further assessment and delayed definitive excisional surgery on an elective basis. Resection and primary anastomosis can usually be performed if sepsis and fecal loading are not prominent, usually with a defunctioning proximal stoma.

If there is a frank perforation with purulent or fecal peritonitis, primary resection of the involved segment is the procedure of choice, with extensive peritoneal lavage. A Hartmann's procedure with a left iliac fossa sigmoid colostomy and oversewing of the rectal stump is the procedure of choice for fecal peritonitis, but a case can be made for primary anastomosis in purulent peritonitis. Primary excisional surgery may be technically demanding, and the availability of a suitably trained and competent surgeon is essential.

The formation of a mucous fistula through the lower end of the abdominal incision facilitates locating the rectal stump at the second procedure, but almost always requires rectal mobilization to bring the proximal rectum to the abdominal wall, and can complicate matters enormously by forming extensive pelvic adhesions. Simply oversewing of the rectum, therefore, has much to recommend it, with the rectal stump marked with a non-absorbable suture.

Solitary cecal diverticula are adequately managed by simple excision and closure, but in the emergency situation in which the diverticulum is acutely inflamed and possibly perforated, it is often impossible to differentiate it from a cecal carcinoma. It is therefore wiser to carry out a formal right colectomy if there is any doubt about the diagnosis, with primary ileocolic anastomosis.

Acute diverticulitis

- Inspect the chest radiograph for subdiaphragmatic gas indicating perforation.
- In the absence of perforation, treat with broad-spectrum antibiotics initially.

INTESTINAL OBSTRUCTION

The clinical approach to intestinal obstruction follows well-established lines, and may be summarized in a series of short questions, the answers providing a suitable framework for subsequent management.

A STEP-BY-STEP APPROACH TO INTESTINAL OBSTRUCTION

Is there a Systemic Disturbance?

Hypovolemia may be due to either fluid sequestration in the obstructed gut or fluid lost to the exterior as vomitus. It tends to be more marked if the obstruction is more proximal, and needs to be corrected as quickly as possible if surgical intervention is contemplated.

Is there an Ischemic Bowel?

There is no single investigation that is reliable in this situation. Local tenderness may be the only sign. Raised inflammatory markers and lactate acidosis are unreliable. A high index of suspicion is important because delaying surgical intervention until after an ischemic loop has perforated is to court disaster (Fig. 2.17).

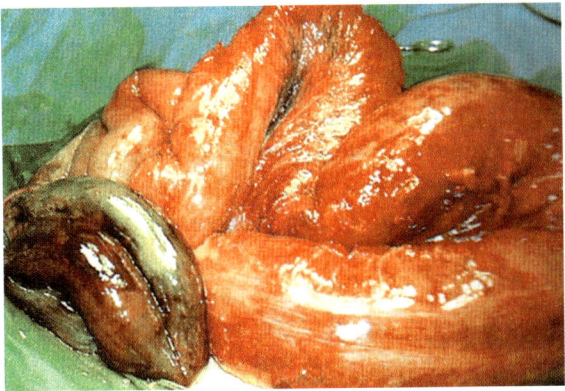

Fig. 2.17: Necrotic small bowel loop discovered at the time of a laparotomy for small bowel obstruction.

What is the Level of the Obstruction?

Proximal obstruction can usually be distinguished from distal obstruction by careful interpretation of plain radiographs, but CT would provide a more definitive answer and is always indicated in this situation.

What is the Probable Underlying Diagnosis?

Adhesions and hernias are the most common causes of small bowel obstruction, and large bowel carcinomas are the most common cause of large bowel obstruction. The precise diagnosis may be relatively unimportant in the initial management because most of these patients should have an early laparotomy and definitive surgery.

Step-by-step approach to intestinal obstruction

- Is obstruction present (based on clinical findings, radiological evidence)?
- Is there evidence of systemic effect (e.g. hypotension, tachycardia or oliguria)?
- Is there evidence of intestinal ischemia?
- What is the level of obstruction?
- What is the cause of the obstruction?

Diagnosis and initial management of intestinal obstruction:

- A CT scan is best to differentiate pseudo-obstruction and mechanical large bowel obstruction.
- Small bowel loops with diameter larger than 2.5 cm or colon with diameter larger than 7 cm together with a paucity of gas distally show a high specificity for a diagnosis of obstruction.
- CT scans will usually reveal the level and possibly also the cause of obstruction.
- It is dangerous to anesthetize an obstructed patient without first placing a nasogastric tube.
- Femoral hernia is still a commonly missed cause of small bowel obstruction especially in elderly females.

Etiology

Adhesions

If the patient has had previous abdominal surgery, adhesions are the most likely cause of small bowel obstruction, but if the original surgery was for a malignant process, recurrent disease causing obstruction should also be considered. It is often not possible to differentiate between these two situations without a CT scan.

If adhesive obstruction is confidently diagnosed and there are no features to suggest ischemia, a 24-h period of conservative measures including nasogastric aspiration, intravenous fluids and regular review is reasonable before reoperating if there is no improvement. The only real exceptions are:
- The patient who has had multiple laparotomies for adhesive small bowel obstruction and has known extensive adhesions, when procrastination beyond 24 h may be justified.
- The patient with known peritoneal metastases for whom surgery will rarely improve the situation.

Hernias

Hernias are the second most common cause of small bowel obstruction, and need to be actively looked for because occasionally the patient is unaware of their presence, particularly the elderly obese female with a small femoral hernia, which can be easily missed. Severe local tenderness, a lack of bowel sounds or cough impulse and a recent change in the character of the hernia such as a rapid enlargement are all features suggesting that the hernia is the cause of the problem.

Internal hernias may occur in natural spaces (e.g. obturator, paraduodenal fossae or sacral foramina) or as postoperative complication (e.g. Petersen's hernia after bariatric surgery) are occasional causes of small bowel obstruction and will not become apparent without CT imaging or at the time of surgery, requiring a high index of suspicion (Fig. 2.18).

Other Causes of Small Bowel Obstruction

The patient presenting with small bowel obstruction de novo, who has had no previous surgery and has no obvious hernia, presents an interesting clinical challenge, which is usually resolved fairly rapidly by surgical intervention.

The range of diagnostic possibilities here is very wide, with common diagnoses being Crohn's disease, a tumor of the small bowel (e.g. a benign polyp, carcinoma, lymphoma or carcinoid) or large bowel (e.g. cecal carcinoma), or an inflammatory process involving the small bowel loops such as appendicitis, acute diverticular disease, gynecological sepsis and endometriosis.

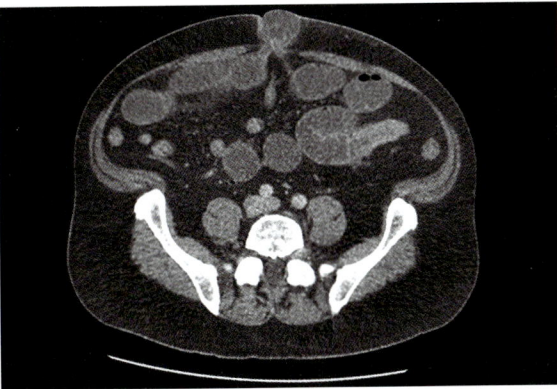

Fig. 2.18: Axial CT showing an umbilical hernia containing small bowel. The afferent limb consists of dilated small bowel, but the efferent limb is collapsed. (CT: Computed tomography.) *Courtesy:* Keegan C.

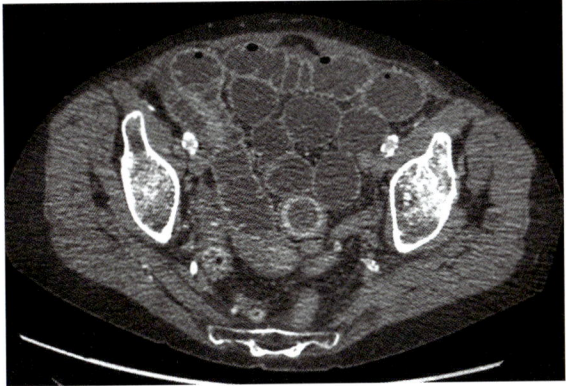

Fig. 2.19: Axial CT demonstrating small bowel dilation to the level of a 2.4 × 4 cm obstructing gallstone at the distal ileum. (CT: Computed tomography.)

Therapeutic abdominal-pelvic irradiation occasionally causes significant small bowel damage, the end results often being extensive stricture formation and small bowel obstruction. This can be a difficult situation to deal with because the damage is often widespread. The combination of small bowel obstruction and gas in the biliary tree on radiological imaging is usually caused by gallstones ileus (Fig. 2.19).

Common Conditions Other than Colorectal Cancer Leading to Large Bowel Constriction

Common conditions other than colorectal cancer leading to large bowel obstruction include volvulus (of the sigmoid or less commonly cecum) and occasionally, acute diverticular disease. Once diagnosed, resection is indicated almost universally. The older procedures of operative detorsion and fixation of large bowel loops (pexy) have fallen from favor because the results of resection are much more successful. Diverticular disease causing large bowel obstruction is usually a good indicator for surgery (if only to exclude a coexisting neoplasm), but it may settle with conservative measures. Occasional rarities such as colonic lipomas may present with large bowel obstruction.

Pseudo-obstruction (Ogilvie's Syndrome)

Pseudo-obstruction is poorly understood and may mimic mechanical large bowel obstruction, both clinically and radiologically. A CT is important to confirm or refute mechanical obstruction before surgery, as surgical intervention will not help a patient with pseudo-obstruction.

Pseudo-obstruction usually occurs in elderly patients who are unwell for some other reason, such as acute myocardial infarction or a recent orthopedic procedure, or who have an underlying biochemical abnormality such as hypokalemia.

Management of Small Bowel Obstruction

Once a diagnosis of intestinal obstruction has been confirmed and the volume deficit replaced, which may require placement of a central venous line and urinary catheter depending on the extent of systemic disturbance, early surgical intervention is the mainstay of treatment, given the few exceptions mentioned earlier.

A midline abdominal incision is most useful for idiopathic and adhesive intestinal obstruction, particularly if this approach was used for the previous surgery. Whatever pathology is found must be dealt with on merit:

- In Crohn's disease, excisional surgery must be kept to a minimum and a case can be made for simply closing the abdomen and instituting maximal medical therapy (including steroids), in the hope that the obstructive element will settle as the inflammatory process is brought under control.
- In inactive previously confirmed Crohn's disease in which short fibrous strictures are the cause of the obstruction, stricture plasty (i.e. a longitudinal enterotomy across the stricture, closed transversely) may be considered in later stages.
- In adhesive obstruction, simple division of adhesions is usually all that is required, and even bowel that appears non-viable on first inspection will usually reperfuse adequately once the obstruction has been dealt with.
- Frankly gangrenous bowel must be resected, but is relatively uncommon.
- Inguinal hernias causing small bowel obstruction are generally dealt with satisfactorily using a standard groin approach and if resection becomes necessary, it can usually be achieved through the same incision, simply

by dilating the neck of the usually indirect hernia sac. Occasionally, a second lower midline incision is needed to carry out the resection.
- If the problem is confidently diagnosed preoperatively as a small bowel obstruction related to a femoral hernia, the authors favor a midline abdominal incision approach from the outset, with an extraperitoneal approach to the femoral canal. Exposure of the femoral canal (bilaterally, if necessary) is far superior from above, facilitating the performance of the repair and the bowel resection through the same incision.
- Management of obstruction related to other pathological processes, such as diverticular disease, volvulus or endometriosis generally involves resecting the obstructed segment, followed by a decision to defunction the bowel or an attempt at primary anastomosis. Leakage from an anastomosis can have disastrous consequences, and there may be a significant disparity between the sizes of the two lumens.

Management of Large Bowel Obstruction

The management of large bowel obstruction is a little more complicated, and depends on the site of the obstruction and the probably underlying pathology. The most common situation involves an obstructing carcinoma in the left colon or sigmoid. Having resected the primary tumors, there are several options:
- A simple end colostomy with closure of the rectal stump (Hartmann's procedure) is usually a safe operation, but commits the patient to a second procedure to close the stoma, or indeed to a permanent stoma.
- Usually the best approach is a subtotal colectomy, anastomosing the terminal ileum to the distal non-obstructed segment, but the functional results in terms of diarrhea and incontinence may not be acceptable if this is carried out for distal tumors in elderly patients.
- For obstructing more proximal colonic tumors, an extended right colectomy with ileocolic anastomosis is a universally acceptable procedure.
- On-table lavage to clear the proximal colon, followed by primary anastomosis, is an alternative strategy, but is relatively time consuming and no longer commonly practiced, though the advantage for the patient is the avoidance of any further surgery.

If tumor recurrence or persistence in the pelvis is thought likely, an anastomosis to the rectum should be avoided in favor of an end-stoma, as the recurrent obstruction that often occurs in the pelvis can be difficult to manage. Colo-colic bypass is occasionally needed for totally unresectable colon cancer, but this is relatively rare.

In sigmoid volvulus, it is often possible to resolve the acute problem by passing a flatus tube (or colonoscope) through the twisted segment to deflate the sigmoid loop. Using a flatus tube at least twice as long as the rigid

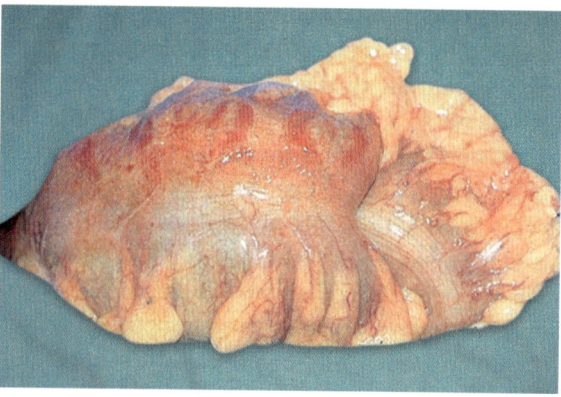

Fig. 2.20: Intussuscepting lipoma of the sigmoid colon causing intermittent large bowel obstruction.

sigmoidoscope to allow the tube to be positioned correctly and left in situ when the sigmoidoscope is withdrawn is of considerable practical importance. A primary resection and anastomosis can be considered at a later time.

In pseudo-obstruction, surgical intervention may be required if the situation fails to resolve to the extent that cecal perforation is imminent. Therapeutic colonoscopic decompression should be attempted first, in the knowledge that the procedure is unlikely to be easy in the unprepared bowel, and that the situation may be exacerbated by the insufflation of air. Furthermore, the procedure may need to be repeated if the situation still does not improve, although it is also possible to place a flatus tube to provide a vent. Finally, it may become necessary to decompress the colon by formal cecostomy; indeed, this is probably the only indication for cecostomy in modern surgical practice, assuming a very unfit patient. Alternatively, a sub-total colectomy may be required in selected patients, and it is fair to say that the natural history of this condition usually involves multiple recurrences, such that ultimately surgical intervention of some sort is likely to be needed (Figs. 2.20 and 2.21).

■ VASCULAR ABNORMALITIES

Ruptured Abdominal Aortic Aneurysm

Natural History

The typical patient is an elderly man with arteriopathy who presents with a sudden collapse and severe abdominal and often back pain. He may have a previous history suggesting the diagnosis and may even have a known aneurysm, which is under surveillance or awaiting a planned repair.

The cardinal feature on examination is a tender pulsatile mass in the epigastrium, but this can be missed relatively easily in the hypotensive patient,

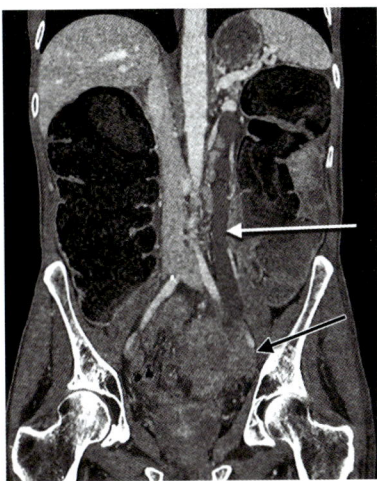

Fig. 2.21: Coronal reformat of a CT in the portal venous phase. There is grossly distended large bowel secondary to a subacutely obstructing sigmoid lesion (black arrow), which has also given rise to significant hydroureter (white arrow). (CT: Computed tomography.) *Courtesy:* Keegan C.

and unless the diagnosis is considered early, it may only become apparent at postmortem. A preoperative assessment of the patency of the leg and pedal pulses must be made to provide a baseline for later comparison.

Management

A plain abdominal radiograph may demonstrate the presence of an aneurysm, which shows up as a curvilinear area of calcification in the left upper quadrant, but a bedside ultrasound scan offers better sensitivity and specificity. CT angiography is the gold standard, allowing for diagnostic confirmation, surgical planning and potential endovascular intervention. Occasionally, there may be a place for symptomatic treatment in a very elderly unfit patient.

Once the diagnosis is made, there should be a prompt discussion with the vascular unit and preparation made for surgical intervention without undue delay. Placement of wide-bore intravenous cannula and a urinary catheter are essential and must be completed before anesthesia. Extras such as an arterial line and central venous line can be placed during surgery. The transfusion department should be notified of the problem, and a massive transfusion protocol initiated, with eight units of whole blood crossmatched, platelets and fresh-frozen plasma made available.

For an open repair of an infrarenal aneurysm, the abdomen is opened through a long midline incision after including both groins in the sterile field. Assuming that the diagnosis is confirmed, the small bowel is reflected to the right and the duodenal–jejunal flexure mobilized to expose the aorta above the aneurysm. The left renal vein is reflected upward and an arterial clamp placed above the neck to control the aorta. Both common iliacs are controlled below the bifurcation and the aneurysm is opened. Intraluminal thrombus is evacuated, and vessels such as the lumbar arteries and the inferior mesenteric artery are controlled, usually from within the sac. Usually, the ruptured aorta can be replaced with a straight graft, placed between the neck of the aneurysm and the aortic bifurcation. Alternatively, an aorto-bi-iliac or aorto-bifemoral graft is occasionally necessary.

For endovascular repair, access to both common femoral arteries is required. An angiogram is performed intraoperatively to ascertain the position of the renal arteries. With the aid of a guidewire, a stent graft is introduced. Under angiographic guidance, the endograft is positioned and deployed with the upper margin aligned with the lower border of the renal artery. Then, the guidewire is passed into the contralateral limb to deploy the second limb into the short leg. A complete angiogram will confirm the position of the graft and identify any endoleaks.

Mesenteric Vascular Occlusion

Natural History

The typical patient is elderly, often with a history of vascular disease, who presents with severe abdominal pain and colic, which are later associated with vomiting and diarrhea. An abdominal film may demonstrate the classical sign of "thumbprinting," due to intense mucosal edema in the ischemic segment. In the early stages, there may be a low-grade pyrexia, elevated inflammatory markers and lactic acidosis. A CT angiogram would confirm the diagnosis, and potentially differentiate between an emboli or venous thrombosis against other intra-abdominal pathology.

Often there is little in the way of abnormal physical signs initially. As the pathological process progresses a combination of endotoxemia and hypovolemic shock follows relatively rapidly, and the outlook becomes more bleak as time progresses. The development of peritoneal irritation usually signifies full-thickness necrosis and a worsening of prognosis.

Etiology and Pathogenesis

Acute intestinal ischemia not involving mechanical intestinal obstruction can have a variety of causes including arterial emboli and thrombosis, venous thrombosis, small vessel disease (as occurs in polyarteritis) and a low flow state (as might be seen after cardiac surgery) in an already compromised mesenteric vascular supply.

Management

Management before laparotomy involves aggressive resuscitation, but the longer the delay, the more advanced will be the extent of damage, and an

early operation is important. Broad-spectrum antibiotics are administered and the patient is fully heparinized postoperatively. Once a laparotomy has been undertaken, there are three surgical options:
- To do nothing (close the abdomen and let nature take its course)
- To revascularize the gut
- To resect.

The first option is obviously reserved for irremediable situations when the patient is extremely unwell for other reasons or because the extent of infarction is incompatible with life.

Many techniques for revascularizing the gut include catheter embolectomy, formal thrombectomy, reimplantation of visceral arteries and bypass procedures. All are difficult as gaining access to the origins of the visceral arteries involves a tedious dissection, particularly in obese patients. There has been an increasing interest in endovascular techniques as an alternative, and a discussion with a tertiary vascular center is warranted.

The usual operative finding of grossly ischemic gut would obviously require a resection of all non-viable segments. In such a situation, it is a folly to attempt an anastomosis, and suitably placed stomas are the safest alternative, with the possibility of reversal at a later date. Even patients who have had a massive small bowel resection can survive using long-term home parenteral nutrition, although their quality of life is often relatively poor. The chances of success with enteral nutrition are greatly increased if the ileocecal valve can be preserved.

Mesenteric venous occlusion is rare, but important, because it occasionally complicates hypercoagulable states such as antithrombin III deficiency, which must be actively and urgently searched for; further thromboses are almost inevitable unless the hypercoagulable state is adequately treated, usually with long-term anticoagulation (Figs. 2.22 and 2.23).

Finally, as infarction is often patchy in this condition, a second-look laparotomy 24–48 h after the first is often indicated.

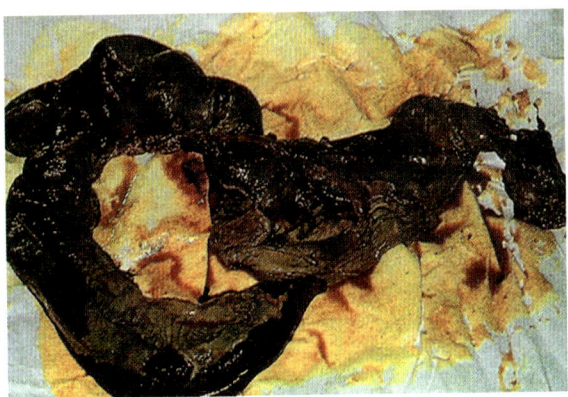

Fig. 2.22: Known arteriopathy showing almost total infarction of the small bowel.

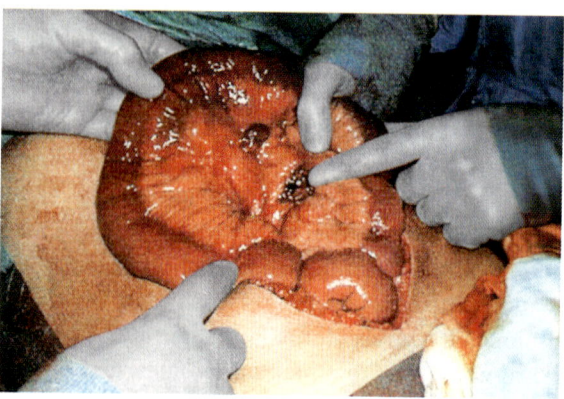

Fig. 2.23: Mesenteric venous thrombosis in a patient with antithrombin III deficiency.

> **Diagnosis and management of abdominal vascular crises**
> - A patient with cardiovascular disease or atrial fibrillation and significant abdominal pain has intestinal ischemia until proved otherwise.
> - Consider stomas and a "second-look" strategy at 48 h in intestinal ischemia.
> - Palpate carefully for an aortic aneurysm, particularly when the femoral arteries are aneurysmal.
> - Investigate for underlying hypercoagulable states in mesenteric venous infarction.
> - Anticoagulation postoperatively is crucial.

Acute Intermittent Porphyria

Acute intermittent porphyria in fact belongs to a group of eight metabolic disorders characterized by defects in heme synthesis. The major clinical features of acute intermittent porphyria (acute abdominal pain, tachycardia, vomiting, constipation, epilepsy, confusion, psychosis, motor neuropathy and hypertension) correlate with, but are not necessarily due to, the high porphobilinogen (PBG) levels. Many of the clinical and biochemical features closely mimic those of lead poisoning.

Etiology and Pathogenesis

Acute intermittent porphyria is almost unique as an example of an enzyme defect (porphobilinogen deaminase) inherited as an autosomal dominant condition. As a result of the enzyme defect, there is an accumulation of porphobilinogen, which can be detected in the urine, and of its precursor delta-levulinic acid. This in turn is synthesized from succinyl CoA and glycine. The end products of the synthetic chain are the porphyrins, which are the precursors of heme and cytochromes.

In the liver, which is the site of the main problem in acute intermittent (hepatic) porphyria, the cytochromes are the main end products of porphyrin synthesis. Any situation that induces cytochrome enzymes, particularly drug therapy, is therefore likely to increase porphyrin synthesis and consequently exacerbate porphyria.

The diagnosis is readily made during an acute attack by detecting PBG in urine, which goes dark red on standing.

Management

The first and most important step is to make an early diagnosis. Often the first case in any family is fatal because of delayed diagnosis. A common and tragic course is for acute abdominal pain leading to laparotomy using barbiturates for inducing anesthesia, which is followed by status epilepticus and even more barbiturate therapy. Barbiturates are one in a long list of drugs that can exacerbate porphyria.

A list must be obtained, if not already in the patient's possession, of those drugs that may safely be prescribed.

Main principles of therapy are:
- High carbohydrate intake (>300 g/day)
- Narcotic analgesia
- Controlling hypertension, usually with beta blockers such as propranolol
- Monitoring and correcting electrolyte abnormalities, especially hyponatremia and hypomagnesemia
- Controlling seizures with diazepam
- Controlling vomiting with ondansetron or chlorpromazine
- Using intravenous heme therapy with consultation at a specialized unit.

Attacks are more common in women in whom they often coincide with ovulation. Ovulation-suppressive therapy may occasionally be considered. The long-term prognosis is variable, but should be good with careful management, although some may progress to requiring liver transplantation.

Screening of family members is essential and needs to be done in collaboration with major referral centers.

FURTHER READING

Appendicitis
1. Alvarado A. A practical score for the early diagnosis of acute appendicitis. Ann Emerg Med. 1986;15(5):557-64.
2. Bhangu A, Søreide K, Di Saverio S, et al. Acute appendicitis: modern understanding of pathogenesis, diagnosis, and management. Lancet. 2015;386(10000):1278-87.
3. Doria AS, Moineddin R, Kellenberger CJ, et al. US or CT for diagnosis of appendicitis in children and adults? A meta-analysis. Radiology. 2006;241(1):83-94.
4. Duke E, Kalb B, Arif-Tiwari H, et al. A systematic review and meta-analysis of diagnostic performance of MRI for evaluation of acute appendicitis. AJR Am J Roentgenol. 2016;206(3):508-17.
5. Ebell MH, Shinholser J. What are the most clinically useful cutoffs for the Alvarado and pediatric appendicitis scores? A systematic review. Ann Emerg Med. 2014;64(4):365-72.e2.

6. Yu CW, Juan LI, Wu MH, et al. Systematic review and meta-analysis of the diagnostic accuracy of procalcitonin, C-reactive protein and white blood cell count for suspected acute appendicitis. Br J Surg. 2013;100(3):322-9.

Acute Abdomen in the Elderly

7. Desserud KF, Veen T, Søreide K. Emergency general surgery in the geriatric patient. Br J Surg. 2016;103(2):e52-61.

Acute Cholecystitis

8. Ansaloni L, Pisano M, Coccolini F, et al. 2016 WSES guidelines on acute calculous cholecystitis. World J Emerg Surg. 2016;11:25.
9. Ambrosetti P, Becker C, Terrier F. Colonic diverticulitis: impact of imaging on surgical management—a prospective study of 542 patients. Eur Radiol. 2002;12(5):1145-9.
10. Hinchey EJ, Schaal PG, Richard GK. Treatment of perforated diverticular disease of the colon. Adv Surg. 1978;12:85-109.
11. McDermott FD, Collins D, Heeney A, et al. Minimally invasive and surgical management strategies tailored to the severity of acute diverticulitis. Br J Surg. 2014;101(1):e90-9.
12. Morris AM, Regenbogen SE, Hardiman KM, et al. Sigmoid diverticulitis: a systematic review. JAMA. 2014;311(3):287-97.

Acute Pancreatitis

13. Banks PA, Bollen TL, Dervenis C, et al. Classification of acute pancreatitis—2012: revision of the Atlanta classification and definitions by international consensus. Gut. 2013;62(1):102-11.
14. Johnson CD, Besselink MG, Carter R. Acute pancreatitis. BMJ. 2014;349:g4859.
15. Van Baal MC, van Santvoort HC, Bollen TL, et al. Systematic review of percutaneous catheter drainage as primary treatment for necrotizing pancreatitis. Br J Surg. 2011;98:18-27.

Acute Porphyria

16. American Porphyria Foundation. Drug Database. <http://www.porphyriafoundation.com/drug-database> [accessed 01.10.16].
17. Besur S, Schmeltzer P, Bonkovsky HL. Acute porphyrias. J Emerg Med. 2015;49(3):305-12.
18. Puy H, Gouya L, Deybach JC. Porphyrias. Lancet. 2010;375(9718):924-37.

Gynecological Emergencies

19. McWilliams GD, Hill MJ, Dietrich CS. Gynecologic emergencies. Surg Clin North Am. 2008;88(2):265-83, vi.
20. Ramphal SR, Moodley J. Emergency gynaecology. Best Pract Res Clin Obstet Gynaecol. 2006;20(5):729-50.

Intestinal Perforation

21. Crofts TJ, Park KG, Steele RJ, et al. A randomized trial of nonoperative treatment for perforated peptic ulcer. N Engl J Med. 1989;320(15):970-3.
22. Søreide K, Thorsen K, Søreide JA. Strategies to improve the outcome of emergency surgery for perforated peptic ulcer. Br J Surg. 2014;101(1):e51-64.

Laparoscopy

23. Agresta F, Ansaloni L, Baiocchi GL, et al. Laparoscopic approach to acute abdomen from the Consensus Development Conference of the Società Italiana di Chirurgia Endoscopica e nuove tecnologie (SICE), Associazione Chirurghi Ospedalieri Italiani (ACOI), Società Italiana di Chirurgia (SIC), Società Italiana di Chirurgia d'Urgenza e del Trauma (SICUT), Società Italiana di Chirurgia nell'Ospedalità Privata (SICOP),

and the European Association for Endoscopic Surgery (EAES). Surg Endosc. 2012;26(8):2134-64.
24. Paterson-Brown S. Emergency laparoscopic surgery. Br J Surg. 1993;80(3):279-83.

Radiology
25. Coyle JP, Brennan CR, Parfrey SF, et al. Is serum C-reactive protein a reliable predictor of abdomino-pelvic CT findings in the clinical setting of the non-traumatic acute abdomen? Emerg Radiol. 2012;19(5):455-62.
26. Gans SL, Atema JJ, van Dieren S, et al. Diagnostic value of C-reactive protein to rule out infectious complications after major abdominal surgery: a systematic review and meta-analysis. Int J Colorectal Dis. 2015;30(7):861-73.
27. Maddu KK, Mittal P, Shuaib W, et al. Colorectal emergencies and related complications: a comprehensive imaging review—imaging of colitis and complications. AJR Am J Roentgenol. 2014;203(6):1205-16.
28. Stoker J, van Randen A, Laméris W, et al. Imaging patients with acute abdominal pain. Radiology. 2009;253(1):31-46.
29. Valentin L. Characterising acute gynaecological pathology with ultrasound: an overview and case examples. Best Pract Res Clin Obstet Gynaecol. 2009;23(5):577-93.

Vascular Abnormalities
30. Acosta S, Björck M. Modern treatment of acute mesenteric ischaemia. Br J Surg. 2014;101(1):e100-8.
31. Azhar B, Patel SR, Holt PJ, et al. Misdiagnosis of ruptured abdominal aortic aneurysm: systematic review and meta-analysis. J Endovasc Ther. 2014;21(4):568-75.
32. Badger S, Bedenis R, Blair PH, et al. Endovascular treatment for ruptured abdominal aortic aneurysm. Cochrane Database Syst Rev. 2014;7:CD005261.
33. Kent KC. Clinical practice. Abdominal aortic aneurysms. N Engl J Med. 2014;371(22):2101-8.
34. Ryer EJ, Kalra M, Oderich GS, et al. Revascularization for acute mesenteric ischemia. J Vasc Surg. 2012;55:1682-9.
35. Schermerhorn ML, Giles KA, Hamdan AD, et al. Mesenteric revascularization: management and outcomes in the United States, 1988–2006. J Vasc Surg. 2009;50(2):341-8.

CHAPTER 3

Diarrhea

Her Hsin Tsai

■ REACHING A DIAGNOSIS

Is it Diarrhea?

Patients often have a different idea of what constitutes diarrhea from their doctors. The patient should be asked directly whether he/she is passing liquid feces or merely has frequent but mainly formed bowel movements. A Bristol stool chart may be used to facilitate clarity as to type of feces produced and in cases of doubt, patients could be encouraged to take a picture on their mobile devices and present it at consultation.

Is it Infective?

Symptoms

The duration of the diarrhea often gives a helpful clue. Most infective causes of diarrhea resolve after a few days or 2–3 weeks at the most. Exceptions, which may cause more prolonged diarrhea, include pathogenic amebae, *Giardia, Campylobacter jejuni* and *Yersinia* spp. Often the patient with infective diarrhea will give a history of sudden onset of abdominal pain and vomiting and there may be a history of other family members or acquaintances who have been similarly affected. A history of ingesting a suspect item of food like a cold chicken salad may be obtained. A history of travel particularly to less developed nations should alert the clinician. Outbreaks of infective diarrhea particularly on cruise ships or institutions and hotels are often caused by norovirus infection.

Microscopy

Stool microscopy and culture is essential to confirm the diagnosis and allow identification of the source. If amebic dysentery is suspected because of recent travel to endemic areas, the stools should be transferred rapidly to the laboratory while still warm so that motile amebae-containing phagocytosed red cells can be identified (feces commonly contain non-pathogenic *Entamoeba coli* which do not ingest red cells).

Microscopy is important not only for the diagnosis of parasites such as amebae and *Giardia* but also for the identification of pus cells (neutrophils) which may aid in the diagnosis. Infectious diarrhea may be classified as inflammatory or non-inflammatory according to the presence or absence of neutrophils in the feces.

Inflammatory infective diarrhea results from organisms such as *Salmonella, Campylobacter* and *Shigella* which tend to infect the distal ileum and colon. The diarrhea may then be bloody and is often accompanied by fever. In the absence of positive stool, microscopy or culture inflammatory bowel disease (IBD) or ischemic colitis should be considered as differential diagnoses.

Non-inflammatory infective diarrhea is usually more voluminous and is watery rather than bloody and contains few pus cells. It is associated with infection of the small intestine by agents such as rotavirus (particularly common in children), norovirus, *Cryptosporidium* and toxigenic *Escherichia coli*. Cholera is another classic example of this type of infective diarrhea.

If microscopy and culture is negative, then viral cause should be suspected. Norovirus is now the leading cause of diarrheal illness worldwide. In nations with colder climates, it is often seasonal peaking in winter months. Diagnosis is by immunoassay of feces or more specifically by polymerase chain reaction of virus.

Is the Diarrhea Watery or Fatty?

If the diarrhea is not infective, the next step in diagnosis is to establish whether it is predominantly watery or fatty. A mistake at this stage will result in a completely inappropriate series of investigations. The patient's description of feces can often be misleading and it is essential to inspect the feces. Voluminous, fatty stools suggest steatorrhea. Although classically described as floating, this is often inaccurately described by patients. Patients can be encouraged to take a picture of the feces with their mobile devices. Any patient with diarrhea that has persisted for more than a few days should have a rigid of flexible sigmoidoscopy and this allows an opportunity to inspect the feces in addition to the rectal mucosa. If diarrhea is prolonged (more than a month) and watery, it may be justified to proceed to colonoscopy where direct visualization of the whole colon and terminal ileum is possible. Biopsy of the right colon of macroscopically normal mucosa may pick up microcytic and collagenous colitis. In most cases, the history and inspection of the feces will give a clear guide as to whether the diarrhea is likely to be due to malabsorption, but in some cases, a further test will be required. The standard test is the fecal fat estimation. This must be one of the least popular tests for patients and laboratory staff, but gives reliable information if properly carried out. Feces need to be collected over at least a 3-day period and the fat intake should at least be "average" during this period. If there is genuine malabsorption, then there may be signs of nutritional deficiencies, weight loss and hypoalbuminemia. A number of fat absorption tests have been promoted such as the measurement of blood fat after ingestion of a test sample (usually butter on toast) or the ^{14}C-trioleate breath test but they have limited reliability and largely abandoned. It is a more useful test for specific conditions and excludes them individually. Hence:

- Celiac disease: Simple celiac antibody test is highly sensitive and specific.
- Small intestinal/bowel bacterial overgrowth (SIBO): Hydrogen (or methane) hydrogen breath test
- Bile salt malabsorption: SeHCAT scan
- Pancreatic insufficiency: Fecal elastase is a measure of pancreatic exocrine function but this may be falsely positive if fecal collection is inadequate or diluted. If suspected, imaging with computed tomography (CT) would be helpful.

Watery Diarrhea: Functional or Organic?

Having established that the diarrhea is predominantly watery, the next step is to decide whether it is likely to be functional or organic. This can largely be based on the history. If the patient is aged <40, gives a history of bloating, alternating diarrhea and constipation without weight loss or bleeding and without nocturnal diarrhea, then a functional cause—the irritable bowel syndrome (IBS)—is most likely. If sigmoidoscopy reveals a normal rectal mucosa (which should include rectal biopsy because of the possibility of missing microscopic colitis or Crohn's disease) and fecal calprotectin and occult blood is negative and the full blood count and erythrocyte sedimentation rate and serum C-reactive protein (CRP) are normal, then the patient can be reassured and treated symptomatically without further investigation. The IBS is so common (affecting up to one in three) that it is more appropriate to attempt a positive diagnosis, particularly in the younger patient, rather than making the diagnosis by exclusion after endoscopy and/or barium studies. Some patients with diarrhea predominant IBS (IBS-D) do however have more persistent diarrhea and these require more extensive investigation, usually including colonoscopy, to exclude organic causes such as IBD. Bloody diarrhea, weight loss, nocturnal diarrhea and continual diarrhea that is not interspersed by normal bowel actions or diarrhea that occurs for the first time over the age of 40 should always be assumed to be due to an organic cause and thoroughly investigated.

Watery Diarrhea: Drug-related?

Mistakes are often made as the result of failing to obtain a complete drug history from the patient. Many drugs occasionally cause diarrhea, while others such as colchicine or magnesium trisilicate will inevitably do so if given in sufficient dosage. Any drugs that are not essential should be stopped. Drugs that commonly cause diarrhea include lansoprazole, metformin, thiazide diuretics, theophylline and digoxin. Diarrhea is common following treatment with broad-spectrum antibiotics. This can be due to overgrowth in the bowel of the toxin-producing *Clostridium difficile* which in its most severe manifestation results in pseudomembranous colitis. The diagnosis can be confirmed by testing for *C. difficile* toxin in feces.

Ampicillin rarely causes a hemorrhagic colitis that is thought to be a toxic effect of the drug itself. Nicorandil is known to cause an inflammatory colitis. The chemotherapeutic agent ipilimumab which is a monoclonal antibody that is used in melanoma treatment and works by activating the immune system and may result in a severe colitis. Erythromycin has a prokinetic activity on the gut via its motilin receptor agonist effect. Some drugs rarely cause an ischemic colitis; contraceptive pill and antihypertensives have been blamed and also the drug alosetron, which was initially withdrawn because of it. Purgatives will of course always produce diarrhea if taken in excess and some disturbed patients may complain of diarrhea while going to great lengths to conceal their abuse of purgatives. Stool or urine can easily be screened for phenolphthalein by the addition of alkali (e.g. a pellet of sodium hydroxide) and most laboratories can arrange a screen for anthracene or senna derivatives.

Is it Due to Colonic Disease?

If infection and drugs have been excluded and the diarrhea seems unlikely to be simply functional, then the colon should be investigated. A history of erythema nodosum, acute arthritis of medium-sized or large joints or anterior uveitis is suggestive of (but not specific for) IBD. The perianal area should be inspected for skin tags or fistulae suggestive of Crohn's disease. A fecal calprotectin test is a simple way of excluding inflammatory bowel conditions, although may be normal in collagenous colitis, bowel malignancy and mild Crohn's disease.

Rigid/Flexible Sigmoidoscopy

Rigid sigmoidoscopy can be a useful part of the examination in a patient with unexplained diarrhea. It can easily be done as an outpatient procedure taking only 1 or 2 min and allows direct inspection and biopsy of the rectal mucosa and often allows simultaneous inspection and sampling of feces for culture and occult blood testing. Unfortunately, the technique is somewhat neglected in the modern gastroenterology (GI) unit in favor of the flexible sigmoidoscopy or directly to colonoscopy. It remains a question of easy access to such facilities. Some units have dedicated "suspected colon cancer" pathways where patients are directly channeled to a flexible sigmoidoscopy. Notwithstanding the costs of such an exercise, it deprives many trainee doctors the very useful skill of a simple low-cost outpatient investigation. It is true that if a more proximal view is deemed useful, a flexible sigmoidoscopy should be performed. This can be done with minimal bowel preparation using an enema. In a patient with diarrhea, a view of the rectal mucosa is all that is needed initially and a rigid sigmoidoscopy with a view of the rectal mucosa will suffice. If the more proximal colon needs endoscopic examination (e.g. to exclude polyps or carcinoma), a flexible sigmoidoscopy or colonoscopy should be performed. Suffice to say if flexible sigmoidoscopy is readily available without delay then it is preferred. Inspection and biopsy of the rectal mucosa can easily be performed without distress to the patient and there is no need for sedation or anesthesia.

The normal rectal mucosa appears pale pink and shiny with blood vessels visible beneath the thin mucosa. In any case of chronic diarrhea, whatever be the cause, there is usually some reddening of the mucosa (and often evidence of mild inflammation on rectal histology). In ulcerative colitis (UC), the mucosa is more frankly granular with loss of visible vessels and easy contact bleeding and there may be obvious mucosal ulceration in more severe colitis. Crohn's disease often "spares" the rectum but if it is involved, there may be either small "aphthoid" or serpiginous "snail track" ulcers, separated by more healthy mucosa. In pseudomembranous colitis, a characteristic yellowish membrane of sloughed-off superficial epithelium may be seen. The rectal mucosa ought to be biopsied even if it appears macroscopically normal since microscopic granulomata may be present in a normal appearing mucosa in Crohn's disease and clinically significant microscopic or collagenous colitis will also be missed without a biopsy. Biopsy should probably only be carried out at a hospital setting since it carries a slight risk of perforation or bleeding. This risk approaches zero if the posterior rectal wall is biopsied using sharp well-designed endoscopic forceps (Figs. 3.1 to 3.5).

Histology

Rectal histology may yield one of several results: it may show diagnostic features of Crohn's disease, i.e. non-caseating granulomata, chronic inflammation penetrating deep to the muscularis mucosa and relative goblet cell mucus retention, it may be normal or it may show features that are highly suggestive of UC, e.g. acute and chronic inflammation which is predominantly mucosal with crypt abscess formation, mucus depletion and sparsity or branching of crypts. Commonly, however, the findings will be non-specific: crypt abscess

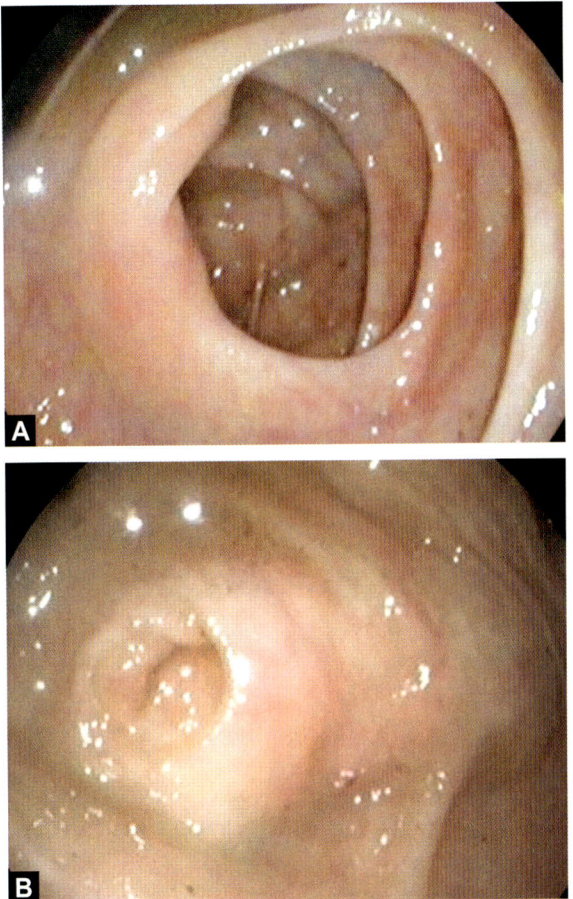

Figs. 3.1A and B: Normal colonoscopy showing the ileocecal valve (A) and the appendix orifice (B).

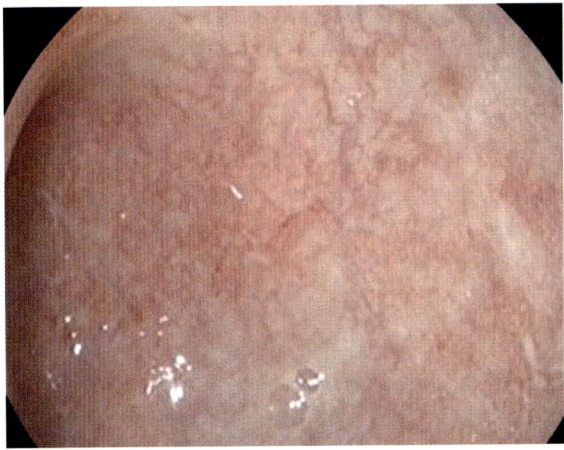

Fig. 3.2: Mild inflammation with reddening of mucosa with blood vessels injected. This is mild ulcerative colitis.

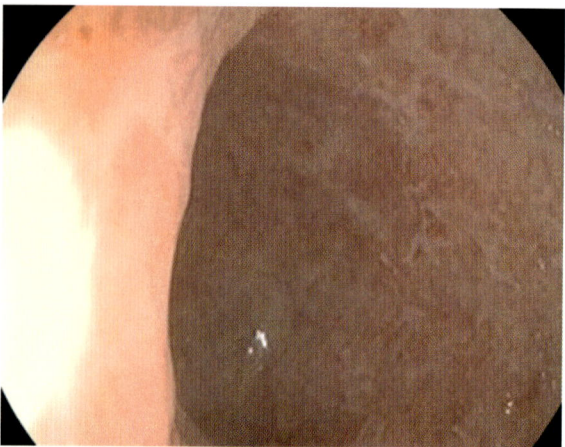

Fig. 3.3: The blood vessels are not visible and there is confluent inflammation of moderate ulcerative colitis.

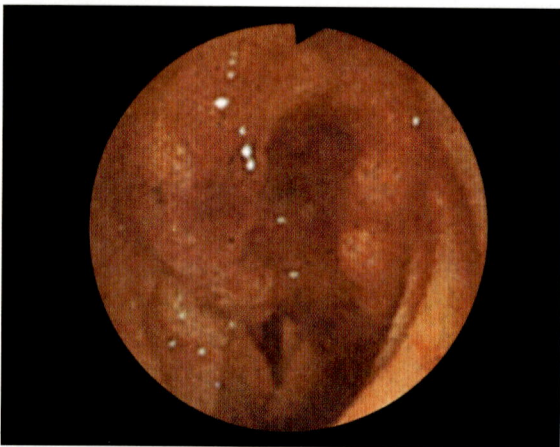

Fig. 3.4: In severe colitis, there is contact bleeding or spontaneous hemorrhage.

formation without crypt branching or sparsity, increased lamina propria mononuclear cells and mild mucus depletion. These findings will be compatible with either UC or an inflammatory type of infective diarrhea such as *Campylobacter enteritis*. Patchy focal areas of inflammation are particularly suggestive of an infective cause (Figs. 3.6 to 3.9).

Which Investigation?

In the examination of the colon, there are three options: colonoscopy, CT colography or barium enema. A plain abdominal film can be also very helpful in specific situations, as well as a standard CT of the abdomen.

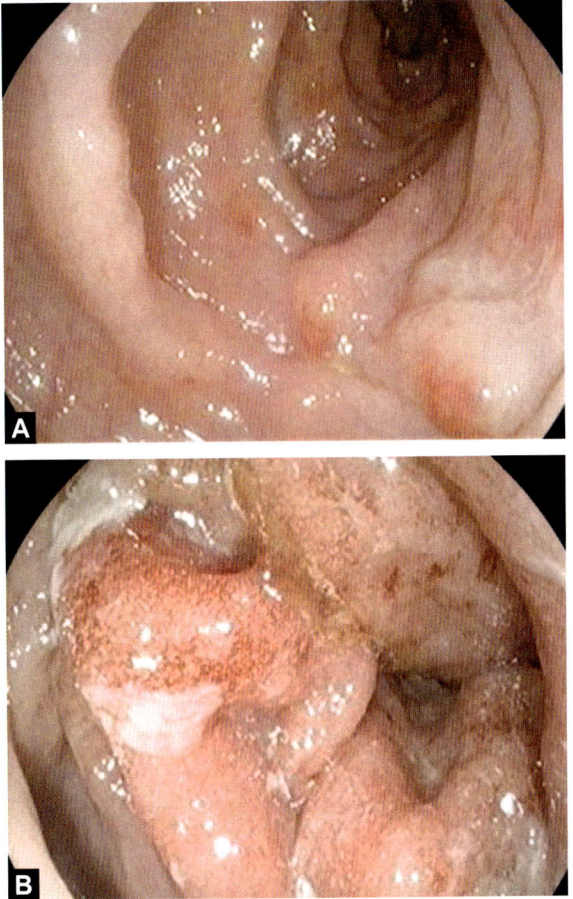

Figs. 3.5A and B: Inflammation around sigmoid diverticula suggests diverticulitis not UC. (UC: Ulcerative colitis.)

If rigid or flexible sigmoidoscopy and rectal biopsy have not given a definitive diagnosis, the remainder of the colon will then need studying by either colonoscopy or barium enema. Flexible sigmoidoscopy with a well-performed double contrast barium enema is a cost-effective investigation that will pick up majority of major pathologies. In the investigation of rectal bleeding or anemia (*see* Chapter 6) colonoscopy is by far the investigation of choice but in the investigation of altered bowel habit, a good case can be made for either investigation. However, a colonoscopy of a well-prepared bowel carried by a competent endoscopist is the best investigation for diarrhea. Apart from directly visualizing colonic pathologies, it is possible to remove polyps and take biopsies of lesions as well. When the number of patients who had barium enemas who subsequently require colonoscopies is added to the cost, the two approaches show little cost difference. Colonoscopy is clearly

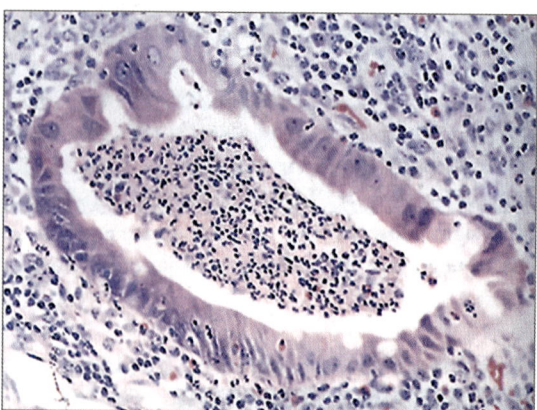

Fig. 3.6: A crypt abscess, where inflammatory cells pack the colonic pits.

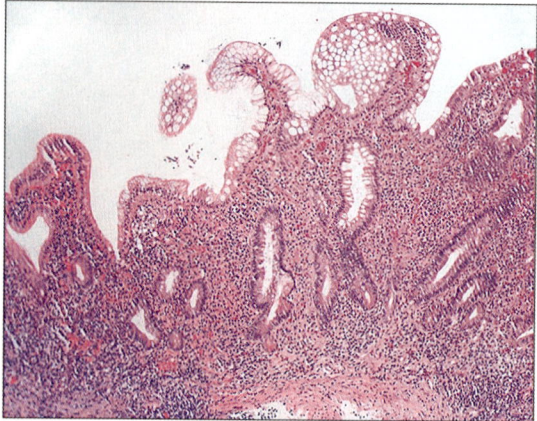

Fig. 3.7: Marked inflammatory cell infiltration is found in ulcerative colitis, along with crypt branching.

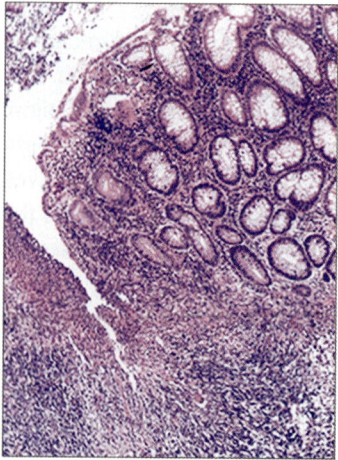

Fig. 3.8: Deep fissuring ulcers in Crohn's disease: there is marked inflammation.

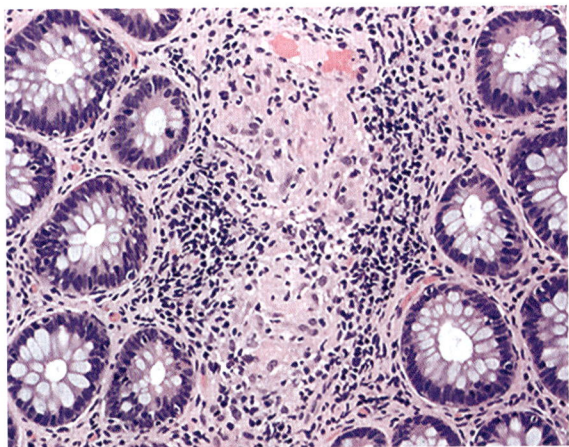

Fig. 3.9: Granulomas in the submucosa can be found in Crohn's disease and it is the histological distinguishing factor from ulcerative colitis.

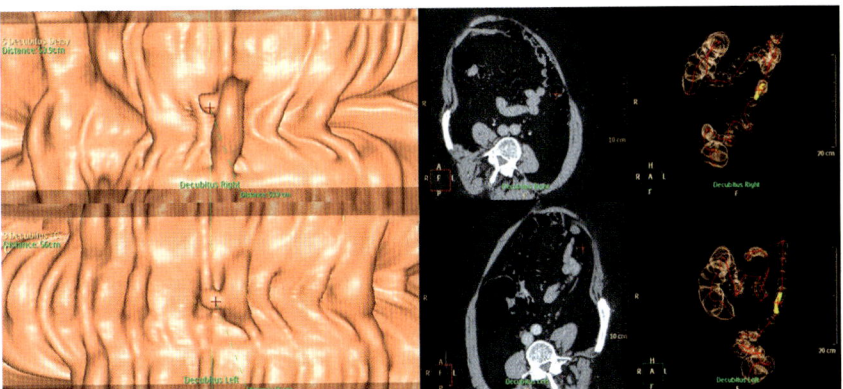

Fig. 3.10: Computed tomography colography (virtual colonoscopy): sophisticated software showing a polyp in the descending colon.

the investigation of choice; and in most institutions, it is down to availability and timeliness that influence the choice of investigation.

For patients who are very frail or for any reason a colonoscopy is unsafe or refused, a CT colography (virtual colonoscopy) is a very good alternative. Like a barium enema, a colonoscopy is still required if a biopsy is required, so best reserved for cases where a biopsy or polypectomy is unlikely to be required. A high-resolution helical CT image of a bowel that is distended with gas via a rectal tube is captured in a single breath-hold. The air is the contrast media and also inflates the colon (Fig. 3.10).

Neither colonoscopy nor barium enema is safe or necessary in a patient with severe acute colitis. If this diagnosis is suspected, a plain abdominal X-ray will give valuable information: in particular whether the colon contains

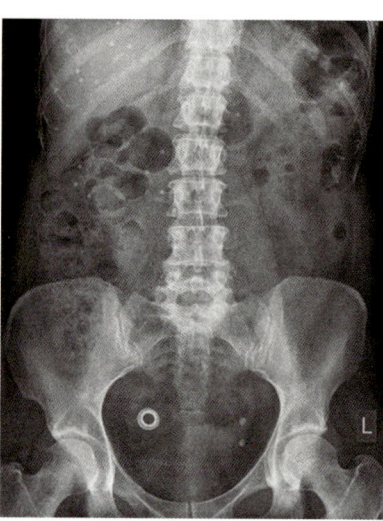

Fig. 3.11: This patient with distal ulcerative colitis presenting with diarrhea and rectal bleeding but has severe proximal constipation which a plain X-ray quite easily picks up.

feces (i.e. is relatively healthy) or is dilated. A plain abdominal X-ray may be diagnostic in ischemic colitis where massive mucosal edema is reflected by the appearance of "thumbprinting" of the colonic mucosa. Barium enema or colonoscopy should generally be deferred until the patient's condition has improved with treatment, a diagnosis having been reached on the basis of sigmoidoscopy, rectal histology and stool culture. In the situation of a patient with acute severe colitis, a CT of the abdomen usually provides with all the imaging information required to manage the problem and urgent treatment should be the immediate concern (Fig. 3.11).

While most colonic lesions are diagnosable by a combination of rigid sigmoidoscopy and double-contrast barium enema, there is a significant miss rate. A full and complete colonoscopy remains the best investigation, and in the investigation of diarrhea, terminal ileum should ideally be inspected as well. Ulcerative colitis with superficial confluent ulceration and rectal involvement is usually readily distinguished from colonic Crohn's disease with deep fissure ulcers, skip lesions and rectal sparing but in up to a third of cases with colitis, the distinction between the two conditions is difficult even with histology. These patients are often labeled as having "indeterminate colitis." The distinction between UC and Crohn's disease is of particular importance when surgery is contemplated (Figs. 3.12 to 3.15).

Behçet's disease (oral and genital ulceration, arthritis, uveitis and venous thrombosis) can rarely cause a colitis which mimics UC or Crohn's disease (Fig. 3.16).

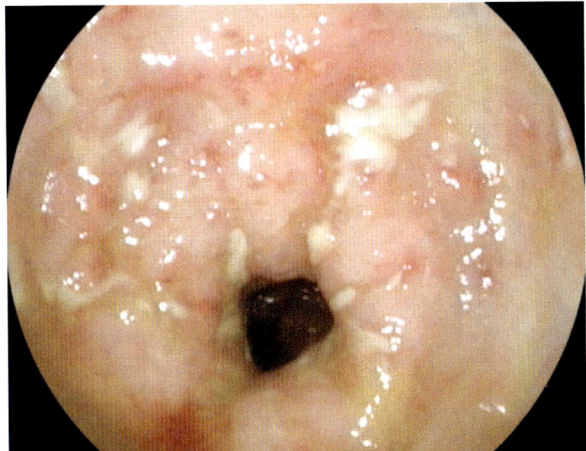

Fig. 3.12: Deep "serpiginous" ulcers often patchy are suggestive of Crohn's disease. Often the endoscopic appearance and MRI are more useful than histology in establishing diagnosis. (MRI: Magnetic resonance imaging.)

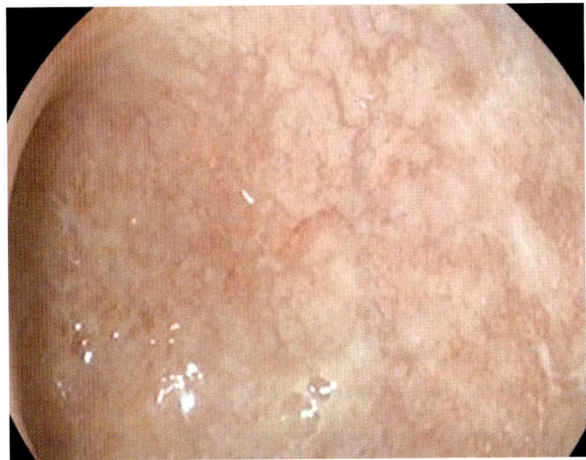

Fig. 3.13: A confluent inflammation with loss of vascularity is mild ulcerative colitis.

Although diagnosis of colonic carcinoma can often be made confidently on the basis of barium enema, this is largely superseded by colonoscopy. CT colography has a place, especially if there is some uncertainty as to the site of the lesion as colonoscopy can be inaccurate in mid-colonic lesions. However, only endoscopy can provide histological verification of the tumor with biopsies. Colonoscopy should also be performed in patients with persistent diarrhea who have a normal barium enema. Lesions not uncommonly missed on barium enema include the serpiginous or aphthoid ulcers of

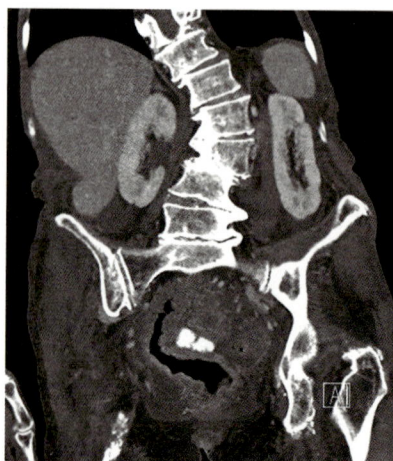

Fig. 3.14: Computed tomography can be very helpful as this shows a sigmoid that is inflamed and thickened.

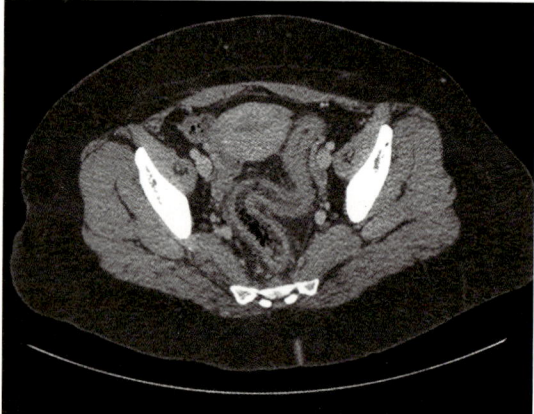

Fig. 3.15: Pelvic section of CT showing sigmoid inflammation. (CT: Computed tomography.)

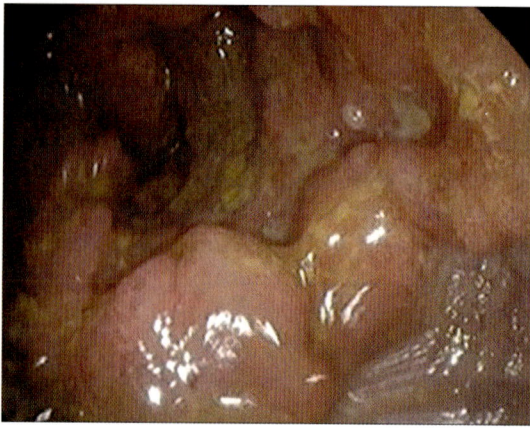

Fig. 3.16: Colonic cancer can manifest as a plaque-like lesion, a central ulcerated lesion with heaped edges, an annular, stricturing or a polypoidal lesion.

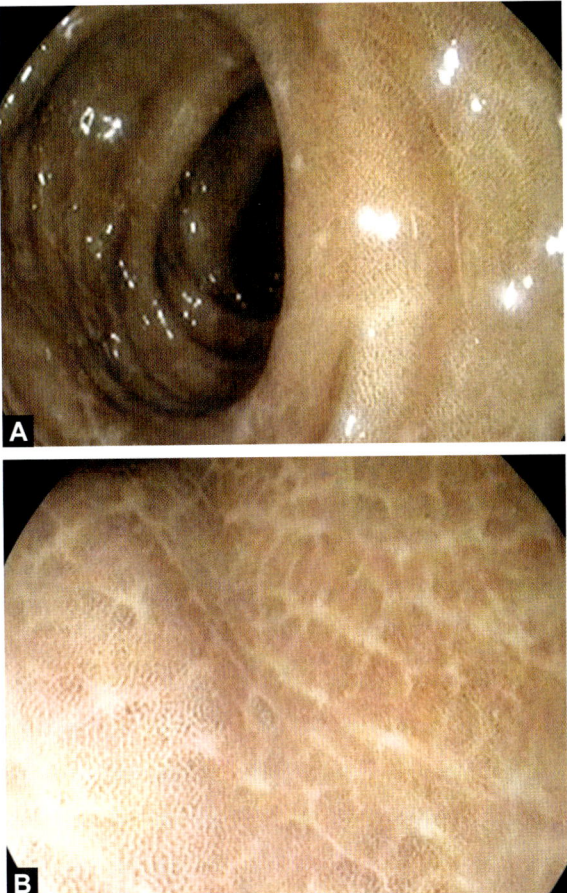

Figs. 3.17A and B: Melanosis coli on colonoscopy is seen in patients with laxative abuse.

colonic Crohn's disease, small carcinomas (particularly in a sigmoid colon that is affected by diverticular disease) and more rarely a villous adenoma. Occasionally, colonoscopy will reveal extensive melanosis in patients with purgative abuse (Figs. 3.17A and B).

Radiation enteritis should be considered as a possible diagnosis whenever patients have been given previous pelvic radiotherapy. This could be from previous prostate cancer treatment. This could be early, soon after irradiation with nausea, diarrhea and tenesmus or after many months or years, usually presenting with rectal bleeding or anemia. Colonoscopic appearance is characteristic. There is an atrophic looking mucosa with fragile telangiectatic lesions that bleed easily. Biopsies reveal narrowed arterioles, bizarre "irradiation" fibroblasts and extensive fibrosis (Fig. 3.18).

Pneumatosis cystoides intestinalis is an uncommon condition where multiple gas-filled cysts occur in the submucosa or subserosal tissue of the colon and small bowel (Figs. 3.19 and 3.20).

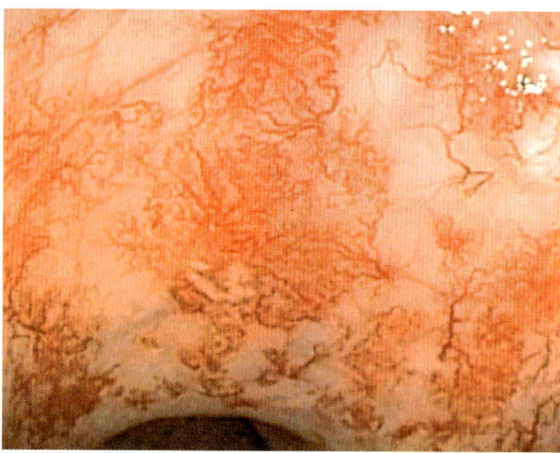

Fig. 3.18: Radiation proctitis: colonoscopic appearances showing fragile telangiectatic vessels.

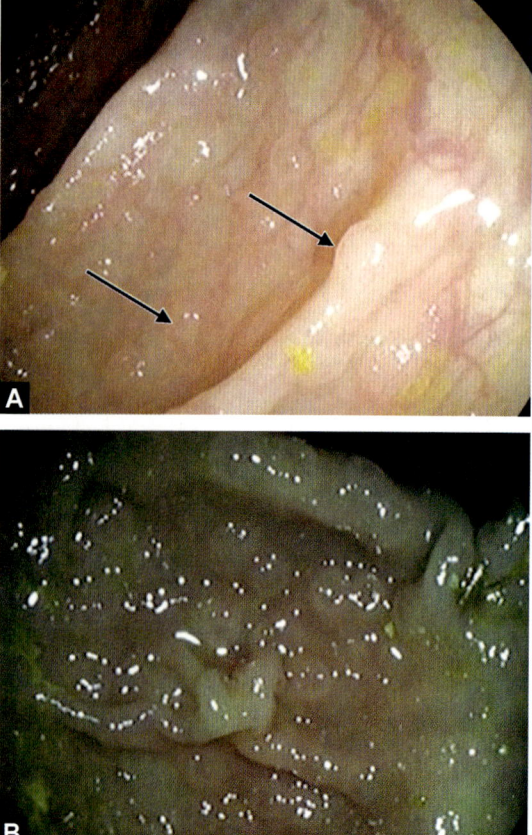

Figs. 3.19A and B: Pneumatosis cystoides intestinalis as seen on colonoscopy.

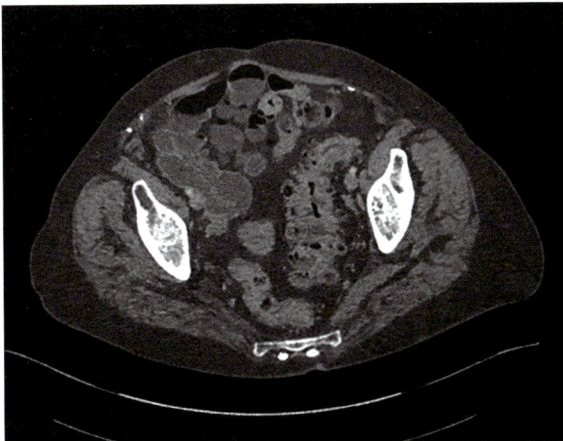

Fig. 3.20: Computed tomography scan showing gas-filled cysts in both mucosa and subserosal surface of colon in pneumatosis. On histology, the cysts are lined with columnar epithelium and may show epithelioid cells which can form giant cell granulomas. They can be symptomless or present with abdominal pain and diarrhea and even rectal bleeding.

Watery Diarrhea: Secretory?

Large volume diarrhea of 1 L or more per day usually implies active secretion of salt and water into the intestine rather than simply exudation or a failure of absorption. This suspicion can be confirmed if the diarrhea continues at a similar rate when nothing is taken by mouth. This should only be done in hospital as intravenous (IV) fluid and electrolyte replacement will be needed. Cholera is the commonest cause of secretory diarrhea worldwide but unfortunately purgative abuse is probably the commonest noninfective cause in the "civilized" world.

If these conditions can be excluded, then the rare syndromes associated with hormone or peptide-secreting tumors should be sought. They include the secretion of vasoactive intestinal polypeptide (VIP) by a pancreatic tumor "vipoma" which results in watery diarrhea, hypochlorhydria and alkalosis (Verner–Morrison's syndrome) and the watery diarrhea that is associated with a calcitonin-secreting medullary carcinoma of the thyroid. Serum assays for VIP and calcitonin are available. CT scanning, magnetic resonance imaging (MRI) or positron-emission tomography scanning may be needed to localize the tumor and to assess resectability.

Zollinger–Ellison's syndrome (gastrin-secreting pancreatic tumor) may be associated with watery diarrhea resulting from the massive hypersecretion of gastric acid although some degree of fat malabsorption is commonly present.

Carcinoid syndrome (diarrhea, flushing and wheezing due to malignant carcinoid) only occurs if there is considerable metastatic spread of tumor to the liver which is usually enlarged. Urine should be screened for 5 hydroxyindole acetic acid (5HIAA), the metabolite of 5 hydroxytryptamine.

Watery Diarrhea: Osmotic?

Measurement of fecal osmolality may be very useful in the patient with watery diarrhea. If the osmolality in mOsmol/L exceeds by >50 mOsmol/L, the sum of the sodium and potassium (in mEq/L) multiplied by 2, it is likely that there is an osmotic cause for the diarrhea. Possibilities include magnesium, lactose (in patients with hypolactasia) and sorbitol (commonly used as a filler in mints and also present in some packaged fruit juices).

Watery Diarrhea: Endocrine Disease?

Thyrotoxicosis may occasionally present with diarrhea although other features will usually be present.

Diabetic patients sometimes get a puzzling and troublesome intermittent watery diarrhea which is sometimes nocturnal. Its etiology is uncertain but it is probably due to a combination of the effects of autonomic neuropathy on the gut and bacterial overgrowth.

Adrenal failure (Addison's disease) commonly presents with prolonged diarrhea, vomiting and hypovolemia, and palmar crease and buccal pigmentation should be sought and the plasma cortisol checked before and after Synacthen or adrenocorticotropic hormone challenge.

Watery Diarrhea: Bile Salt-related?

Bile salts are normally recirculated efficiently with 95% reabsorption in the distal ileum. If the ileum is diseased or has been resected, conjugated bile salts will pass into the colon, causing stimulation of mucosal adenyl cyclase resulting in a secretory diarrhea. Since the small bowel is not involved, the volume of diarrhea is not usually as massive as with other secretory diarrheas but may be considerable (500–1000 mL per day). There is usually a clear history of surgical resection of the small intestine, e.g. for Crohn's disease, or of irradiation to the lower abdomen causing irradiation ileitis. However, it has recently been shown that some patients without any such predisposing cause may have chronic bile salt diarrhea and this probably accounts for a significant proportion of patients previously labeled as having the IBS. The diagnosis may be confirmed by measuring the absorption of an isotopically labeled bile acid (SeHCAT scan) but in practice, a therapeutic trial of oral cholestyramine is a cheaper and simpler way of establishing the diagnosis. Cholestyramine is an ion exchange resin which chelates bile acids and prevents them having a stimulatory effect on colonic adenyl cyclase. Response is usually immediate if the diagnosis is correct (Fig. 3.21).

Fatty Diarrhea—Steatorrhea—Which Approach?

There are two possible approaches to the diagnosis of fat malabsorption: a logical approach and a practical approach. The logical approach is to assess

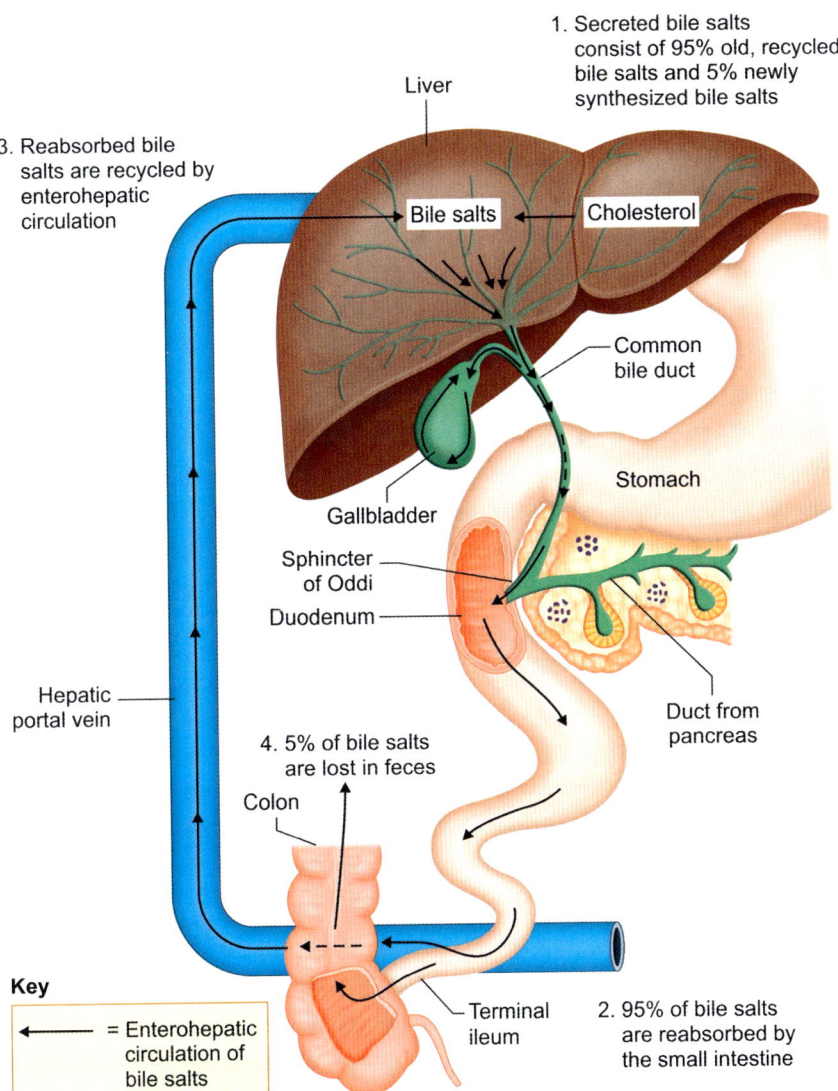

Fig. 3.21: Enterohepatic circulation.

the total fat excretion after a standard fat containing diet. This involves a 3-day stool collection and measurement of fat content, an exercise that is likely to be unpopular both to the patient and the laboratory staff. A simpler version of measuring fat absorption after a fatty meal by measuring lipids in blood is quite unreliable.

A more direct approach is to test for the presence of the disease thought most likely to be present. This approach usually leads to a diagnosis with fewer tests and is more practical even if less intellectually satisfying.

Steatorrhea: Intestinal Disease?

Celiac Disease?

In a young person with iron and/or folate deficiency and steatorrhea, celiac disease is highly probable. Other features which suggest the diagnosis include short stature, secondary amenorrhea and a blood film with features of hyposplenism (abnormally shaped red cells and Howell–Jolly bodies) or even infertility in women. Hyposplenism may also occur in IBD so this collection of clinical features is not specific for celiac disease.

The discovery of the diagnostic value of serology makes this an easy diagnosis to make. There are several available antibodies to measure. The most popular being the test for immunoglobulin A (IgA) tissue transglutaminase (tTG). Most laboratories would offer the total IgA as well because a significant number of celiac patients have IgA deficiency. If the IgA anti-tTG is mildly raised or indeterminate, IgA endomysial antibodies (EMA) can be performed con confirm positivity. In IgA-deficient individuals, then alternatives like IgG EMA, IgG-deamidated gliadin peptide or IgG tTG can be performed. These tests are remarkably reliable high specificity and sensitivity.

However, most authorities still consider that a histological diagnosis requires a jejunal or duodenal biopsy. The traditional method is jejunal biopsy using a Crosby capsule—a spring-loaded suction-activated rotating knife inside a metal capsule now thankfully obsolete. Duodenal biopsy using an endoscope is now the method of choice. The typical findings in a duodenal or jejunal biopsy from a patient with untreated celiac disease are villous atrophy with an increased number of lymphocytes within the epithelium and crypt hyperplasia. While there are other causes of partial villous atrophy or epithelial lymphocytes, in the context of an elevated celiac antibody, the diagnosis can be definitively made (Fig. 3.22).

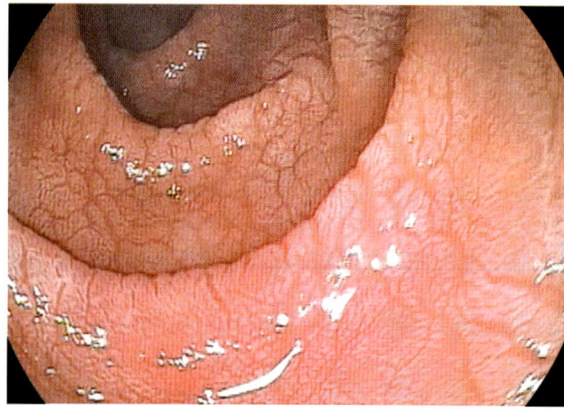

Fig. 3.22: Endoscopic appearance of untreated celiac disease can be characteristic.

Other Causes of Malabsorption

A duodenal or jejunal aspirate can be obtained at the same time as the biopsy and this, together with the biopsy, can be examined for parasites—*Giardia lamblia* and *Strongyloides* in particular. Rarer causes of malabsorption may be diagnosed from intestinal biopsy and include Whipple's disease, intestinal lymphoma and intestinal lymphangiectasia. Whipple's disease is a bacterial infestation of the small intestine which results in villous atrophy and macrophages-containing periodic acid Schiff (PAS) positive "foamy" remnants of dead bacteria accumulate within the lamina propria. It typically affects middle-aged men and as well as malabsorption causes arthritis, usually of large joints, and central nervous system involvement which may be present as a slowly progressive encephalopathy. If Whipple's disease is suspected, it is important to specifically request a PAS staining on the duodenal biopsy sample.

In patients from the Middle East or Africa with finger clubbing and malabsorption, alpha chain disease should be considered. This is a form of intestinal lymphoma in which a malignant clone of IgA-producing cells develops in the intestine. These cells produce the IgA heavy chain (alpha chain) in excess with little or no light chain. Alpha chains are shed into the plasma and excreted in urine. Diagnosis is confirmed by immunoelectrophoresis of serum or concentrated urine and may also be made by immunohistochemistry of intestinal biopsies with staining for alpha chains and light chains.

Imaging the Small Bowel

The upper GI endoscope can provide views of the upper GI tract up to the third part of the duodenum. Longer enteroscopes are available and may offer views of the jejunum but are difficult to use. The terminal ileum can usually be viewed by a colonoscope. The rest of the small bowel remains difficult to image, but thankfully, pathology here is rare. Capsule endoscopy involves swallowing a disposable capsule incorporating a light source with a chip camera and a radio transmitter sending images as it transits the gut under peristalsis. While it sounds like an ideal method, there is little control over the capsule and trolling over the hours of images is tedious. Clever software is available to assist in this task. It is expensive as the capsule is disposed in the feces and its value is chiefly in diagnosing obscure GI bleeding.

Some information can often be gained by "barium enteroclysis" or "small bowel enema." In this technique, a nasoenteral tube is passed into the duodenum under X-ray screening and dilute barium is run rapidly into the intestine. Excellent views of the mucosa can be obtained using this technique. However, this technique is increasingly being replaced by magnetic resonance enteroclysis (MRE). By using an osmotic solution polyethylene glycol

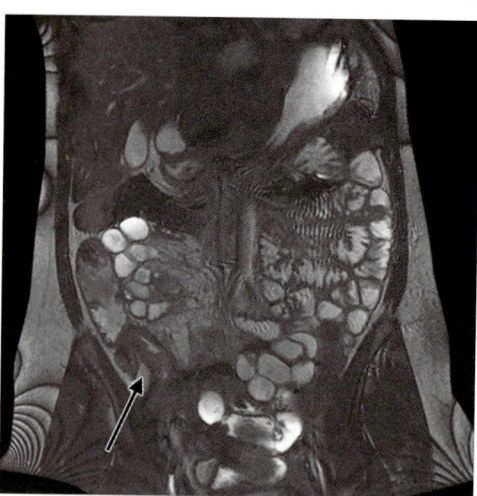

Fig. 3.23: Terminal ileum inflammation and stricture shown on MRE. (MRE: Magnetic resonance enteroclysis.)

(PEG) as a water contrast and MR performed, remarkably good pictures of the small bowel can be obtained (Fig. 3.23).

Diagnoses that could be made or excluded at this stage include Crohn's disease, tuberculosis and intestinal lymphoma. Histology may be required to make the diagnosis with certainty. Gastrointestinal tuberculosis most commonly affects the ileocecal region and there is commonly but not invariably evidence of concomitant pulmonary disease. If the lesion can be reached by colonoscopy or terminal ileoscopy, it should be biopsied and cultured for tuberculosis but laparotomy may be necessary to obtain a tissue diagnosis. In a Caucasian patient with typical radiological appearances of Crohn's disease with stricturing and skip lesions separated by unaffected bowel, it may be considered reasonable to base the diagnosis and treatment solely on the radiological findings but in patients from a population with a high incidence of tuberculosis histological confirmation is the only safe policy and tuberculosis should be strenuously excluded before commencement of steroid or anti-TNF (TNF, tumor necrosis factor) biologic therapy. This may include tuberculosis tuberculin skin tests but these have recently been largely replaced by surrogate markers like the commercial QuantiFERON-TB Gold In-Tube test.

Steatorrhea: Pancreatic Disease?

A history of excessive alcohol ingestion can be obtained in at least 90% of cases of chronic pancreatitis and impaired glucose tolerance is present in one third, so the presence of either of these factors in a patient with steatorrhea necessitates investigation of the pancreas.

Pancreatic Imaging

A plain abdominal X-ray should be performed first. Calcification of the pancreas will be visible in about one-third of cases of chronic pancreatitis and is diagnostic, if present. Further investigation of the pancreas is notoriously difficult. The "best" test is probably endoscopic pancreatography (ERCP) which will produce a pancreatogram in approximately 90% of cases and will give a correct diagnosis in approximately 90% of these. However, it is a complicated and expensive test with a significant risk of causing acute pancreatitis which fortunately is usually mild. Ultrasonography in skilled hands can be a very useful way of selecting patients who need ERCP. The pancreas can be adequately visualized in about 90% of cases and a correct diagnosis is reached in approximately 80% of these. The test, however, is very dependent on the skill of the operator and the reliability of scanning may vary considerably from one center to another. Computerized tomography (CAT scanning) is superior to ultrasound and less operator-dependent and it is readily available in most centers. CT or MRI is now probably the modality of choice if chronic pancreatitis or pancreatic cancer is suspected. Endoscopic ultrasound is also very useful if small lesions in the head of pancreas are encountered. Lesions can be sampled using a fine-needle aspirate and sent for histological examination. Autoimmune pancreatitis may be suspected if uniform swelling of the pancreas is encountered. IgG4 levels would be raised in this uncommon condition, so samples should be sent for this specific assay (Figs. 3.24 and 3.25).

Pancreatic Function Tests

Assessment of pancreatic exocrine function is useful in quantifying the problem but will not reliably discriminate benign from malignant

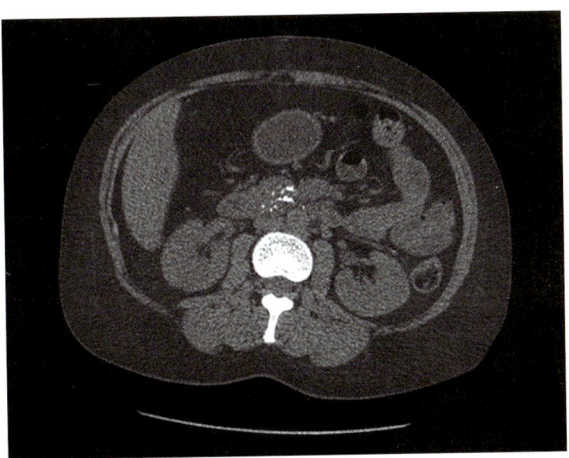

Fig. 3.24: Computed tomography of pancreas showing calcification of chronic pancreatitis.

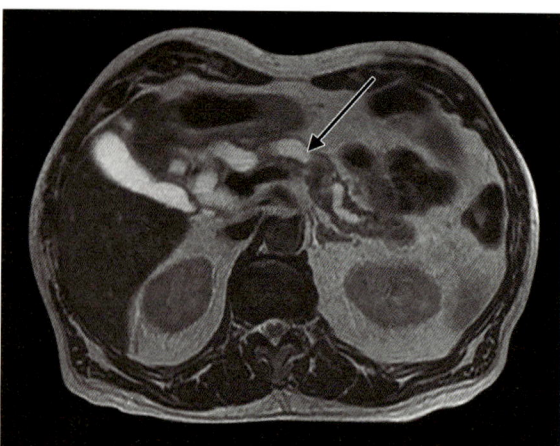

Fig. 3.25: Magnetic resonance imaging of the pancreas showing dilated pancreatic duct of chronic pancreatitis.

pancreatic disease. The standard test for pancreatic function has been the secretin test but in routine clinical practice, this has largely been superseded by "tubeless" tests. The secretin test requires intubation of the duodenum under X-ray screening with a second tube aspirating the stomach to prevent contamination of the duodenal aspirate with acid. IV secretin lu/kg is given, sometimes followed 30 min later by cholecystokinin/pancreozymin. Duodenal juice is collected in aliquots over the hour following secretin and assayed for volume, bicarbonate concentration and enzyme concentration (trypsin, lipase or amylase). Volume, maximal bicarbonate concentration and enzyme concentration are all usually reduced in significant benign or malignant pancreatic disease but in carcinoma, there is a tendency for bicarbonate and amylase concentrations to be less markedly depressed than in chronic pancreatitis. This distinction, however, is not reliable and the test is mainly of use either in quantifying function in patients with known pancreatic disease or in discriminating between the normal and the diseased pancreas.

Tubeless Function Tests: Patients never like swallowing tubes and the secretin test is time-consuming for both doctor and patient. "Tubeless" alternative tests have become available. The two most widely used are the *N*-benzoyl-L-tyrosyl-*p*-amino-benzoic acid (NBT-PABA) test and the fluorescein dilaurate test. NBT-PABA is split by pancreatic chymotrypsin with release of para-aminobenzoic acid (PABA) which is then absorbed and excreted in the urine. In order to exclude the possible effects of intestinal and renal function on the test, a second part of the test involves the measurement of the absorption and excretion of PABA alone. A ratio is calculated between excretion of PABA (1) following ingestion of PABA and (2) following ingestion of NBT-PABA. This can either be done as a 2-day test or in 1 day if C14 PABA is used to check absorption. Concurrent treatment with furosemide, thiazides, sulfonamides and paracetamol has to be avoided as these drugs interfere with the assay for PABA.

But these tests are difficult to perform and indirect tests are increasingly being used. The commonest is fecal elastase assay. Fecal collection is made and elastase measured. As the enzyme is largely undigested, significant levels are present in the feces. If this level is very low, it would suggest impaired pancreatic function. The major problem with this test is its poor reliability in measuring pancreatic exocrine function, and is best used to exclude obvious pancreatic exocrine failure in the right clinical context. These tests should be supported by imaging before the diagnosis is made.

Steatorrhea: Bacterial Overgrowth?

Small intestinal bacterial overgrowth (SIBO) is increasingly recognized as a primary as well as a secondary cause of diarrhea. Overgrowth of the small intestine with anaerobic bile salt deconjugating bacteria may result in fat malabsorption. Deconjugation of bile acids results in a failure of the entero-hepatic recirculation and depletion of the bile acid pool results. There may also be microscopic changes in the gut epithelium. Significant contamination of the small intestine usually only occurs if there is an anatomical abnormality, either a surgically constructed "blind loop" such as the afferent loop of a Polya gastrectomy or if there is diverticulosis or stricturing of the small intestine. Bacterial overgrowth of the small intestine may also occur spontaneously in elderly patients without any anatomical abnormality and in patients with diabetes mellitus. At least some patients with IBS-D have an element of SIBO.

The clinical presentation is either with steatorrhea which may be intermittent and severe or with vitamin B12 deficiency. The mechanism of the B12 deficiency is not clearly understood. Although fat malabsorption always seems to be the result of overgrowth with anaerobic bacteria, it is thought that aerobic bacteria may sometimes cause vitamin B12 malabsorption. There are several possible explanations: firstly the bacteria may consume vitamin B12, secondly they may break the bond between intrinsic factor and vitamin B12 and thirdly they may adhere to the B12/intrinsic factor complex and prevent its uptake in the terminal ileum.

The most direct approach to diagnosis is by sampling the small bowel contents but this is often unreliable as anaerobic bacteria may be difficult to culture and the siting of the sampling tube may also be critical, particularly if bacterial overgrowth is localized to a short section of the small intestine.

If the main problem is fat malabsorption, then the most logical test for bacterial overgrowth is the C14 glycocholate breath test. In this test, a small amount of C14 labeled glycocholate is taken by mouth. The radiolabel is sited in the glycine molecule and in a healthy person approximately 95% of the C14 glycocholate is taken up intact in the distal ileum and recirculated via the liver into the bile without breakdown. In a patient with SIBO, the glycocholate is deconjugated by anaerobic bacteria into glycine and cholic acid; the glycine is then absorbed and metabolized by the liver and one of the metabolites formed is C14 labeled carbon dioxide which is then breathed out via the lungs. This process is fairly lengthy and as a result the test has to be performed over 7 or 8 h but it is very simple and non-invasive apart from the small dose of radiation. A known molar quantity of carbon dioxide is collected by asking the patient to breathe out through a trap containing an indicator and the proportion of the carbon dioxide that is radiolabeled is estimated by scintillation counting. The main drawback of this test apart from its length is that patients with small intestinal disease (e.g. Crohn's disease) will fail to absorb the C14 glycocholate which will then pass into the colon and be deconjugated by the colonic bacteria. Because of the time taken to metabolize the glycine, it is not possible to distinguish malabsorption of the C14 glycocholate from bacterial overgrowth.

An alternative test, which avoids this problem, is the lactulose hydrogen breath test. In this test, 20 mL of lactulose syrup (containing approximately 8.5 g of lactulose) is taken by mouth and breath hydrogen sampled at 5-min intervals for half an hour and then at 15-min intervals for 3 h. Almost all the hydrogen in the breath comes from carbohydrate fermentation by bacteria in the intestine and in the fasting, patient breath hydrogen levels are usually <20 parts per million (ppm). In the normal patient, the lactulose will pass through into the cecum with a transit time varying between 30 and 120 min and hydrogen will be identifiable in the breath within 5–10 min of the transit time. In a patient with SIBO hydrogen (a rise of >20 ppm is significant) can be detected in the breath in the first 5–15 min after swallowing lactulose. Glucose can also be used, but is less reliable due to early absorption of glucose in the duodenum, and thus distal small bowel overgrowth may be missed.

If the patient has B12 deficiency, then a Schilling test for B12 absorption will typically show malabsorption of B12 that is not corrected by the addition of intrinsic factor but this also occurs in patients with disease of the small intestine.

An alternative to the performance of these tests is a therapeutic trial of antibiotics, either tetracycline or metronidazole. The non-absorbable antibiotic rifaximin has been touted as a possible alternative. The breath tests are however very easy to perform and give a more certain diagnosis.

CONDITIONS CAUSING DIARRHEA: NATURAL HISTORY AND MANAGEMENT

Ulcerative Colitis

Epidemiology

Surveys in Europe and North America have shown an incidence of new cases of UC of between 2 and 8/100,000 per year and a prevalence of between 40 and 80 per 100,000. There is no convincing evidence of any change in frequency over the last 30 years. Between 10 and 20% of patients will have a first-degree relative with IBD. This will not necessarily be UC as there is also an increased risk of Crohn's disease in first-degree relatives of patients with UC (and vice versa). This has led to speculation that UC and Crohn's disease might represent different ends of a spectrum of IBD with a common etiology. Genetic association studies have identified multiple loci, including some that are associated with both UC and Crohn's disease; one recently identified locus is also associated with susceptibility to colorectal cancer.

Etiology

The etiology of UC remains unknown. However, there are genetic factors that probably affect immune reactions to environmental factors. Epigenetic factors which govern the expression of key genes play an important role and may be affected by environmental factors like low levels of antioxidants, psychological stress factors, a smoking history and consumption of milk products. Chromosomes are thought to be less stable in patients with UC, with shortened telomeres in colonocytes of patients with UC, suggesting premature aging and conferring cancer risk. There is a very striking association between non-smoking and UC with up to 95% being non-smokers or ex-smokers. This is in contradistinction with Crohn's disease where smoking is associated with the disease and poor clinical course. Also ex-smokers with UC are at a higher risk of colonic cancer. Appendicectomy appears to protect against development of disease and suggest that immune processing by the juvenile appendix may be a factor.

Histologically, it resembles the inflammatory types of infectious diarrhea but although attacks may occasionally be precipitated by gastroenteritis, there is little microbiological or epidemiological evidence to support an infective cause. However, the colon is packed with bacteria and there is a close relationship between colonic immune cells and the luminal bacteria. There are several protective barriers including the mucus layer and tight junctions. There is increasing interest in the colonic bacteria flora ("biotome") and alterations are found in patients with active UC. Other environmental factors include NSAID usage, low levels of antioxidants and dietary factors although the only foods that have been implicated are milk products. Psychological

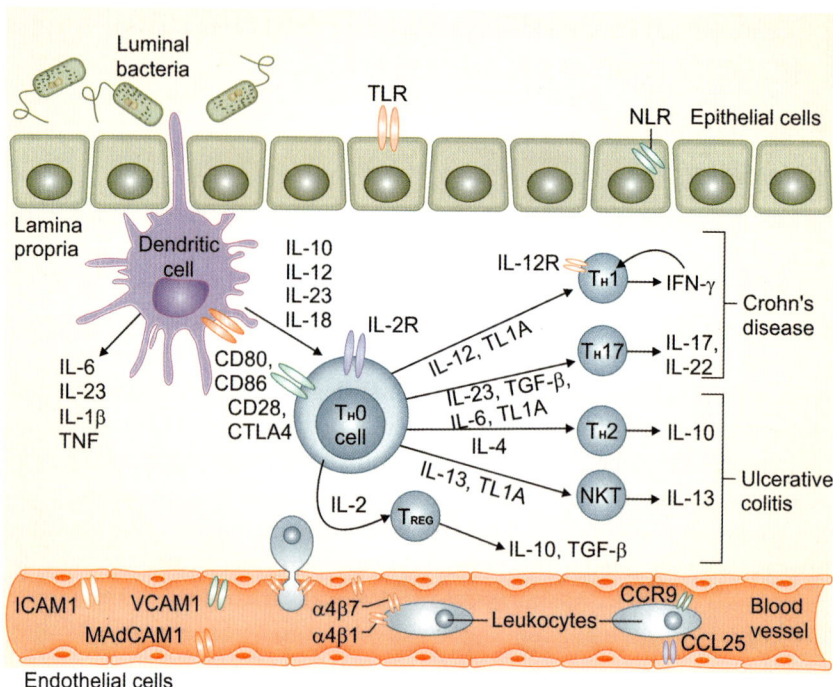

Fig. 3.26: Proposed gut immune responses in ulcerative colitis and Crohn's disease.

stress affects the immune system and may trigger or stimulate the immune system in the colon.

Whatever the trigger may be, and there may be many, the main control of the gut immune system is the dendritic cell which senses any eminent "danger" signals. This leads to expression of important cytokines that leads to stimulation of the immune response. The current proposed mechanism is pictured (Fig. 3.26) with the differentiation of the T-helper lymphocyte results in whether the resultant inflammatory process resembles a UC or Crohn's pattern. These inflammatory cytokines include some of the targets for therapy and include anti-TNF, IL-12 and IL-23. Recruitment of peripheral leukocytes from the blood vessels is mediated by adhesion molecules (MadCAM1 and VCAM1).

Clinical Course

Ulcerative colitis can affect patients of any age from early childhood onward but the incidence is highest in early adulthood. Usually, an acute attack is followed by a long period of remission but unfortunately relapse is almost inevitable at some stage. In one series only 4% remained free from attacks after 15 years of follow-up. In about one-third of cases, the disease fails to go into a clear-cut remission but continues to grumble on. The severity of attacks is very variable and is closely linked to the extent of colonic involvement. If the disease is limited to the rectum (proctitis), symptoms usually consist of passage of mucus and blood per rectum with annoying tenesmus but little diarrhea. More extensive ulceration causes diarrhea which is often bloody and if ulceration extends deeper into the mucosa pain and fever develop. In such a severe attack, there is an appreciable risk of perforation and before modern surgery and corticosteroid therapy were available such attacks had a mortality of approximately 1 in 3. In a survey from Oxford, the risk of needing surgery during the first 5 years after the onset of proctitis was 1 in 50, with colitis of intermediate severity 1 in 20, with severe colitis 1 in 3 and in another study the overall likelihood of needing surgery was 15% in the first 10 years.

Recent cohort studies in European centers showed approximately a third have proctitis, another third have left-sided disease and the remainder third have extensive disease on presentation. There is a reported a 10-year cumulative colectomy risk of 9%. In a pediatric cohort study of children aged 0–17 years, the calculated cumulative rate of colectomy was as high as 20% at 5 years.

In a meta-analysis of >10,000 patients with UC in 10 studies there was a slightly greater mortality risk in patients UC as compared with the respective background population (RR: 1.2, 95% CI 1.0–1.5, $p = 0.047$) if proctitis is excluded. This is largely due to increased risk of colorectal cancer. Another large meta-analysis, patients with UC were also found to be at an increased risk of cancer of the liver and biliary system (RR: 2.58, 95% CI: 1.58–4.22), probably related to primary sclerosing cholangitis (PSC) in patients with UC.

In a longitudinal study only 25% of patients in the 5 years after first diagnosis were in remission, 57% of patients had intermittent and 18% had continuous activity. Within a median observation period of 3 years, 77% of the patients had at least 1 second flare. In the Norwegian cohort study of 423 patients with UC, they were asked to categorize their clinical course for the previous 10 years using 1 out of 4 predefined curves (Fig. 3.27). About 12% of patients could not choose a curve because they had already colectomies. The remaining patients selected curve 3 or 4 in 43% of the cases, which means that about 50% of the patients had an unfavorable course of the disease (either colectomy or chronic continuous or chronic intermittent symptoms).

Extraintestinal Manifestations

Ulcerative colitis and Crohn's disease both have a number of extraintestinal manifestations which occur particularly when the bowel disease is active. Erythema nodosum (painful red nodules usually on the lower legs), non-erosive arthritis usually of medium- or large-sized joints—particularly the knees and episcleritis or uveitis all occur not uncommonly. Although troublesome at the time they all resolve when the underlying bowel disease is effectively treated. Similar problems occur in infective diarrheas and it is

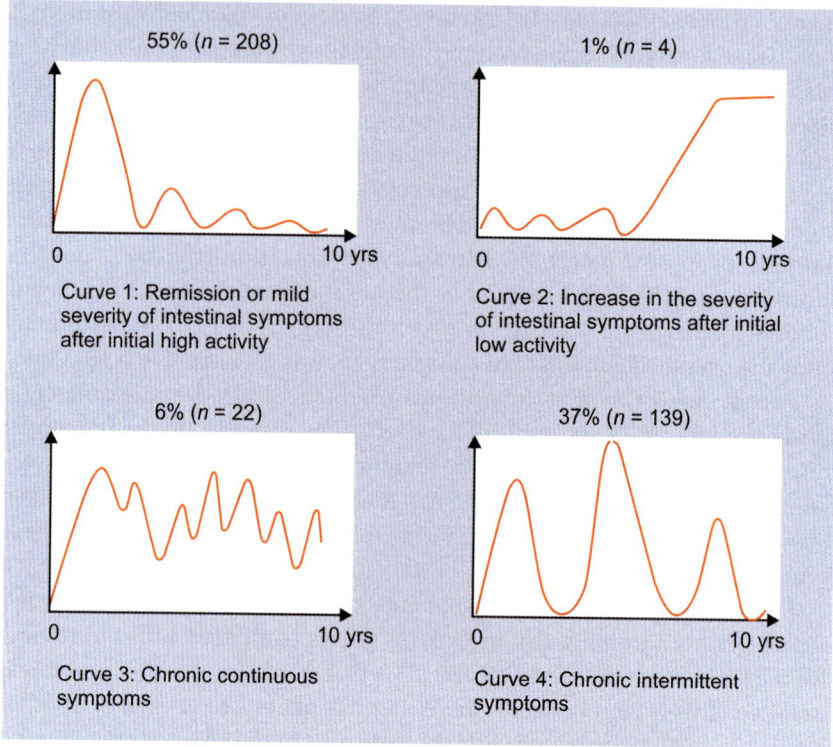

Fig. 3.27: Patterns of behavior of ulcerative colitis over a 10-year course.

likely that they are related to the presence of circulating immune complexes formed as a result of antigens, probably bacterial in origin, leaking in through the ulcerated intestine. Ulcerative colitis and Crohn's disease are also associated within a 20–30-fold increased risk of ankylosing spondylitis which affects between 2 and 6% of patients. This is associated with HLA-B27 (in approximately 65%) although not as strongly as in ankylosing spondylitis in the absence of IBD (HLA-B27 >90%) and bears no relation to the activity of the underlying bowel disease which it may antedate.

Pyoderma gangrenosum is an unpleasant chronic ulcerating skin disease with lesions usually starting on the limb or trunk. It occurs in 1–5% of patients with UC and nearly half the patients with pyoderma have colitis. Its presence bears little relationship to the activity of colitis and in several cases it has developed some time after colectomy. Finger clubbing is not uncommon in UC but usually very mild (Figs. 3.28 and 3.29).

Primary sclerosing cholangitis is a rare chronic stricturing disease of the intra and extra hepatic bile ducts that is associated with UC in over 70% of cases. The colitis may be mild or even subclinical and colectomy has no effect on the course of the liver disease which ultimately leads to secondary biliary cirrhosis and portal hypertension. Bile duct carcinoma is also associated with

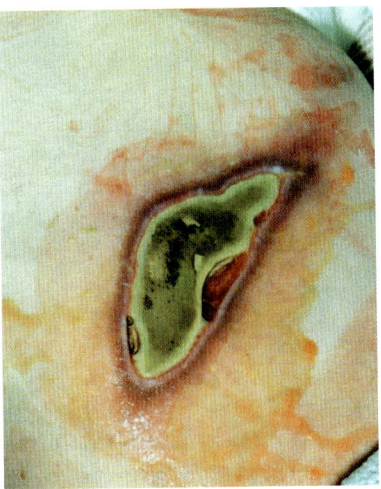

Fig. 3.28: Pyoderma gangrenosum with adherent slough.

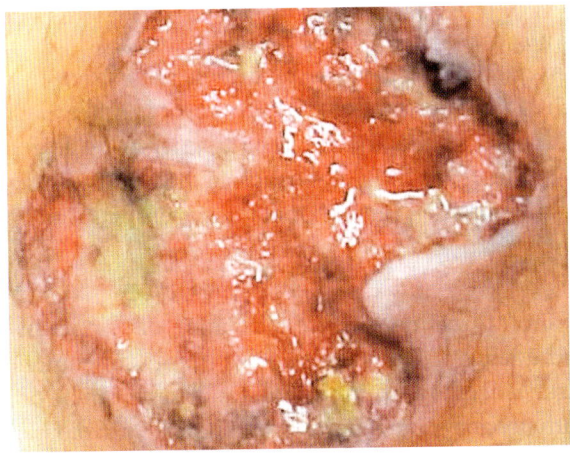

Fig. 3.29: Pyoderma gangrenosum.

UC and although the incidence is low (approximately 1%), the relative risk for a patient with UC developing this cancer is increased 22-fold compared with an age-matched control population (Fig. 3.30).

Colorectal Cancer

Colonic cancer is the long-term complication of UC that gives most concern. The size of the increased risk correlates with the extent of the disease and degree and persistence of inflammation. Patients with disease limited to the rectum and sigmoid have little or no increase in risk and recent data from three centers in the United Kingdom and Sweden have shown that patients

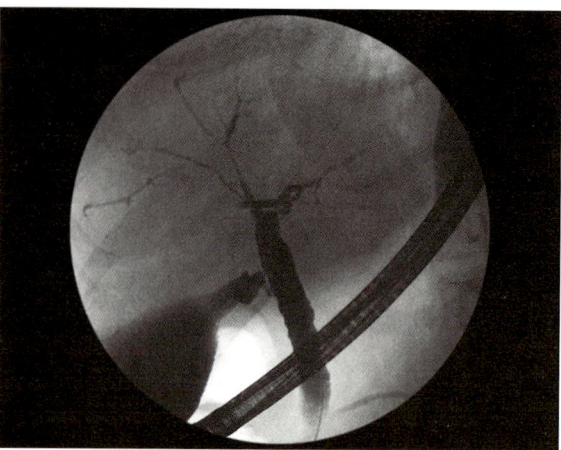

Fig. 3.30: Primary sclerosing cholangitis: multiple stricturing of the secondary and tertiary ducts give "beading" effect as seen on this ERCP. (ERCP: Endoscopic retrograde cholangiopancreatography.)

with extensive colitis have a 0.6% risk of developing colonic cancer in the first 10 years after diagnosis, 7.1% in the first 20 years and 16.4% in the first 30 years. The association with disease duration is not as simple as it seems as the age-matched relative risk remains fairly constant after the first 5 years so it is possible to speculate that there may be an underlying defect that simultaneously predisposes to both UC and cancer rather than a simple progression from chronic inflammation through metaplasia, dysplasia and cancer.

Management

The primary aim of treatment is the alleviation of symptoms and restoration of a good quality of life. Prevention of long-term complications especially colorectal cancer is also important. Colectomy can be difficult to cope with, even with ileoanal pouch surgery and hence its avoidance should also be a therapeutic goal. With the advent of new biological therapies, complete remission from disease could be achieved with medical therapy. Objective measures of remission like mucosal healing can be ascertained with endoscopy and fecal calprotectin measurement is also increasingly used. Hence, it is now not unreasonable to strive for endoscopic remission with the early use of biological therapy.

However, it is difficult at diagnosis to ascertain which patients are going to have a poor prognosis. A full assessment is required in order to ascertain the severity and extent of the disease. Clinical assessment includes a detailed history. Bowel frequency is often difficult to ascertain and may not correlate with endoscopic severity. More objective measure would include blood tests like CRP, full blood count and if available, a fecal calprotectin. A full colonoscopy is required unless the patient has severe disease, when a limited flexible sigmoidoscopy is preferred with a plain abdominal film or CT scan. The disease may thus be broadly classified as mild, moderate or severe and extent classified as proctitis, left-sided or extensive (pancolitis). A variety of scoring systems are available such as the Mayo score which is a combination of patient symptoms and endoscopic appearance and physicians' overall impression. These scores are highly subjective and perhaps the only objective markers are CRP, endoscopic appearance and fecal calprotectin levels. Endoscopic scoring systems have also been devised to standardize endoscopic reporting.

Treatment Options for UC

There are many available drug therapies for UC. Selection of the appropriate treatment depends on severity and extent of the disease. A brief discussion of the drugs available and management of specific groups of patients is discussed later.

Corticosteroids are the most effective treatment in the acute attack. They may be given rectally, orally or intravenously depending on the extent of the colitis. If the disease is localized to the rectum, local steroids are the best form of treatment. They may be given either as a twice daily enema or as a hydrocortisone or prednisolone rectal foam which many patients find easier to manage. If the colitis is more extensive, in which case diarrhea will be more prominent a symptom, systemic corticosteroids should be used. Controlled trials suggest that prednisolone 40 mg/day is the optimum dose in adults. The dose should be tailed down gradually over the next 6–8 weeks.

Corticosteroid use is limited by its well-recognized adverse effects like hypertension, diabetes, infections, moon face and osteoporosis and while they are effective in short courses of up to 8 weeks, prolonged use should be avoided. Recently a delayed-release version of budesonide (Cortiment) and beclometasone dipropionate (Clipper) have been introduced. They are released in the colon and any absorbed steroid undergoes a rapid first pass metabolism and hence systemic effects of steroids are minimized. They may be useful in limited patients who need more prolonged steroid therapy.

Sulfasalazine and the related 5-Aminosalicylates (5-ASA, mesalazine/mesalamine) are widely used in UC. Sulfasalazine consists of a sulfonamide (sulfapyridine) linked by an azo bond to 5-amino salicylic acid (5-ASA). It was first developed in the 1940s for the treatment of rheumatoid arthritis but found fortuitously to improve colitis. The 5-ASA component seems to be the active moiety, the sulfapyridine serving to carry the 5-ASA through the colon in high concentration. The majority of the sulfasalazine is then split by bacteria with release of the 5-ASA. It is this molecule that is the active moiety. Its mode of action is uncertain but seems to be unrelated to prostaglandin inhibition (and other prostaglandin inhibitors tend to make colitis worse). It has a number of immunological effects including the suppression of chemotactic leukotriene production by leukocytes. It has a mild effect in acute colitis but is most useful as maintenance therapy to prevent relapse of the disease.

Maintenance treatment with sulfasalazine 2 g/day reduces the risk of relapse by two-thirds. Unfortunately about 20% of patients are unable to tolerate the drug in adequate dosage. The main reason for this is intolerance to the sulfapyridine some of which gets absorbed and causes nausea and headaches. This is particularly a problem in patients who are slow acetylators. This problem can be got around by using one of several alternative preparations in which the 5-ASA is either linked to a different carrier molecule (balsalazide), dimerized via an azo bond (olsalazine) or contained in a delayed-release capsule (mesalazine). These delayed-release 5-ASA products are the most popular. They are either pH-dependent released or a slow-release formulation. Allergy is less commonly a problem and may be due to either the sulfonamide or salicylate component. Headaches and rashes are the main adverse effects and usually minor and renal impairment is a rare idiosyncratic reaction.

Mesalazine is also available as rectal preparations from suppositories to foam enemas. There is good evidence that combination of oral and rectal treatment is more effective than either alone. A very reasonable treatment strategy for mild-to-moderate left-sided disease is combination therapy for induction of remission and oral maintenance therapy for prevention of relapses.

Azathioprine and 6-Mercaptopurine

Azathioprine is the pro-drug which is converted in the body to 6-mercaptopurine and then into thioguanine. This is an antimetabolite which is incorporated into replicating DNA and halting transcription. Thus, it stops the proliferation of immune cells like lymphocytes. It is effective as a steroid-sparing agent. It may take up to 3 months before its effects become manifest and hence patience is required. A dose of 2.5 mg/kg body weight is recommended. The main adverse effect of concern is leukopenia and hence careful monitoring of blood count is required. The accumulation of the active drug is dependent on the patient's ability to metabolize the drug. There is a genetically determined variant where levels of the enzyme thiopurine S-methyltransferase (TPMT) are lacking, hence the active drug accumulates. TPMT levels can be measured and the rare group (<2% in the United Kingdom) of patients who lack the enzyme can be picked out and their azathioprine dose adjusted down accordingly.

However, despite its undoubted usefulness, up to 25% of all patients cannot tolerate the drug due to GI side effects like nausea, vomiting, headaches and rashes. Pancreatitis and liver toxicity are also well recognized, with a cholestatic jaundice being the main pattern.

Antidiarrheal Drugs

Antidiarrheal drugs such as codeine and loperamide should generally be avoided, firstly because they may make it difficult to assess whether the colitis is responding adequately to treatment, secondly because there is anecdotal evidence that they increase the risk of colonic dilatation and thirdly because they have little effect on bowel frequency in colitis. Their use may be necessary in the occasional patient with chronic low-grade colitis.

Biological Therapy

The 21st century has seen the rise of a number of treatments targeting specific pathways of the immune system. The most successful of these drugs include antibodies to tumor necrosis factor (anti-TNF) of which there are several, currently in the market licensed for use in UC. TNF is an important cytokine involved in signaling of T-helper lymphocytes to differentiate into activated T-helper cells. These drugs are antibodies that can bind to both soluble and membrane-bound TNF thus suppressing their function. They include infliximab, adalimumab and golimumab; the former required an IV infusion, while the latter two are self-injecting subcutaneous preparations. Infliximab (now a number of generic "biosimilar" products are available) was the first to be introduced and is a chimeric antibody, being 75% human and 25% mouse antibody. Adalimumab and golimumab are humanized version, while certolimumab is a pegylated antibody. Despite being humanized, all are proteins "foreign" to the patient and thus may produce an antibody response. This can be measured and also trough drug levels can be monitored and are useful tools in deciding on dose and dosing intervals for these drugs. Trials have shown them to be effective in moderate-to-severe UC. The main side effect is infections and particularly important to exclude active or dormant tuberculosis as it can be fatal. Screening is mandatory before commencement of therapy, and should include a chest X-rays, and tuberculin or QuantiFERON test for TB.

Also available for UC is vedolizumab, an antibody against the α4β7 integrin. It blocks the interaction of α4β7 integrin with mucosal addressin cell adhesion molecule-1 (MAdCAM-1) and inhibits the migration of memory T-lymphocytes across the endothelium into inflamed gastrointestinal tissue. The blocking of lymphocyte recruitment thus limits inflammation.

Antibodies are complex proteins that require parenteral administration. All proteins may invoke an antibody response which may attenuate the drug's efficacy. Combination of azathioprine and these biologics appear to enhance its efficacy, probably be the suppression of antibody production. In most cases, patients are likely to be already on azathioprine anyway when the biologic is added to treatment.

Parenteral medication is tedious and orally active agents thus would be advantageous. One such agent is tofacitinib, a JAK-inhibitor. JAK (Janus Kinase) are important proteins that affect cell signaling when a cytokine binds to its active site which transmits extracellular information into the cell nucleus, influencing DNA transcription of active T-lymphocytes. They are promising agents which have recently been available (Fig. 3.31).

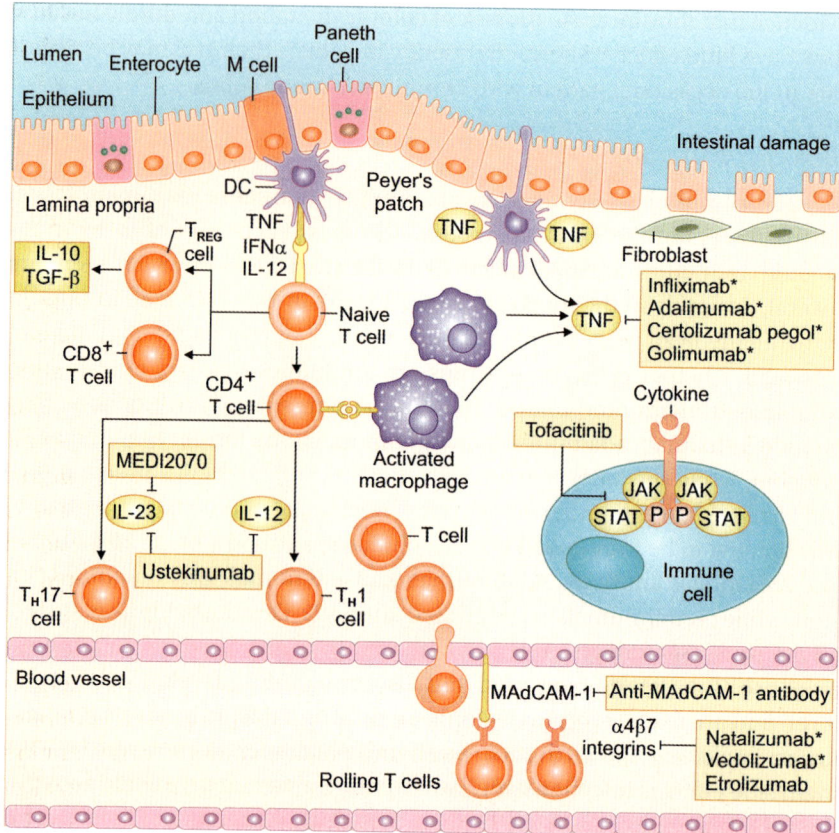

Fig. 3.31: New drugs in IBD treatment. (IBD: Inflammatory bowel disease.)

Diet

Diet seems to have little effect on the course of UC. Bowel rest and IV feeding have no beneficial effect although may be necessary in the severely ill, malnourished patient. About one in five patients will benefit from avoiding milk and it is sensible in any case to advise a low milk diet in all patients with active colitis because hypolactasia is common during attacks and milk is therefore likely to exacerbate the diarrhea. Patients should otherwise be encouraged to eat a normal diet.

Clinical Scenarios

Approach to Treatment: With a wide choice of medical treatment and the option of surgery available, it is reasonable to adopt a pyramidal structure of treatment, starting with the least potent and adding on therapy until satisfactory control of symptoms is achieved. So a physician could start with oral mesalazine, then adding rectally administered mesalazine or steroids.

For exacerbations, steroids could be used and if that fails or if they become steroid dependent, then azathioprine is used as a steroid-sparing agent. If disease continues to flare, then anti-TNF treatment is given and if they are non-responders or if they lose response, then vedolizumab or tofacitinib is worth trying. At the top of the treatment, pyramid is colectomy. However, it is important that the clinician tailors the treatment to the patient's needs. It is also important to achieve genuine endoscopic remission as continued inflammation is associated with poor outcome and increased cancer risk.

The New Diagnosis: When a patient is first diagnosed, there is often a degree of apprehension and fear. Hence, patients require good information and reassurance that good treatment is available. A patient information pack should be made available, and patient be given access to an IBD nurse practitioner and a telephone consultation "hot line". As soon as an infective cause is excluded, or when typical features on endoscopy confirm the diagnosis, patients should be treated immediately. If the disease is mild, then oral mesalazine alone may be all that is required. If the disease is any more severe than that, then oral steroids are usually required. It is necessary to give a full dose of prednisolone 40 mg/day for at least 4 weeks to achieve satisfactory remission and the dose can be tailed off over the following 3–4 weeks. Blood testing for TPMT levels will help in preparing for azathioprine introduction if required. Patients with moderate-to-severe disease will require a full course of prednisolone and consideration for early introduction of azathioprine and the addition biologic therapy like infliximab if they fail to respond or have frequent relapses. In patients who have severe disease or are unresponsive to steroids, there should be an early discussion of surgery to prepare them for this possibility (Fig. 3.32).

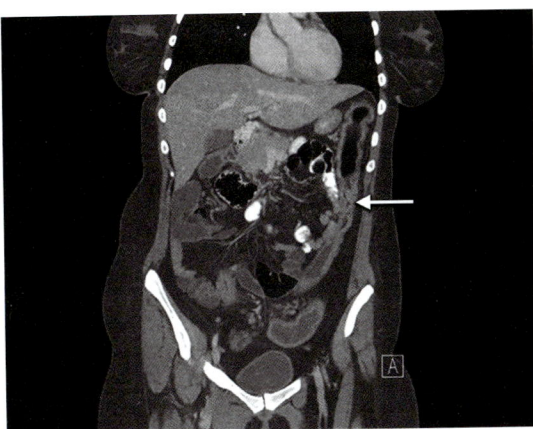

Fig. 3.32: Computed tomography of a patient admitted with acute severe disease. The sigmoid and descending colon is shown with thickening of the colonic mucosa.

Acute Severe Disease: If there is no convincing response to treatment within 2 weeks or if the patient is ill with abdominal pain, vomiting, fever or anemia, the patient should be admitted to hospital. As absorption may be unpredictable, corticosteroids should then be given intravenously. This is usually in the form of hydrocortisone at a high dose of 300 mg/day. A plain abdominal X-ray should be performed and repeated daily if the patient is unwell or if the initial X-ray shows evidence of colonic dilatation (a diameter of >6 cm in the transverse colon). Dilatation almost always implies that inflammation has spread through the muscle layer of the colon and is associated with a high risk of perforation which has a significant mortality. Patients should be examined daily and if there is signs of an acute abdomen, then surgical opinion should be immediately sought. If the dilatation fails to resolve within 1 or 2 days, colectomy is indicated and it may be unwise to delay even this long if the patient is toxic and tender over the colon.

If toxic megacolon and perforation is excluded, the patient should remain under close supervision and IV steroid. Daily blood test including full blood count and CRP should be performed. At day 3 of IV steroid, if the CRP is >50 mg/L, there is a significant chance that colectomy will be required. There are two possible medical "rescue" therapies available: cyclosporine or infliximab. Both have shown some promise of reducing risk or at least postponing the need for colectomy. This may be important as colectomy in the acute setting carries a poorer outcome. Cyclosporine is usually administered intravenously at least until response then patient may be discharged on oral cyclosporine. It carries a risk of renal impairment and in patients who have major comorbidity, infliximab may be favored.

Apart from drug therapy, it is vital to provide adequate nutritional support. It is also important to give adequate veno-thromboembolic disease prevention measures with fractionated heparin in all admitted patients as thromboembolic risk is high in all admitted IBD patients (Fig. 3.33).

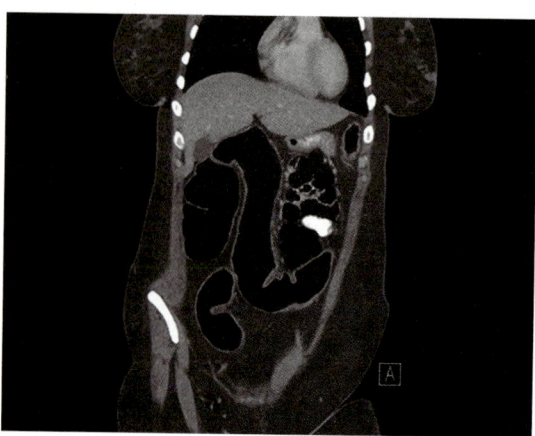

Fig. 3.33: Colonic dilatation on CT abdomen. (CT: Computed tomography.)

Prevention of Relapses and Flares: After response to initial induction of remission, more than half of all patients with a new diagnosis of ulcerative will relapse within a year. In mild-to-moderate disease, continuation of 5-ASA products is recommended as they are shown to reduce the frequency of flares. If patients have >2 flares a year, then the use of steroid-sparing agent like azathioprine is advised. If the patient is intolerant of azathioprine, then 6-MP, its active metabolite could be tried, but there is cross-reactivity of some adverse effects, especially of liver abnormalities. In these situations, monotherapy with a biologic is justified.

Proctitis: There is a distinct group of patients who have a persistent inflammation of the rectum only or with distal sigmoiditis. Although the inflammatory extent may appear trivial, the patient often experience marked symptoms or urgency, tenesmus and rectal bleeding. They can be frustratingly difficult to treat, and the idea of using expensive biologic or surgery to tackle a small area of inflammation appears too drastic. In these situations, it is best to use as much local therapy as possible. Combination of oral and rectal mesalazine (suppository or foam/liquid enema) is advised and when remission is achieved, the patient should be encouraged to continue on the oral preparation and introduce the rectal product as soon as a flare occurs. Retention of enemas can be difficult, and is best given at night just before sleep. Local steroid foam enemas or liquid retention enemas can also be tried. One of the oldest forms of therapy which still has an occasional role is arsenic in the form of acetarsol suppositories. Finally, abdominal examination and abdominal film should be performed as many have a proximal constipation, and remission can be achieved by clearing this constipation with a laxative (Fig. 3.34).

Surgery

The main indications for colectomy in UC are failure of medical treatment and the development of cancer or severe dysplasia. In a patient hospitalized with severe colitis failure to respond after 1 week of high dose IV corticosteroid therapy should usually be taken as an indication for surgery, especially if there is no response infliximab. Colonic dilatation in an acute colitis that has not settled within 48 h should also be taken as an indication for surgery. Perforation is of course an indication for emergency colectomy but it carries a significant mortality.

There remains a group of patients who have persistent symptoms despite treatment. Patients would have multiple medical treatments which could include mesalazine, immunosuppressive agents and biologic therapy. Various biologics could be tried and if the first (usually an anti-TNF) fail, vedolizumab may be tried followed by tofacitinib if that fails. Despite this, some patients continue to have active disease either a primary non-responder (never responded) or secondary loss of response to multiple biologics.

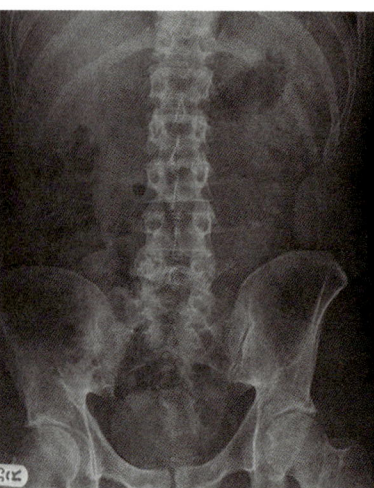

Fig. 3.34: A plain X-ray of the patient with distal colitis affecting the rectum to descending colon demonstrated considerable constipation in the right colon. A good laxative-induced rapid remission of symptoms.

Some patients may consider surgery preferable to endless cycles of drug therapy. Colectomy is not an appropriate treatment for the extraintestinal manifestations of colitis. Sclerosing cholangitis and ankylosing spondylitis both continue unchecked and although colectomy has been recommended for patients with intractable pyoderma gangrenosum, the response is very unreliable and there have been several reports of the skin lesion appearing for the first time after colectomy.

Types of Colectomy: The conventional operation is total colectomy with ileostomy. If the patient is ill, many surgeons prefer to perform this as a two-stage procedure leaving behind a rectal stump at the first operation. However, this should not be left indefinitely as continuing proctitis is likely to be very troublesome. Occasionally, an ileorectal anastomosis is performed and surgeons vary considerably in their views on this. Most people would only consider the operation worthwhile either in the elderly or as a temporary measure in the young nulliparous patient with relative rectal sparing.

The most commonly performed procedure is a pan-proctocolectomy and an ileoanal pouch. This is usually done as a two-stage procedure. A pouch is fashioned out of the distal ileum, usually a J-shaped receptacle and anastomosed to the anus leaving only a tiny cuff. This may leak and hence an ileostomy to divert feces and thus protecting while the pouch heals. This is usually only done in the elective setting. The ileostomy is closed usually after 6 months or so. The functional results are good, although bowel frequency may still be of the order of 4–6 times a day. There is also a risk of reduced fertility in young women (Fig. 3.35).

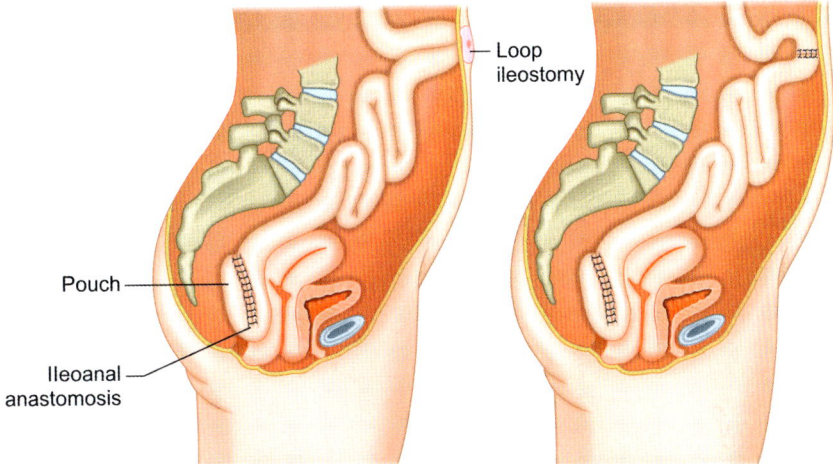

Fig. 3.35: Two-stage ileoanal pouch operation.

The main problem with ileoanal pouches is pouchitis. This is associated with bacterial colonization of the pouch and a troublesome persistent inflammation leads to frequency and bleeding. Treatment with metronidazole may be helpful. Addition of probiotics like VSL-3 may be helpful. Infliximab has a role in persistent pouchitis, but conversion to end-ileostomy may be necessary.

Screening for Cancer

The increased risk of colon cancer in UC arguably justifies regular colonoscopic surveillance. The risk of colorectal cancer increases with duration of disease, extent of disease and persistence of active inflammation. Hence, a patient with longstanding active pancolitis is at the highest risk, and a mild distal proctitis has the lowest risk. There is evidence that patients with PSC have an additional increased risk of colorectal cancer. Age of patient itself is a risk factor. Hence, it is usual to try to stratify risk of cancer and effort is put into screening of the most vulnerable groups (Table 3.1).

If available, chromoendoscopy is the preferred modality, where an application of a dilute contrast dye like indigo-carmine is sprayed on the mucosa to enhance its features and can pick up areas of flat dysplasia. Modern videoscopes have digital image enhancement and select light wavebands that can help. Abnormal areas can be sampled and if there is dysplasia, then these patients are carefully followed up and offered colectomy if there is high-grade dysplasia. If there is a dysplasia with raised lesion or mass (DALM), then the probability of actual cancer is high and colectomy is indicated.

Table 3.1: Risk of developing colorectal cancer in people with IBD.

Low risk:
- Extensive but quiescent UC or
- Extensive but quiescent Crohn's colitis or
- Left-sided UC (but not proctitis alone) or Crohn's colitis of a similar extent

Intermediate risk:
- Extensive ulcerative or Crohn's colitis with mild active inflammation that has been confirmed endoscopically or histologically or
- Postinflammatory polyps or
- Family history of colorectal cancer in a first-degree relative aged 50 years or over

High risk:
- Extensive ulcerative or Crohn's colitis with moderate or severe active inflammation that has been confirmed endoscopically or histologically or
- PSC (including after liver transplant) or
- Colonic stricture in the past 5 years or
- Any grade of dysplasia in the past 5 years or
- Family history of colorectal cancer in a first-degree relative aged under 50 years

Source: NICE Guidelines, 2011.

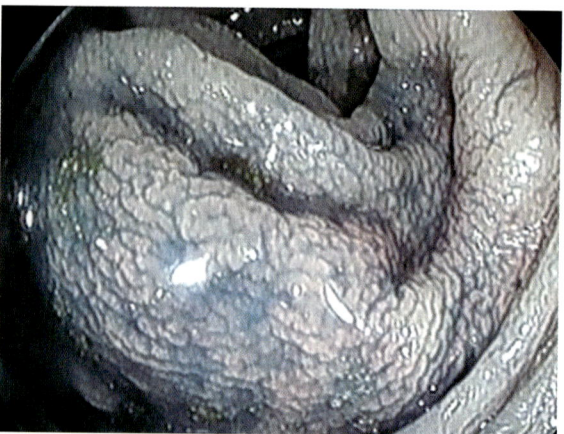

Fig. 3.36: A dilute dye is used to enhance surface features in colonoscopy.

If after a base-line colonoscopy, it is deemed a low risk patient, then colonoscopic surveillance interval can be increased to every 5 years or not at all. Intermediate risk group may have surveillance intervals every 3 years and those with high risk offered yearly surveillance (Fig. 3.36).

Crohn's Disease

Epidemiology and Etiology

The incidence of Crohn's disease is about 83 per million people per year in the United Kingdom (about half that of UC). The incidence of Crohn's disease increased about three-fold between 1968 and 1993. The reasons for this increase are unknown, but it may be due to environmental factors. Worldwide, there is a considerable variability in incidence, it is rare in Far East and Southeast Asian countries and in Europe, there is a higher incidence in the Northern European countries compared to the Southern and Mediterranean countries.

The prevalence of Crohn's disease is about 145 per 100,000 people in the United Kingdom and similarly rising. The commonest age of presentation is in adolescence and early adulthood—the median age at diagnosis is about 30 years. Crohn's disease occurs in men and women at approximately equal rates. A general practice serving 2000 people can expect to have about 6–7 people with IBD (Crohn's disease and UC), and to see a new case of Crohn's disease every 5 years on average.

Genetic and environmental factors are probably both important in the etiology. Approximately 25% of patients have a relative with IBD which in about 1 in 3 cases is UC rather than Crohn's disease. This has led to speculation that Crohn's disease and UC may represent opposite ends of a spectrum of one IBD rather than being separate diseases. Siblings of an individual with Crohn's disease are 17–35 times more likely to develop the condition than the general population. Twin studies show only a 50% concordance with monozygotic twin siblings suggesting other environmental triggers. Genetic studies show a complex and diverse picture and not fully understood. At least 200 genes have been found to be associated with Crohn's disease. Many of these genes are involved in immune modulation or the regulation of the intestinal epithelium integrity. Epigenetics, which decides if certain genes are expressed or not, are likely to be important but currently poorly understood.

As Crohn's disease has a propensity to affect areas where there is bacterial colonization like the colon, rectum and terminal ileum, the role of intestinal bacteria especially bacteria in the mucus layer have come under scrutiny but remain speculative. The principal intestinal cell that triggers the inflammatory response is the stellate cell and immune cytokines are released that starts the process of T-helper cell differentiation into activated cell, possibly via the Th1 and Th17 pathways (Fig. 3.37).

It is also logical to assume that dietary habits may play a role, particularly as childhood diets can affect epigenetic expression of genes. Some dietary surveys have shown that patients with Crohn's disease tend to have a high pre-illness intake of refined sugar and a low intake of vegetable fiber although recent studies have been inconclusive.

Other epidemiological studies have shown other risk factors apart from genetics. The most important being smoking. The risk of Crohn's disease is almost twice in smokers than in non-smokers. This is the opposite of that in UC, for which the risk is decreased. Another curious contradistinction from UC is appendectomy. The risk of Crohn's disease increases early after

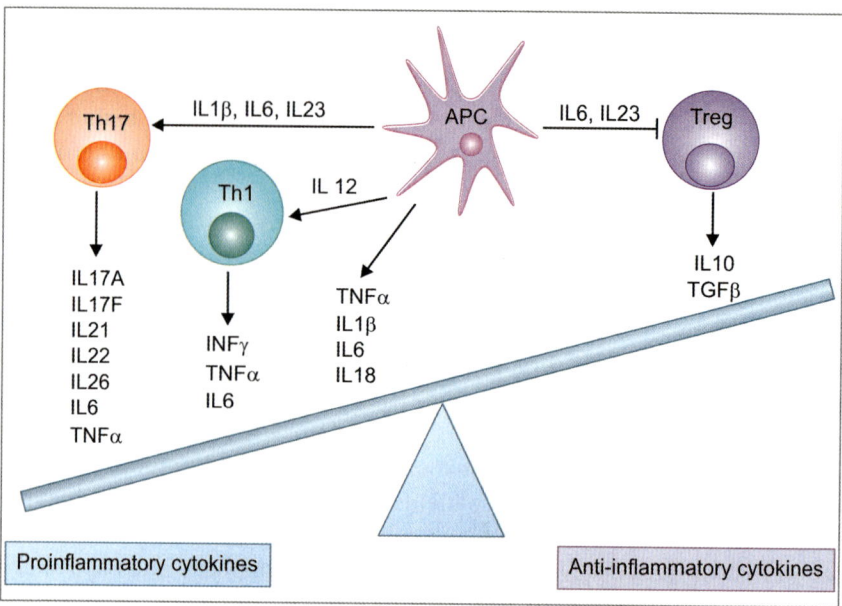

Fig. 3.37: An imbalance of pro- and anti-inflammatory cytokines leads to inflammation.

an appendectomy and then decreases to that of the general population after about 5 years. In the first year after appendectomy, the relative risk could be as high as 7 times the normal population. Drugs including nonsteroidal anti-inflammatory agents have been implicated in the flare of Crohn's disease. Although it appears in some studies to be associated with Crohn's disease, it can itself cause isolated ulceration of the terminal ileum or colonic strictures, particularly the delayed-release medication, which can be misdiagnosed as Crohn's disease. There is probably an association between oral contraceptive usage and a form of colitis that mimics Crohn's disease and this may account for a small proportion of cases of colonic Crohn's disease.

Although Burrill Crohn and his colleagues only described terminal ileal disease and its complications in 1922, it is now known that the disease can affect any part of the gastrointestinal tract from mouth to anus. The most common site for disease is the ileocecal region followed by the colon alone, small intestine alone and much more rarely stomach, mouth and very rarely esophagus. Inflammation runs deep into the layers of the intestine in distinction with UC where it rarely breaches the muscularis mucosa. As a consequence, strictures, fissures and fistulae are hallmarks of the disease. Fistulae are particularly disabling and may lead from one segment of intestine to another and from intestine to bladder, vagina or skin. Malabsorption is common and if the disease occurs in childhood, growth is likely to be inhibited and this may even be the presenting symptom if intestinal symptoms are mild (Figs. 3.38 to 3.40).

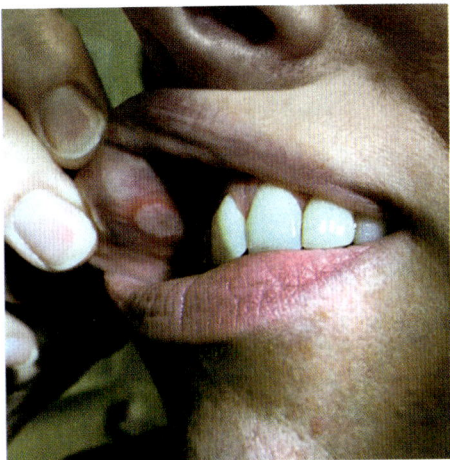
Fig. 3.38: Oral ulcer is in the common buccal position.

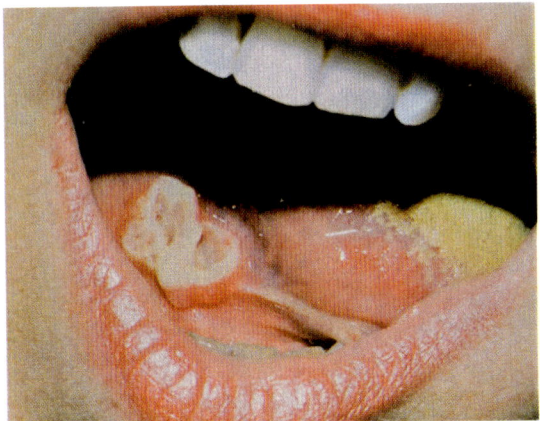
Fig. 3.39: Large oral ulcers are common in Crohn's disease.

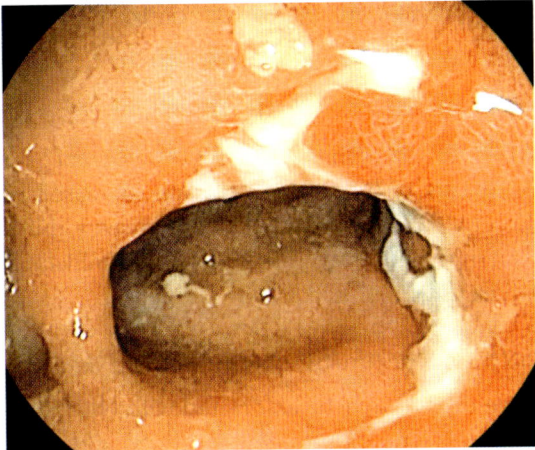
Fig. 3.40: Terminal ileum with serpiginous ulcers.

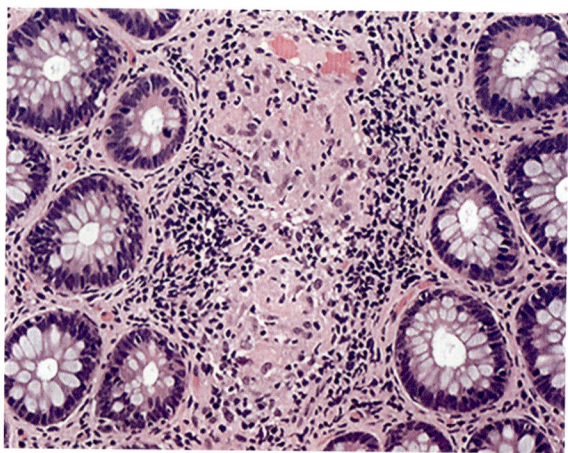

Fig. 3.41: Non-caseating granulomata are the classic hallmarks of Crohn's disease.

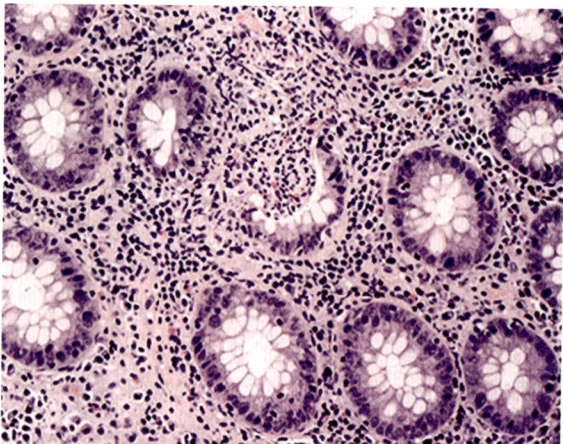

Fig. 3.42: Inflammatory infiltration and crypt abscess formation in the colonic lamina propria.

Pathology

Histologically, the hallmark of the disease is the occurrence of non-caseating granulomata. All layers of the mucosa contain increased chronic inflammatory cells. Crypt abscesses occur in colonic disease, but mucus is usually retained even in the presence of inflammation unlike UC where mucus depletion is marked (Figs. 3.41 and 3.42).

Extraintestinal Manifestations

As with UC, active disease may be associated with "reactive" inflammation outside the intestine in the form of acute arthritis, anterior uveitis or erythema nodosum.

Extraintestinal manifestations occurs roughly at the same rates in Crohn's disease and UC, except for arthritis, which is more common in Crohn's disease which affects some 10–35% of people with Crohn's disease. Patients with Crohn's colitis are most likely to have extraintestinal manifestations.

Some of these extraintestinal manifestations are related to disease activity. These include pauciarticular arthritis, erythema nodosum, apthoid ulceration and episcleritis.

Pauciarticular arthritis affects fewer than five large joints, such as the ankles, knees, hips, wrists, elbows and shoulders. It is usually asymmetric, acute and self-limiting (lasting for weeks rather than months) and joints tend not to be permanently damaged. There is often associated enthesitis (inflammation where a tendon attaches to a bone), tenosynovitis (inflammation of a tendon and its sheath) or dactylitis (inflammation of an entire finger or toe).

Erythema nodosums are tender, red or violet subcutaneous nodules, 1–5 cm in diameter which typically occur in the anterior tibial area or extensor surfaces of the legs or arms. Aphthous ulcers occur in the mouth or underside of the tongue and less commonly in the genitals. Episcleritis presents as painful red eye with injected sclera and conjunctiva.

Metabolic bone disease (osteopenia, osteoporosis and osteomalacia) is remarkably prevalent in Crohn's disease. Osteoporosis could be regarded as both a complication and an extraintestinal manifestation of IBD because contributing factors include age, corticosteroid treatment, smoking, low physical activity (including that from hospitalization), inflammatory cytokines, extensive small-bowel disease or resection, and nutritional deficiencies.

Some of the extraintestinal manifestations are not related to disease activity. These include polyarticular arthritis pyoderma gangrenosum and uveitis. Hepatobiliary conditions, including PSC, pericholangitis, steatosis, chronic hepatitis, cirrhosis, and gallstones also show increased incidence in Crohn's disease, although PSC is more associated with UC and gallstones more with Crohn's. Abnormal liver function tests may be due to the drugs used to treat Crohn's disease rather than due to liver disease. Azathioprine can cause a cholestatic jaundice and infliximab can cause an autoimmune hepatitis-like reaction.

There is an increased venous thromboembolism risk, especially in hospitalized patients. Amyloidosis may rarely complicate Crohn's disease and may occasionally present early in the course of the disease. It is probably linked with the very marked "acute phase response" associated with active Crohn's disease. One of the acute phase proteins produced by the liver as part of this response is the amyloid A protein. Other proteins produced in increased quantity include orosomucoid (serum acid glycoprotein) and CRP, measurement of which gives a useful guide to the activity of Crohn's disease.

Clinical Course of Disease

Crohn's disease is a lifelong condition, with unpredictable episodes of relapses and remissions. The consequences of the disease depend on the site of bowel involvement and the age at onset. Ileal disease typically causes colicky pain, diarrhea and, if untreated, weight loss while colonic disease causes diarrhea and sometimes rectal bleeding usually with relatively little pain. Perianal disease causes painful abscess and discharge from fistulating disease.

Typically in the disease starts with a predominantly inflammatory phase. This inflammation can be transmural and may heal with stricturing of the bowel. Deep fissures may cause fistulation which can occur with another part of the bowel as in an entero-enteric fistula, to another organ like a colovesical or rectovaginal fistulation or to the skin as an external fistula. This may eventually heal with fibrosis or patients may have undergone surgical intervention leading to more fibrosis and eventually to loss of function (Fig. 3.43).

A review of population-based studies of the natural history of Crohn's disease found that the location of the disease (ileitis, colitis or ileocolitis) remained broadly stable over time. About 30% of people had an intestinal stricture or fistula when diagnosed. About 10% of people had prolonged clinical remission. Each year, about 20% of people were admitted to hospital. About 50% of people underwent surgery within 10 years of being diagnosed. About 50% of people undergoing surgery had a recurrence of symptoms within 10 years after surgery. Mortality is higher than in the general population and has not changed significantly over 30 years (standardized mortality ratio 1.52, 95% CI: 1.32–1.74).

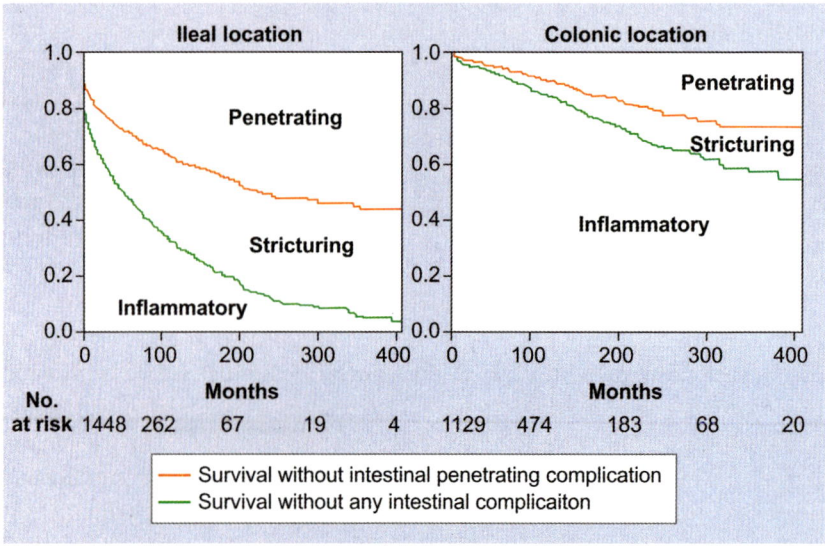

Fig. 3.43: Natural history of Crohn's disease over time.

In the course of the disease, the majority will require some sort of surgical intervention, some are minor like abscess drainage to major resection and permanent ileostomies. Hence, there is increasing move toward early aggressive therapy to improve what is still a largely dismal long-term outlook for the disease.

Goals of Treatment

The primary goal of therapy is to induce remission and to maintain disease-free state for as long as possible. The long-term objective is to alter the natural history of the disease. This laudable goal is at present not fully achievable with current treatments but with a few key principles, it is possible to optimize therapy. These include:
- Early recognition of disease and recognition of the poor prognosis group that will require rapid escalation of treatment
- Induce remission and maintaining remission using the most effective and least toxic therapy available
- Ensure that patients are able to maintain normal daily family, social and employment lives
- Provide and maintain the best nutritional state possible.

Hence, treatment may be a combination of drug, surgical and nutritional interventions.

Management

Much of the management of Crohn's disease has until recently been empirical and in no other condition can the Hippocratic principle "if you cannot do any good at least do no harm" be more appropriate. Common mistakes in clinical management have in the past included inappropriate maintenance corticosteroid therapy with all its inherent risks, excessive resection of diseased intestine and inadequate attention to nutrition.

Suppression of Active Disease

Drug Therapy
Corticosteroids: Corticosteroids are effective at suppressing symptoms but there is no evidence that they improve the prognosis. It is reasonable to treat active disease with short courses of corticosteroids starting with prednisolone 20–40 mg/day in an adult, and tailing off over 2–3 months. Unfortunately, the symptoms frequently recur when the corticosteroids are tailed off. Maintenance corticosteroid therapy should be avoided. Rectal Crohn's disease may be treated with limited success by corticosteroid enemas but corticosteroid therapy in Crohn's disease that affects other sites needs to be systemic.

Delayed-release steroid budesonide may also have a minor role in mild terminal ileal or ileocolonic disease. Budesonide has a high first-pass metabolism in the liver and hence minimizes its systemic adverse effects. A dose of 9 mg for induction and 6 mg for maintenance of remission for up to 6 months may be used but its effects are modest and should be used only in mild disease, or as a bridge to immunosuppressive.

Sulfasalazine, Other 5-Aminosalicylates and Antibiotics: Mesalazine and sulfasalazine are of doubtful value in Crohn's disease. Trials have shown conflicting results in both small intestinal and colonic Crohn's disease. It probably has a mild beneficial effect and is worth trying in patients with troublesome disease. There is a theoretical advantage of using a delayed-release mesalazine such as Pentasa as opposed to a pH-dependent release product as it is more likely that mesalazine is released into the terminal ileum and not the colon.

Metronidazole has a role in perianal disease. Treatment usually has to be prolonged (e.g. 400 mg bd orally for 2–3 months). More lengthy courses carry a high risk of drug-related peripheral neuropathy. Combination with ciprofloxacin for its wide spectrum can be used for treatment of abscesses but this drug is prone to cause severe *C. difficile* infection.

Immunomodulators: Azathioprine (2.5 mg/kg/day) or its active metabolite 6-mercaptopurine (at half the dose of equivalent azathioprine) are important immunosuppressive agents in the control of inflammation in Crohn's disease. As in the treatment of UC, it is useful as a steroid-sparing agent and in combination with biologic therapy, will enhance effect, and reduce the likelihood of antibody formation in drugs like infliximab. However, the drug has two major shortcomings. Firstly, it may take several weeks and up to 3 months before its effects kick in, and many patients and some inexperienced physicians may lose confidence in the drug. Secondly, it has major side effects and poorly tolerated by some patients. Major side effects are pancreatitis, liver abnormalities from mild liver enzyme changes to cholestatic jaundice and marrow suppression. The latter is dose-related and careful monitoring of blood count and prior TPMT measurements is required. Up to 25% of patients simply cannot tolerate the drug due to nausea and vomiting, although reducing the dose may help. Another long-term concern with azathioprine is malignancy potential. It is linked to a rare but fatal hepato-splenic T-cell lymphoma in children and young adults (Fig. 3.44).

Biological Therapy: These have been discussed earlier for the treatment of UC. All the major classes of antibodies used in UC have similar effects in Crohn's disease. These include infliximab, adalimumab and vedolizumab. Another drug licensed for use in Crohn's disease is ustekinumab. This is an

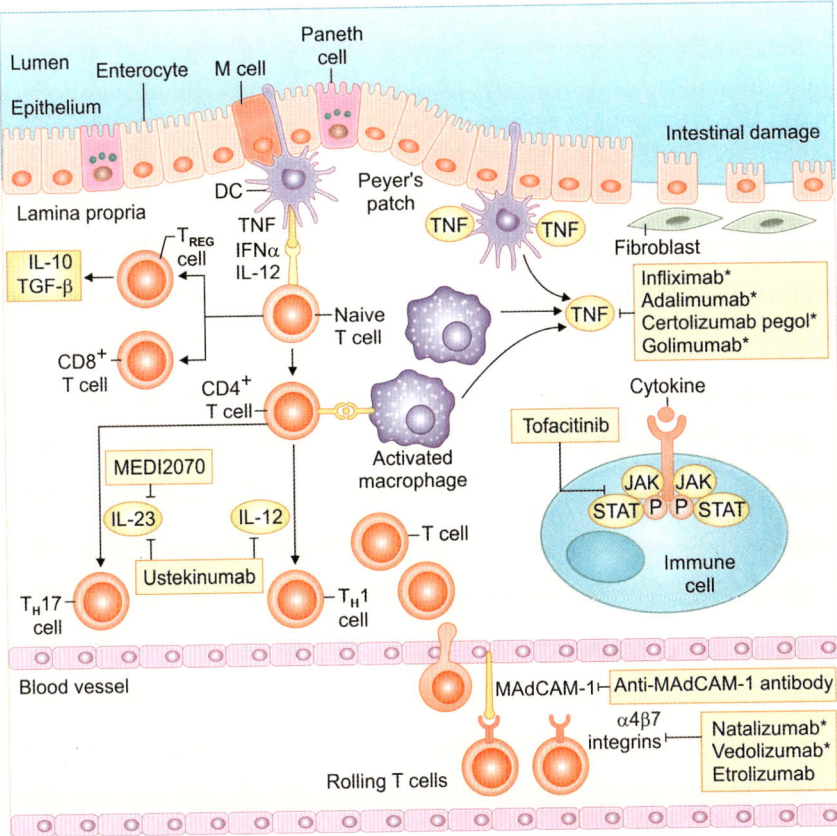

Fig. 3.44: Biologics used in Crohn's disease and their mode of action.

antibody against a common P40 protein in IL-23 and IL-12, two important cytokines that stimulates Th1 and Th17 responses. In general, these drugs are most effective when there is significant inflammatory load and least effective in later stages of fibrotic or fistulating disease. Combination with an immunosuppressive, especially in the first few months of usage will help reduce antibody formation and have synergistic effects. Similar to UC treatment, screening for infections especially TB is important.

Based on the natural clinical course of the disease, it seems logical that patients could be treated early and aggressively in order to avert the late sequelae of the condition. These drugs are expensive and care providers have to avoid wasteful wanton use. But in the right patient, they are highly valuable in inducing and maintaining remission in patients with Crohn's disease.

The methods of administration vary but they are all parenteral and involve an induction dose and then only in responders a maintenance dose is given. While the anti-TNFs generally induce a response within 6 weeks, vedolizumab usually takes longer, perhaps 10–12 weeks to respond. However, these drugs fail to work in about 40% of Crohn's patients. Failure may be "primary," that is the patient never responded to treatment or "secondary," when patients respond initially then relapsed while on treatment. In both situations, trough drug levels (if available) can be measured and dose or frequency can be increased if drug levels are low. Compliance of self-injected drug may be a cause of low drug level. If drug levels are adequate, then a switch to another drug, preferably a different class is indicated. Typically thus, infliximab may be used as the first-line biologic and vedolizumab or ustekinumab used as second or third line drugs.

The field is evolving, and guidance from health organizations like NICE (National Institute of Clinical Excellence) are regularly updated to include the latest clinical evidence and should be consulted.

Dietary Therapy: Very good results have been reported with various forms of dietary therapy. These are used not just to improve nutrition but also to suppress active disease. Three main forms of dietary treatment have been used: IV feeding, enteral feeding with an amino acid based "elemental" feed and exclusion diet therapy. Enteral elemental feeding with an amino-acid based liquid feed (e.g. EO28) as the sole feed has been shown to be as effective as corticosteroids in suppressing active disease. Subsequent studies have shown equally good results with some whole protein liquid feeds (e.g. Triosorbon) but there are interesting discrepancies between some of these studies, and further studies are required to determine what essential features are required in an enteral feed to obtain a remission of Crohn's disease. IV feeding may be necessary in occasional patients with intestinal obstruction or severe malabsorption but is several times more expensive and carries the risks of central venous line sepsis. It is no more effective than enteral feeding and should only be used when enteral feeding is impossible, e.g. because of fistula formation or obstruction.

The great advantage of enteral feeding is that it is almost totally without risk to the patient. It is particularly useful in the short-term therapy of the ill patient with extensive Crohn's disease. Unfortunately, the disease tends to relapse when normal food is introduced (50% relapse within 6 months). In one interesting study, this problem was avoided by step-wise reintroduction of foods with exclusion of any that were subsequently found to induce symptoms. The mechanism for the therapeutic effect of dietary treatment is quite unclear. Some studies have shown similar benefit from supplementing an otherwise normal diet with enteral feeds and it has been shown that improved nutrition produces changes in the immune response, particularly enhanced cellular immunity that might also be responsible for a therapeutic response.

Induction of Remission

Crohn's disease presents with such a diversity of severity and extent that it takes considerably skill and experience to treat every patient optimally. The increasing array of drugs adds to the level of complexity. Thus, all Crohn's patients should be treated in the secondary care environment preferably by gastroenterologists with an interest in the disease. A multidisciplinary team comprising of radiologist, pathologist and surgeon supporting the gastroenterologist as well as a pediatrician, dietitian and IBD specialist nurses should meet regularly to discuss the cases and optimize treatment. In general, for mild-to-moderate disease, treatment may be non-drug, like dietary or in symptomatic patients, steroids with azathioprine introduced early in patients who relapse on withdrawal from steroids. In more severe patients or in those that fail to respond to azathioprine (after at least 3 months), introduction of a first biologic is indicated. If this fails to induce remission from the disease, then surgical or second/third-line biologic is considered. This step-wise approach is logical but some argue for mare rapid use of biologics to improve the clinical course of the disease.

Maintenance of Remission

Whichever drug is successful in inducing remission is usually chosen as the maintenance drug of choice. Occasionally, biologics are used to "bridge" patients till immunomodulators like azathioprine's effects kick in. It is possible to assess patient's state of remission with regular fecal calprotectin measurements and in low colonic disease, a flexible sigmoidoscopy allows the physician to assess treatment success. Assessment of perianal disease is by clinical inspection, a simple squeeze test to see if lesions are still discharging. If patient remains continuously well after a year, withdrawal from biologics can be considered although almost half will relapse in the following year.

Surgical Treatment

Surgery for Crohn's disease is never curative and should be conservative. However, it is still a valuable resource and best results are achieved by specialist surgeons who have specific experience in dealing with Crohn's disease. Surgery may be used in the primary treatment of Crohn's disease or after failure of medical therapy. It may also be for the treatment of complications of Crohn's. Primary resection can be considered in patients with short segment or limited terminal ileal disease, especially those with obstructive symptoms. A resection and primary anastomosis can achieve remission without the use of drugs. In these patients treated by surgery, the median interval between resections is about 15 years. Thus for the fit individual, resection is a good treatment for limited terminal ileal disease. However, patients with extensive

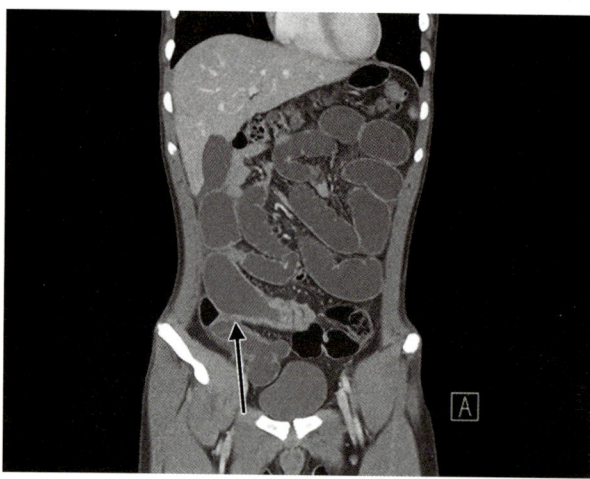

Fig. 3.45: Many patients are complex. Dilated proximal small bowel in this CT scan shows small bowel obstruction from an inflammatory stricture in the distal ileum. Surgery or medical therapy may be considered. There is also an entero-sigmoid fistula (see arrow). (CT: Computed tomography.)

or colonic disease, it is best to optimize medical treatment. Colonic disease of moderate severity or worse, fistulating or perianal diseases all require biologic therapy, infection control and nutritional support. However, despite this, if medical therapy fails, surgery is necessary (Fig. 3.45).

Treatment of Specific Complications of Crohn's Disease

Strictures: Patients with strictures would present with abdominal pain perhaps with nausea or vomiting, weight loss and diarrhea. However, symptoms often correlate poorly with disease appearance on colonoscopy or radiology. MRE is the best imaging modality and along with direct colonoscopic examination will determine whether the stricture is largely inflammatory or fibrotic in nature. The former can respond to medical therapy, while the latter is best treated with surgery (Figs. 3.46 and 3.47).

Where there are multiple strictures, it is best to perform stricturoplasties rather than resection. The bowel is cut lengthwise and stitched circumferentially, thus widening the lumen without resection. Such "bowel-preserving" surgery is best practiced by specialist surgeons who are part of an IBD MDT (Fig. 3.48).

Fistulae: Fistulae in Crohn's disease may be enteroenteral, enterovesical, enterovaginal or enterocutaneous. Treatment can be quite challenging. Enteroenteral fistulae can often be ignored if they do not bypass sufficient

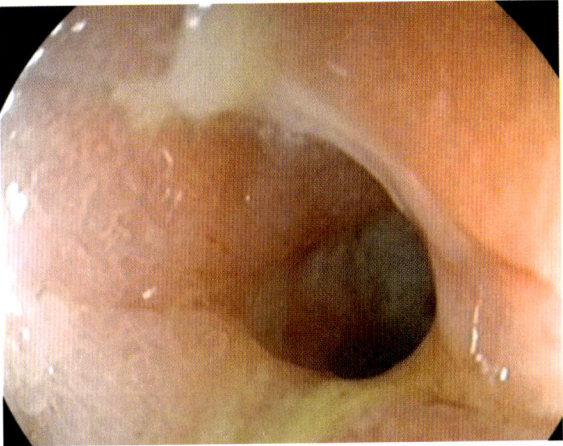

Fig. 3.46: Colonoscopic view of a tight fibrotic stricture.

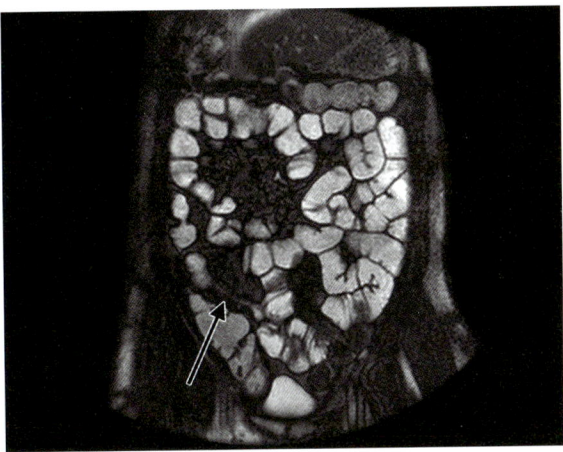

Fig. 3.47: Corresponding MRE showing a fibrotic stricture. (MRE: Magnetic resonance enteroclysis.)

intestine to cause clinically significant malabsorption. All fistulating disease is best managed with combination of azathioprine and anti-TNF like infliximab where there is best evidence that it can achieve healing although some like rectovaginal fistulae are very resistant to medical therapy. Small enterovesical fistulae may cause surprisingly few problems but larger ones do frequent urinary infections or even pneumaturia and will necessitate surgery. Enterovaginal fistulae and enterocutaneous fistulae almost always require surgery, although the type of operation is controversial. Fistulation may lead to nutritional problems and hence careful attention to supplementary feeding will improve chances of fistula closure (Fig. 3.49).

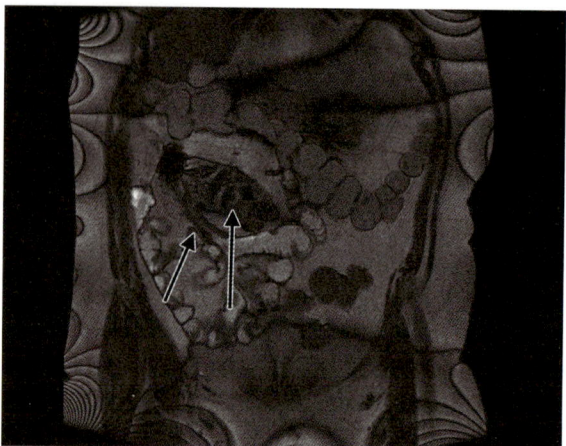

Fig. 3.48: Stricture at previous surgical anastomosis is common and usually fibrotic but often the focus of inflammation. Food debris is seen accumulated above the stricture.

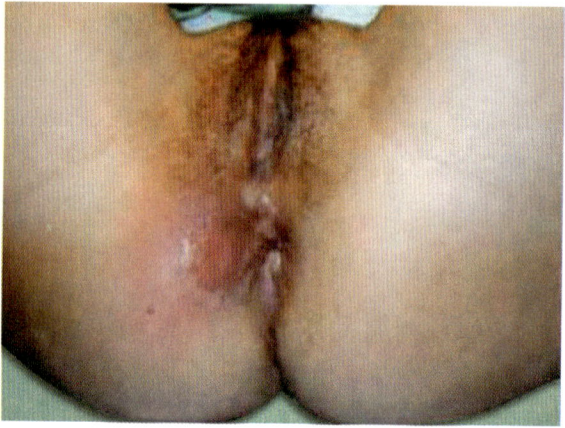

Fig. 3.49: Perianal disease.

Perianal Crohn's disease occurs in up to 70% of patients with Crohn's disease and may be very distressing. Surgery should be kept to the minimum as a conventional approach to fistula excision will often result disastrously in a non-healing ulcer with recurrence of fistula and incontinence. Perianal abscesses may require drainage but this should be achieved simply without excision. The general principle of managing perianal disease is to achieve drainage, clear infection and induce healing with biologic therapy. Steroids should be avoided in perianal disease. Antibiotics, usually a combination with metronidazole and a broad spectrum antibiotic like amoxicillin/clavulanate is given if there is infection (Fig. 3.50).

Magnetic resonance imaging is an invaluable tool in appraising the state of perianal Crohn's disease. This would greatly help the surgeon. An "examination under anesthesia" is then performed. If there is a fistula, then

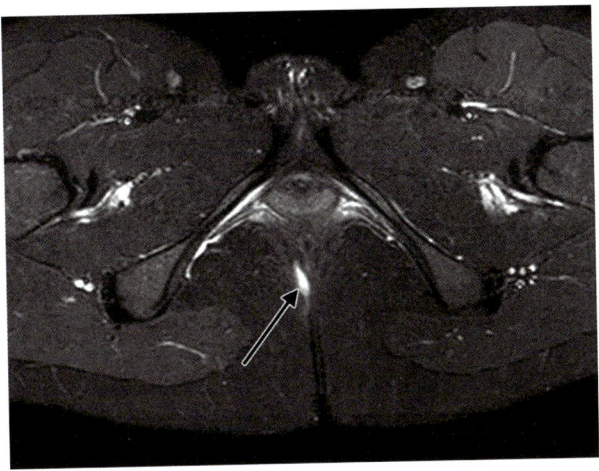

Fig. 3.50: Fistulous track in perianal Crohn's.

the surgeon can probe it and insert a loose suture or "Seton". This Seton keeps the fistula draining and this allows eventual healing. Patients tolerate this remarkably well and may be kept in for many months. Therapy with anti-TNF is indicated. The best evidence for healing of perianal Crohn's is treatment with infliximab. Once good healing is achieved, this Seton may be removed (Fig. 3.51).

Collagenous Colitis and Lymphocytic Colitis

Two conditions associated with diarrhea and normal-looking colonoscopic findings are collagenous colitis and lymphocytic (microscopic) colitis. The former is characterized by deposits of type II collagen in the lamina propria typically of >70 μm in thickness. In the latter, there are increased epithelial lymphocytes. Collagenous colitis presents with watery diarrhea and has a high female preponderance. It may be associated with drugs like lansoprazole. Treatment is with delayed-release budesonide which is very effective but long-term maintenance treatment may be necessary. Symptomatic relief of diarrhea with loperamide and bismuth (Pepto-bismol) may also be helpful. Lymphocytic colitis shows no subepithelial collagen but an increased lymphocyte count in the epithelium. It may be associated with celiac disease which can be excluded by anti-TTG testing. Gluten avoidance may help.

Ischemic Colitis

This can be sometimes confused with Crohn's disease and indeed mimics the condition. History is usually more acute with an episode of abdominal pain urgency and bloody diarrhea which gradually resolves. Colonoscopic appearances show a sharp demarcation between inflamed mucosa and normal

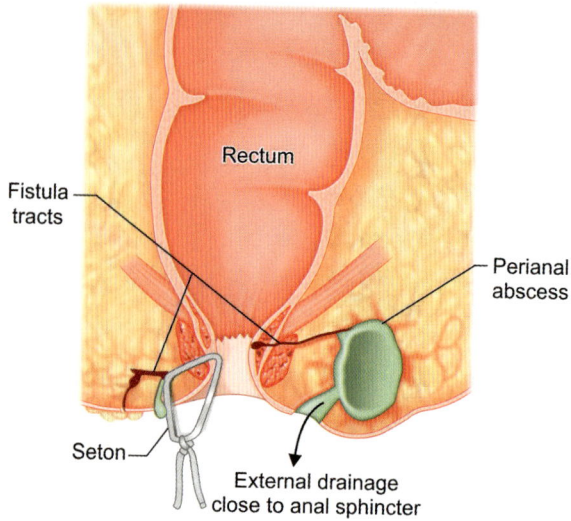

Fig. 3.51: Surgery for perianal Crohn's.

mucosa, usually at the vascular "watersheds" around the splenic flexure. Classically, abdominal film could show "thumbprinting." CT may show thickened bowel at the splenic flexure. There may be a background of vascular disease like abdominal aortic aneurysm or known arteriopath, smoker or atrial fibrillation. In latter stages of the condition, there is scarring of the affected colon.

Radiotherapy to the abdomen or pelvis may cause a radiation enteritis. This may result in bloody diarrhea. Effects may be chronic and lead to malabsorption and malnutrition.

Eosinophilic Gastroenteritis

Eosinophilic gastroenteritis (EGE) is an uncommon disease which is characterized by eosinophilic infiltration of gastrointestinal tissue usually associated with peripheral eosinophilia (50–75%) in the absence of other known causes of eosinophilia.

The etiology of the disease is still poorly understood. However, many patients with EGE have a history of seasonal allergy, atopy, food allergies, asthma and elevated serum IgE levels which may strongly suggest the role of hypersensitivity reactions in the pathogenesis of EGE. Small amount of eosinophils can be found in the mucosa of the gastrointestinal tract of normal healthy individual and they play the role in the host defense mechanism.

The hallmark of eosinophilic enteritis is the histological demonstration of marked inflammation with profusion of eosinophils. CT imaging may show markedly edematous bowel. It may affect any part of the GI tract, although eosinophilic esophagitis is usually regarded as a separate condition.

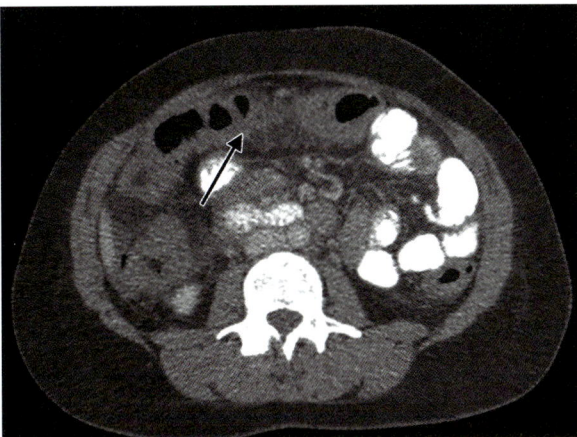

Fig. 3.52: Computed tomography showing thickened inflamed colon of eosinophilic colitis.

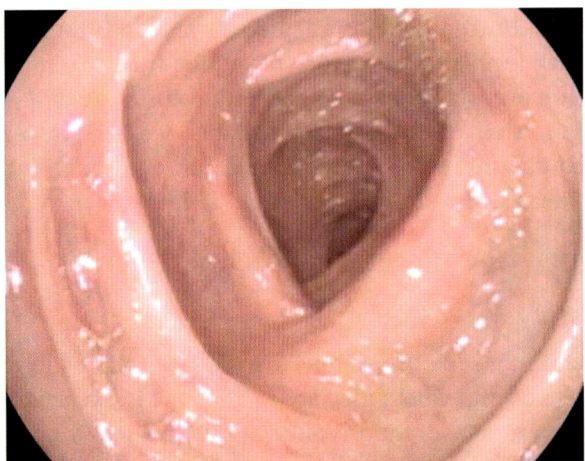

Fig. 3.53: Colonoscopic appearance of patient with eosinophillic colitis.

Depending on the site, the symptoms may vary from abdominal pain and vomiting to severe watery diarrhea (Figs. 3.52 to 3.54).

There are no randomized controlled trials for the treatment of the disease due to its rarity. However, the disease responds to corticosteroids and it is the mainstay of treatment. The best duration of the steroid treatment is unknown and the relapses are common during treatment tapering and may require the long-term treatment in some cases. Sodium cromoglycate (mast cell stabilizer), montelukast (leukotriene receptor antagonist), budesonide, immunosuppressant such as azathioprine are reported to be successful in some case studies. A trial of elimination diets have be tried although the

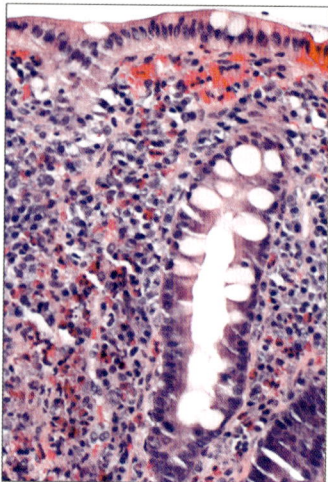

Fig. 3.54: Histology with marked eosinophilic infiltration confirms diagnosis.

results are mixed. Currently, there are studies evaluating the efficacy of the use of mepolizumab (humanized monoclonal antibody against interleukin IL-5) in the treatment of eosinophilic esophagitis and eosinophilic gastrointestinal disorders. Promising results from the studies yield improvement in the eosinophil count and endoscopic findings, however, long-term beneficial effect is still uncertain. There are reports that clarithromycin may be of benefit.

Infective Diarrhea

Natural History

The causes and consequences of infective diarrhea vary widely and depend on who is infected and where they are at the time. It can range from a mild diarrhea to severe dehydration. Worldwide it remains a major killer and remains a global tragedy that dehydration from infective diarrhea especially in children is still a major cause of death. Adults infected in Europe or North America are most likely to have a *Campylobacter* or *Salmonella* infection; travelers in hotter countries are more likely to acquire enterotoxigenic *E. coli*. Viral causes of gastroenteritis include Norovirus which causes episodic outbreaks in cruise ships and military barracks or hotels which mainly affects adults, while children are particularly prone to infection with Rotavirus. The type of infection and severity depends on the infective agent and on host defenses. Classic examples of the relationship between host resistance and infection are found in *C. difficile* infection (pseudomembranous colitis) following the use of broad-spectrum antibiotics, giardiasis in patients with IgA deficiency and cryptosporidiosis in patients with the acquired immune deficiency syndrome.

Diarrhea

Table 3.2: Causes of traveler's diarrhea.	
Bacteria	
Entero-toxigenic *E. coli*	Commonest cause of travel-associated diarrhea
Entero-aggressive *E. coli*	Emerging agent with more severe symptoms
Campylobacter jejuni	Common in Asia
Shigella	
Salmonella	
Viruses	
Norovirus	Associated with cruise ships
Rotavirus	Common in children
Parasites	
Giardia lamblia	Hikers/campers in the countryside drinking from streams. Also in Russia
Cryptosporidium	Water supply as is resistant to chlorine
Entamoeba histolytica	Indian subcontinent

The nature of the illness depends partly on whether the infection causes an inflammatory enteritis or has a predominantly secretory effect. Inflammatory infective diarrheas such as those caused by *Salmonella*, *Campylobacter* and *Shigella* tend to cause more systemic upset with a higher fever (38°C or more) and considerable abdominal pain. Median duration of symptoms is about 10 days. Secretory diarrheas such as that caused by enterotoxigenic *E. coli* ("traveler's diarrhea") usually cause a milder illness with no pyrexia. In most cases, they also have a shorter median duration (about 5 days) with the notable exception of cholera. The degree of debility depends very much on the success with which hydration is maintained (Table 3.2).

Food Poisoning

Contaminated food, provided the inoculum is large enough may cause diarrhea which could vary from mild to severe. A list of common pathogens is given in Table 3.3.

Extraintestinal Manifestations

Extraintestinal manifestations of infective diarrhea may be due either to disseminated infection or immunological reaction. *Salmonella* septicemia is often associated with minimal gastrointestinal symptoms and may result in abscess formation in any part of the body with a particular tendency to cause empyema of the gallbladder. Patients with sickle cell disease are unusually liable to develop *Salmonella* osteomyelitis. Patients with gallstones often fail to clear *Salmonella* even if they avoid empyema and cholecystectomy is then the only way to eradicate the organism. Patients with HLA-B27 are particularly prone to develop a transient reactive non-erosive arthropathy following

Table 3.3: Causes of food poisoning.	
Short incubation 1–6 h	**Food source**
Staphylococcus aureus	Cakes, pastries with cream, cold salads, mayonnaise
Bacillus cereus	Fried rice (from previously cooked overnight)
8–16 h	
Clostridium perfringens	Beef, poultry
>16 h	
Shigella	Salads washed in contaminated water, ice
Salmonella	Poultry and eggs mainly but other meat especially cooked meats contaminated by poor food handling
Campylobacter jejuni	Raw milk, poultry
Vibrio cholerae	Shellfish
Vibrio parahaemolyticus	Prawns, snails

Salmonella or *Yersinia enteritis* (Reiter's syndrome). Erythema nodosum may also occur and cause confusion with IBD. Both the reactive arthritis and erythema nodosum are assumed to be immune-complex-mediated and to reflect antigen leakage through an inflamed gut. Infections associated with the Shiga toxin bacteria like *Shigella dysenteriae* and entero-hemorrhagic *E. coli* can cause a nasty hemolytic-uremic syndrome the hallmarks of which are that of hemolytic anemia, thrombocytopenia and renal failure.

Clostridium difficile Colitis

Clostridium difficile is a spore-forming bacteria that may be a normal commensal but disruption of the normal flora usually by antibiotics lead to colonization of *C. difficile*, release of toxins that cause severe mucosal inflammation which may lead to pseudomembranous colitis, megacolon and perforation. It is an increasing problem as a hospital acquired (nosocomial) infection. In the frail hospitalized individuals are vulnerable to infection and it may be fatal. Infection should be suspected in all patients who develop diarrhea who have received prior antibiotics in the previous 3 months. Other risk factors are the use of proton pump inhibitors and poor hygiene.

Clostridium difficile produces several toxins which include the enterotoxins (toxins A and B). These can be detected in the feces and is the most rapid method of diagnosing the infection. Fluoroquinolone antibiotics such as ciprofloxacin are associated with a particularly virulent strain, the NAP1 hypervirulent strain which is associated with causing severe fulminant colitis. Restriction of prescription of this antibiotic has reduced its incidence (Fig. 3.55).

Treatments include rehydration, usually orally but may require IV fluids. Oral metronidazole is the drug of choice and oral vancomycin in severe cases. Probiotics seem a sensible addition and "fecal transplant" where a donor stool is nasogastrically infused is used in recalcitrant cases.

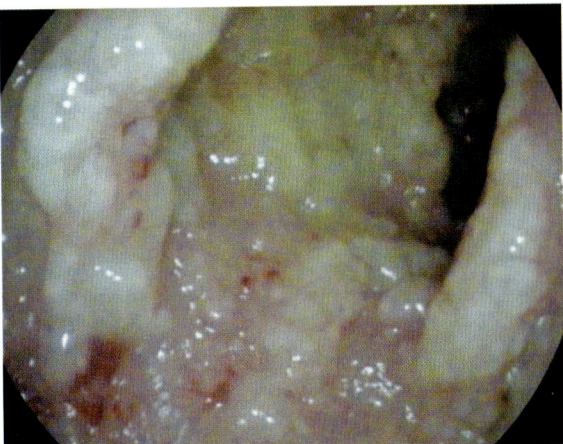

Fig. 3.55: Severe inflammation and formation of "pseudomembranes" in *C. difficile* colitis.

Parasites

Parasites infest most of the world's population but frequently cause no symptoms. Symptoms vary according to the parasite and the degree of infestation.

Amebic Dysentery: In tropical areas, it has been estimated that over 50% of the population harbor the pathogenic ameba *Entamoeba histolytica* and the annual worldwide incidence is estimated to be 10%. The severity of illness that results is very variable. Amebae seem to act synergistically with colonic bacteria and this may explain why previously asymptomatic carriers can suddenly develop symptoms. Infection first occurs as a result of eating food that has been contaminated by feces containing *E. histolytica* cysts. Each cyst divides into eight amebae. On stool microscopy, these are distinguished from non-pathogenic amebae by the presence of phagocytosed red cells.

The main consequence of amebiasis is a colitis that mimics UC. Symptoms include diarrhea with blood and mucus and lower abdominal pain. If the disease is untreated, perforation may ensue and the overall mortality is about 3%. Colonic ulcers tend to be discrete rather than confluent but distinction from UC depends on finding the amebae in feces. Chronic amebiasis may lead to stricturing mass lesions (ameboma) that mimic carcinoma. Approximately 1% of cases will subsequently develop an amebic hepatic abscess, sometimes many years later.

Giardiasis: Giardia lamblia infestation is extremely common but the development of symptoms depends on the dose of infection and the host immunity. In some parts of the world, notably the Rocky Mountains and Leningrad, water is heavily contaminated and clinically important infection is a common cause of travelers' diarrhea. In other places such as the United Kingdom where *Giardia* are much less prevalent in water, symptomatic giardiasis raises a suspicion of immunodeficiency—particularly secretory IgA deficiency is found in common variable immunodeficiency and in nodular lymphoid hyperplasia.

Cysts are swallowed, usually in contaminated water and change into the mature trophozoites in the intestine. Invasion of the mucosa may occur but most of the trophozoites are found adhering to the mucosal surface. Diarrhea results may be watery or fatty. Its mechanism is unclear although sometimes infestation may be so severe as to obscure a considerable proportion of the surface absorptive area. Hypolactasia commonly ensues and contributes to the diarrhea. Extraintestinal disease does not occur.

Schistosomiasis: Schistosomiasis affects over 200 million people and in Egypt the prevalence is over 80%. Three principal species are involved: *Schistosomiasis mansoni, Schistosomiasis japonicum* (in the Far East) and *Schistosomiasis haematobium*. Cercarial forms of the schistosome are secreted into water by the snail intermediate host. Humans become infected by wading barefoot through streams or mud (e.g. paddy fields). The cercaria penetrate the skin and are transmitted via the venous system, right heart and lungs and eventually reach the liver where they mature into the adult worms. They swim upstream in the portal system, *S. japonicum* typically ending up in the small intestine and ascending colon, *S. mansoni* in the descending colon and *S. haematobium* in the bladder and rectum. The worms then mate and produce thousands of eggs which migrate into the surrounding tissues as a result of enzymatic digestion. Multiple small intestinal ulcers develop and a severe dysentery may rarely result. More typically there is diarrhea or rectal bleeding due to chronic inflammation of the intestine which may result in polyp formation. Some ova may be carried back in the portal system and become trapped in the portal tracts of the liver where the ensuing inflammatory and granulomatous reaction results in portal hypertension.

Strongyloidiasis: This parasite also gains entry via the skin. Infective larvae in contaminated soil penetrate the skin, pass via the circulation to the lungs and develop into worms about 2 mm long within the alveoli. Itchy rashes and pneumonitis lasting about 2 weeks result. The worms are then coughed up and swallowed and invade the intestinal mucosa. Symptoms depend on the extent of infestation. Chronic nausea or abdominal pain and more rarely severe diarrhea may result. Fatal dissemination may result in immunosuppressed patients. Self-infection may perpetuate the disease indefinitely.

Ascariasis (Roundworm): Eggs are ingested in fecally contaminated food and hatch into larvae in the small intestine. They invade the mucosa and travel via the portal system and the liver to the lungs where they develop further, are coughed up, swallowed and develop into mature worms up to

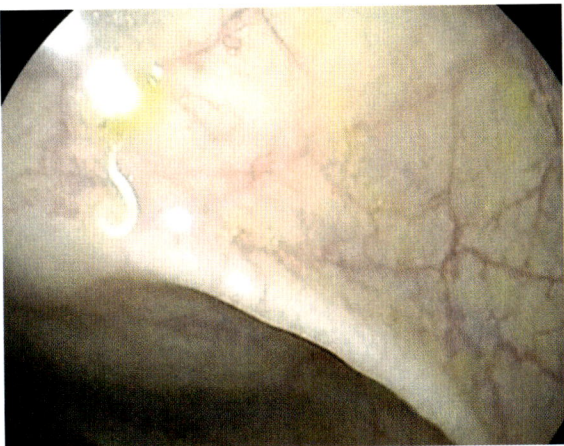

Fig. 3.56: *Enterobius vermicularis* is sometimes encountered on colonoscopy.

20 cm long in their second trip through the intestine. Diarrhea may occur but obstructive symptoms are common. Migration into the bile ducts or appendix may result in jaundice or appendicitis. Pneumonitis occurs during the pulmonary stage.

Trichuris (Whipworm): The adult whipworm is 3–5 cm long and shaped like a whip with a thin anterior portion containing its esophagus and a thick posterior portion. Eggs ingested in contaminated food or water hatch into larvae which mature into adult worms within the colon. Abdominal pain, diarrhea and anemia are the chief symptoms and in severe infection rectal prolapse may occur.

Enterobiasis (Pinworm): This is caused by the 1-cm long worm *Enterobius vermicularis*. It is very common especially in cooler climates. In the United Kingdom, it is estimated what about 1 million individuals may be infected. Spread is from person to person and family members are often affected. Infection is usually asymptomatic but anal pruritus is a cardinal symptom as the worms migrate out to lay their eggs. A sellotape test is helpful. A sticky tape is applied to the anus and put on a slide for the identification of parasite ova. A single dose of mebendazole 100 mg is highly effective but family members should also be treated (Fig. 3.56). A summary of treatments for infestations is given in Table 3.4.

Infective Diarrhea

Management: Most types of infective diarrhea resolve spontaneously and the most important part of treatment is the replacement of water and electrolytes. This has been revolutionized by the discovery that sugars will enhance

Table 3.4 Summary of principal parasitic infestations and treatments.

Parasite	Treatment
Amebae (E. histolytica)	Metronidazole (800 mg tds 5 days)
Giardia lamblia	Metronidazole (400 mg tds 10 days)
Schistosomiasis (S. mansoni, S. haematobium)	Praziquantel 40 mg/kg, single oral dose
S. japonicum	Praziquantel (20 mg/kg, 3 doses in 1 day)
Strongyloides stercoralis	Thiabendazole 25 mg or Mebendazole 2 mg/kg (bd for 3 days, repeated after 2 and 4 weeks)
Ascaris lumbricoides	Piperazine (75 mg/kg as a single dose on 2 consecutive days) or Pyrantel pamoate (10 mg/kg as a single dose)
Trichuris trichiuria	Mebendazole (100 mg bd for 3 days)
	NB: None of these drugs are of proven safety in pregnancy and metronidazole and mebendazole are teratogenic in rats. Their use should therefore be avoided in pregnancy particularly in the first trimester unless the parasite infestation is severe.

salt and water absorption by the intestine. This has allowed even patients with very severe diarrhea to be given adequate replacement therapy by mouth without the need for IV infusion. This has made effective treatment much more readily available in the developing world and has had a major impact on the mortality from infectious diarrhea. The formula recommended by the World Health Organization is sodium chloride 4 g/L, sodium acetate 6.5 g/L, potassium chloride 1 g/L and glucose 9 g/L, but cruder mixtures of salt and sugar are effective in providing a simple measure (such as a double-ended spoon with appropriately sized ends, one for sugar and one for salt) is used to obtain the correct ratio of sugar to salt.

Antidiarrheal drugs such as loperamide are useful in mild diarrhea but have little or no effect in more severe diarrhea and may prolong the course of the illness. Suspensions of bismuth subsalicylate (peptobismol) 30 mL every 30 min until diarrhea settles are effective and have an inhibitory effect on some *E. coli* toxins.

Antibiotics should generally be avoided as they normally have little effect on the course of the illness and may actually prolong the duration of fecal excretion of bacteria.

There are certain specific indications for antibiotics: systemic salmonellosis (high fever, chills and general malaise; usually responsive to cotrimoxazole or ciprofloxacin), severe *Shigella* dysentery (culture and sensitivity needed to decide on antibiotics), prolonged *C. enteritis* (erythromycin), *Yersinia enterocolitica* (usually cotrimoxazole but also sensitive to other antibiotics).

Hypolactasia is a common sequel of severe gastroenteritis and may last several months so a reduction in milk intake is often advisable.

Intestinal Tuberculosis

Natural History and Management

Gastrointestinal tuberculosis is mainly due to infection with *Mycobacterium bovis* contracted from infected milk, but this route of infection has now been abolished by tuberculin testing of cattle. The disease is, however, still not uncommon particularly in Asian immigrants. It is now almost exclusively due to *M. tuberculosis* (hominis) which has usually spread from the lungs via swallowed sputum. Any part of the intestine may be affected but in approximately 60%, the ileocecal region is affected. The radiological, macroscopical and histological appearances closely mimic Crohn's disease, and skip lesions may occur.

Treatment is with triple chemotherapy for 18–24 months unless culture and sensitivity results are available in which case the treatment may be reduced to two appropriate drugs after 3 months.

When the differential diagnosis is in doubt, a trial of antituberculous chemotherapy should always precede a trial of corticosteroids for presumed Crohn's disease as the results of inappropriate corticosteroid therapy in tuberculosis may be disastrous with rapid dissemination. Use of anti-TNF can cause fatal disseminated disease and hence TB should be actively and vigorously excluded before biologic therapy. If uncertainty remains and corticosteroid therapy is felt necessary for presumed active Crohn's disease, antituberculous cover should be given concurrently. Corticosteroid therapy is sometimes used intentionally in combination with antituberculous therapy to reduce the risk of permanent stricturing from tuberculosis.

Approximately 50% of patients with intestinal tuberculosis require surgery at some stage, particularly for the treatment of strictures or fistulae. Sometimes, this can be accomplished without resection by means of a plastic surgical approach to strictures—stricturoplasty—in which the stricture is incised longitudinally and then the incision closed transversely as in a pyloroplasty. Perforation through a tuberculous ulcer may also occur and carries a mortality of 30–50%.

Celiac Disease

Natural History

Celiac disease is a common cause of malabsorption of one or more nutrients in Caucasian populations. Based on population serological studies as many as 1% of the white population in the United Kingdom are affected. The mode of presentation may be very variable. In childhood, it may be subtle, e.g. growth retardation or anemia or more obvious with fatty diarrhea and features of deficiency of fat soluble vitamins. In adults, anemia is the commonest mode of presentation followed by osteoporosis. The hallmark of the condition is the demonstration of duodenal or jejunal villous atrophy plus resolution of these changes with gluten withdrawal. In children a further challenge with gluten should usually be given after resolution since transient villous atrophy due to causes other than celiac disease (particularly following viral gastroenteritis) is common.

The widely available serological markers anti-TTG and endomyosial IgA antibodies make diagnosis easy. However up to 10% of patients with celiac disease have an IgA deficiency and alternative IgG markers are available. Endoscopic biopsies are easy and safe to obtain and sometimes a classic appearance can be discerned on endoscopy (Fig. 3.57).

Gluten is a mixture of water-insoluble cereal proteins which bread its elastic springy consistency. Bread made from gluten free flour unfortunately tends to be bland and crumbly. The gluten can be further subdivided into toxic gliadin fractions and IgA antibodies to gliadin are commonly present in the peripheral blood of celiac patients. The damage to the epithelium is almost certainly cell mediated rather than humoral however. This is reflected by an increase in intraepithelial lymphocytes (predominantly T lymphocytes)

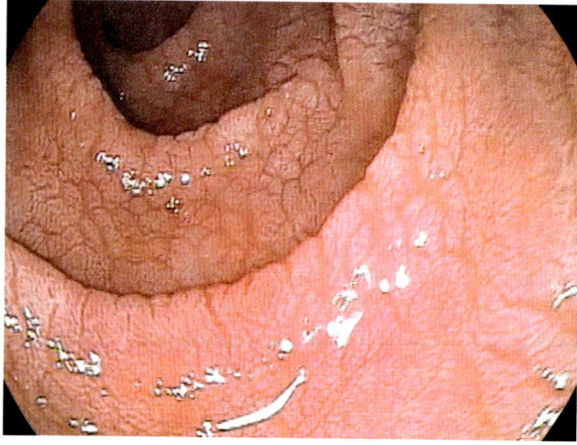

Fig. 3.57: Endoscopic appearance of mid-duodenum of untreated celiac disease. Note the longitudinal ridges, aptly described as "scalloped," similar to the raw scallop.

and an increase in lamina propria mononuclear cells. There is a strong association with the HLA-DR3 antigen and presence of this antigen also correlates with known autoimmune diseases.

There is a close link with the skin condition dermatitis herpetiformis. Itchy vesicles characteristically occur on extensor surfaces of the forearms and other pressure areas. The majority of patients have some degree of small intestinal villous atrophy and in about 50% there is a good therapeutic response to gluten withdrawal. Immunoglobulin A deposits are found at the dermoepidermal junction.

The prognosis is excellent once the diagnosis of celiac disease has been made and treatment by gluten withdrawal initiated. There is, however, an increased risk of carcinoma, particularly of the small intestine but to a lesser extent of other sites particularly the esophagus and an increased risk of an unusual form of intestinal lymphoma. This used to be thought to be of histiocytic origin but subsequent studies using cell-specific monoclonal antibodies showed that it is a T-cell lymphoma and that the histiocytes that are frequently seen in this tumor are probably reactive. Fortunately, the incidence of these tumors as a complication of celiac disease seems to be declining. It is unclear why this should be because there is no convincing link between the risk for these tumors and the degree of control of the celiac disease.

Striking splenic atrophy not uncommonly occurs. Its mechanism is uncertain but may be due to constant bombardment of the reticuloendothelial system with foreign antigens penetrating a leaky intestinal barrier. Changes in the peripheral blood then include abnormally shaped red cells and Howell–Jolly bodies and marked thrombocytosis may occur. There is also an increased risk of sepsis, particularly pneumococcal, which should be remembered if the patient requires surgery for any reason.

Occasionally, patients fail to respond to gluten withdrawal. Ulcerative jejunoileitis, which is arguably a severe form of celiac disease, has a very poor prognosis although some patients will respond to a combination of corticosteroid therapy and gluten withdrawal. Collagenous sprue is another very rare cause of villous atrophy and malabsorption without response to gluten withdrawal. Dense collagen deposition occurs in the lamina propria. The etiology is unknown and prognosis poor.

Management

Toxic gluten is contained in all foods made from wheat, barley or rye. Other cereals including rice, maize and oats are free from toxic glutens. Patients vary considerably in their susceptibility to gluten. In some patients, very small amounts of gluten such as those present in communion wafers are enough to precipitate a relapse, while others seem able to eat gluten-containing foods for several years before relapsing. There are anecdotal reports of patients failing to go into remission following subsequent lapses in diet and the only practical and safe advice to the patient is to avoid gluten indefinitely once the diagnosis is made. Patients should be advised to contact a patient group such as the Celiac Society which is able to give invaluable support and help with recipes and advice about the safety of foods. The Celiac Society, United Kingdom, provides a free application for mobile devices than scanning the supermarket products for gluten-free products. Gluten-free flour, bread and biscuits are also available on prescription in the United Kingdom.

Occasional patients who have otherwise typical features of celiac disease fail to respond to gluten withdrawal. Some of these patients are found to be taking gluten inadvertently, for example in beer. It has recently been shown that occasional "non-responsive celiacs" may respond to avoidance of soy protein. In others there is no explanation but the combination of continued gluten avoidance and corticosteroid therapy may produce a remission.

Patients should be screened for osteoporosis with bone densitometry and treated accordingly. Usually it involves additional vitamin D and calcium supplementation but bisphosphonates are indicated in osteoporotic individual. Follow-up is best done by a dietitian and primary care physician. The increased risk of malignancy is worrying but there is no evidence that any form of screening is going to be effective. Any unexplained deterioration should, however, suggest the possibility of small bowel malignancy, either lymphoma or carcinoma, which should be investigated by CT scan of the abdomen.

Tropical Sprue

Natural History

Tropical sprue is a poorly understood condition presented in much the same way as celiac disease with features of fat and folic acid malabsorption, glossitis and anemia in a patient who has recently been in a hot country. Small intestinal biopsy shows partial or, occasionally, severe villous atrophy. The etiology is unclear but is thought to be due to a combination of bacterial contamination of the small intestine and folate deficiency. Other infections such as giardiasis and strongyloidiasis should be excluded by small bowel sampling. If left untreated, the condition may persist for months or even years.

Management

About 1 g of oral tetracycline per day should be given for 2 weeks and 10 mg of oral folic acid daily until asymptomatic. Vitamin B12 supplementation may also occasionally be needed. Hypolactasia is inevitable and a low milk intake will help to reduce the diarrhea.

Whipple's Disease

Natural History

This unusual disease most commonly affects middle-aged men. Partial villous atrophy and malabsorption result in diarrhea and pigmentation and about two-thirds of patients have joint symptoms, typically an intermittent migratory arthritis affecting large or small joints. Fever and lymphadenopathy are common. A chronic encephalitis with altered behavior, memory loss and cranial nerve lesions may occur and can be the dominant feature. Small bowel biopsy shows diagnostic macrophages within the lamina propria that are packed with foamy PAS positive material, the remains of ingested dead or dying bacteria. The bacterium has been identified as a gram-positive *Actinomycete*, *Tropheryma whippelii*. Cases occur sporadically and infectivity is presumably very low.

Management

Untreated, the disease is usually fatal but fortunately there is usually a good response to antibiotics such as tetracycline, cotrimoxazole or ciprofloxacin but treatment may have to be continued for several months with monitoring by repeated intestinal biopsy (endoscopic duodenal biopsies should suffice). Even with effective antibiotic therapy it may take a year before all the intestinal macrophages are free of the bacteria. Supplementation with fat-soluble vitamins and calcium will also be necessary in cases with severe malabsorption.

Intestinal Lymphoma

Natural History

Lymphoma of the intestine may be either primary or secondary to lymphoma elsewhere. Obstruction, bleeding, perforation, malabsorption and weight loss may all occur. Short primary lymphomatous lesions which have the best prognosis usually are present with obstructive symptoms or as a mass. More extensive involvement is likely to cause malabsorption and anemia. Any part of the intestine may be involved but the distal small intestine is the most common site followed by the stomach.

The cell of origin is often difficult to ascertain with certainty but modern cell marker techniques are beginning to clarify this situation. The majority of primary lymphomas of the intestine are B-cell lymphomas, the main exception being the lymphomas which complicate celiac disease which are T-cell lymphomas. Hodgkin's disease only rarely involves the intestine.

Management

Short primary intestinal lymphomas are best treated by surgical resection and the prognosis is then good with up to 75% 5-year survival.

More extensive primary lymphomas have a worse prognosis but may respond well to chemotherapy. Prognosis in this group is at present very unpredictable. Secondary involvement of the intestine by lymphoma elsewhere has a poor prognosis with a 5-year survival of about 10%; chemotherapy may be useful.

Alpha Chain Disease (Mediterranean Lymphoma)

Natural History and Management

This is arguably premalignant in its early stages and should probably be considered separately from other intestinal lymphomas. There is hyperplasia followed by frank neoplasia of IgA-producing cells within the intestine possibly as a result of chronic antigenic stimulation. The malignant cells produce igA heavy chains in excess without light chains. The chains can be detected in blood and urine. There is a consequent defect in secretory IgA function and bacterial overgrowth or giardiasis, villous atrophy and malabsorption ensue. Patients present with severe malabsorption, anemia, abdominal pain and often have severe clubbing. The disease occurs predominantly in young men in countries around the Mediterranean, in Africa, South America and the Far East. It is thought that poor hygiene and chronic intestinal infestation predispose to it. In its early premalignant phase, improvement and even cure may result from tetracycline therapy but when invasive lymphoma has developed, cytotoxic chemotherapy is usually necessary and the prognosis is poor.

Intestinal Amyloidosis

Natural History and Management

Intestinal involvement occurs in approximately 70% of cases of amyloidosis. Initially, amyloid protein is laid down around submucosal vessels but as the disease progresses the muscle layers and then the mucosa becomes infiltrated. In primary amyloidosis, the proteins deposited are immunoglobulin light chains, while in secondary amyloidosis, the protein is an acute phase reactant, usually amyloid A protein, that has been produced in excess during chronic inflammation or infection.

Because of the muscle involvement, motility problems are common, particularly diarrhea. If involvement is extensive malabsorption and protein losing enteropathy may occur. Bleeding, perforation and ischemic damage are further complications. The treatment is unsatisfactory. Occasional cases of primary amyloidosis respond to cytotoxic drugs such as melphalan and if the cause of secondary amyloidosis can be removed, then regression occasionally occurs.

Chronic Pancreatitis

Chronic pancreatitis is a disease process that leads to irreversible damage to the pancreas. It is best defined by the histological changes of inflammation, fibrosis, ductal damage and progressive loss of function of exocrine and endocrine pancreatic tissue. This eventually leads to the clinical features of abdominal pain diarrhea (steatorrhea) and diabetes.

There are several causes of chronic pancreatitis:
- Alcohol is by far the most common cause in the United Kingdom. Alcohol has direct toxic effects on the pancreas. Recurrent acute attacks eventually lead to pancreatic fibrosis and loss of function.
- Chronic gallstone pancreatitis.
- Cystic fibrosis is the commonest cause in children. As they may, with this genetic defect, live to adulthood, treatment of their chronic pancreatic insufficiency is becoming a major part of their care.
- Idiopathic chronic pancreatitis: A significant number have genetic defects that lead to chronic pancreatitis. There are several genes now known and they include *CFTR* gene which regulate the chloride channel and the *SPINK1* mutation. Individuals with both mutations have a 900-fold risk of developing chronic pancreatitis.
- Hemochromatosis, in late untreated state may lead to chronic pancreatitis ("bronze diabetes").
- Autoimmune pancreatitis: This is an increasingly recognized condition. Patients usually present with mild abdominal pain and jaundice due to swelling of the pancreatic head compressing on the common bile duct. It is often mistaken for pancreatic cancer. The clue is an elevation of immunoglobulins, especially IgG4 in the blood. Patients may have associated autoimmune conditions like Sjögrens' syndrome, PSC, UC and rheumatoid disease. Treatment is with prednisolone (Fig. 3.58).

Pathology

The ductular system becomes dilated and irregular. Proteinaceous plugs may block side branches or even the main pancreatic duct and subsequently calcify. Acinar tissue atrophies and is replaced by fibrous tissue (Fig. 3.59).

Symptoms

Pain is present in the majority of patients and may be severe and intractable. It is typically epigastric with radiation to the back. Duration of pain and association with eating is variable. Weight loss is usual and is often marked if malabsorption is present. Fat malabsorption implies a >90% reduction in pancreatic exocrine function since the healthy pancreas has a large functional reserve. Glucose tolerance tests are abnormal in about two-thirds but clinical

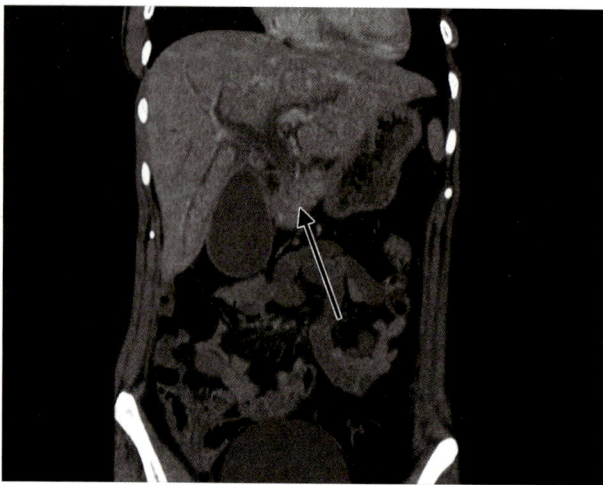

Fig. 3.58: Computed tomography of autoimmune pancreatitis showing a swollen pancreatic head and biliary tree dilation.

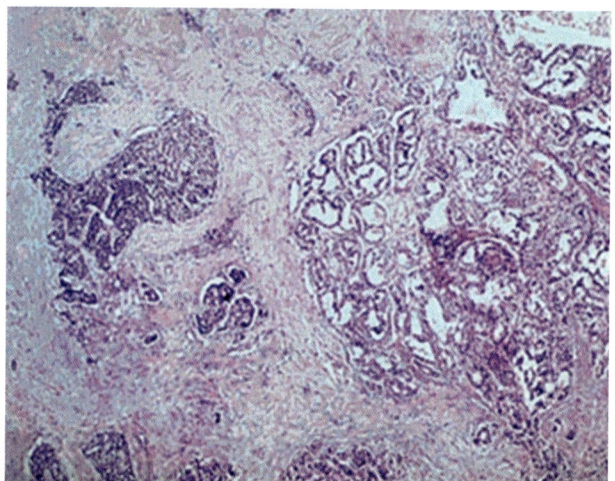

Fig. 3.59: Fibrosis and acinar damage in chronic pancreatitis.

diabetes, which is usually mild, occurs only in about one-third. Jaundice may occur due to biliary obstruction and if left untreated can progress to secondary biliary cirrhosis (Figs. 3.60 and 3.61).

Pancreatic Ascites

Pancreatic ascites is a rare problem which develops insidiously, particularly in patients with alcoholic chronic pancreatitis and presumably results from rupture of a dilated side duct or pseudocyst. Diagnosis is confirmed by finding a high concentration of amylase in the ascitic fluid.

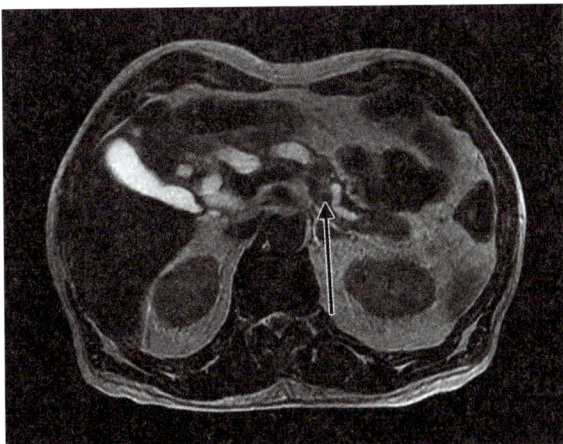

Fig. 3.60: Magnetic resonance imaging shows an atrophic pancreas with a dilated pancreatic duct.

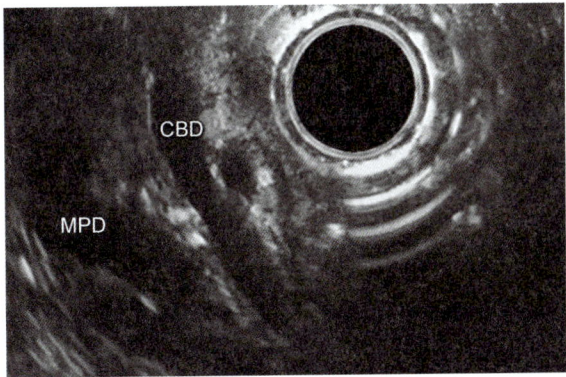

Fig. 3.61: Endoscopic ultrasound (EUS) may occasionally help to show dilated main pancreatic duct. (MPD: Main pancreatic duct; CBD: Common bile duct.)

Management

The most important step is to remove the underlying cause, usually alcohol. If the patient manages to stop drinking, surprising improvement in symptoms and even in radiological appearance of the pancreatic duct system may occur. Pain relief is often difficult and patients frequently become addicted to opiates. Oral pancreatic supplements can sometimes be helpful in reducing pain by suppressing pancreatic secretion. Celiac plexus blocks often produce temporary relief but are not without risk and the pain usually returns within a year or less. Patients with large dilated pancreatic duct could benefit from decompression. This may be achieved with ERCP and pancreatic duct sphincterotomy. If there are gallstones or pancreatic duct stones, they can also be removed. Endoscopic stents may lead to duct damage and best avoided. Octreotide subcutaneous injection may help in a proportion of patients with pain.

Surgery

The role of surgery is uncertain. If a patient is still in pain after 1 year's abstinence from alcohol it is worth performing an ERCP to look for stricturing of the main pancreatic duct with distal dilatation. Occasionally, partial pancreatectomy may be helpful in such cases. Various other operations have been tried including laying open ("filleting") the main pancreatic duct and anastomosing it to jejunum or subtotal or even total pancreatectomy. Opinions vary widely as to their efficacy. Unfortunately, the relationship (if any) between intraductal pressure (or calculi) and pain is unclear and patients left with any residual pancreas often have recurrent pain while total pancreatectomy usually results in very "brittle" diabetes, often in a patient who is already addicted to opiates. The least unsatisfactory course is often a more conservative medical approach emphasizing alcohol abstinence above all else as this carries the only significant hope of long-term improvement (Figs. 3.62A and B).

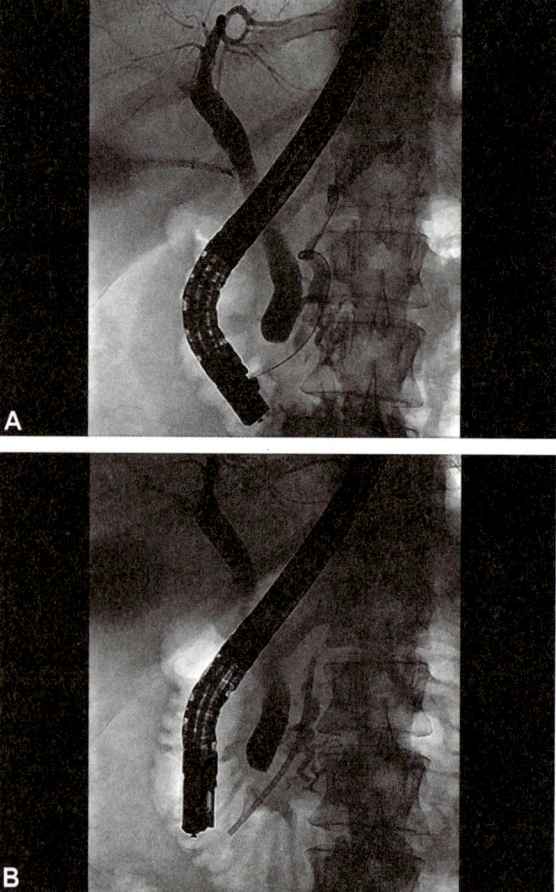

Figs. 3.62A and B: Endoscopic retrograde cholangiopancreatography, showing main duct stricture (A) Sphincterotomy and stent insertion (B) was performed and may help drainage of the pancreatic duct in selected patients.

Malabsorption Due to Chronic Pancreatitis

Malabsorption is much more readily manageable than the pain of chronic pancreatitis. Oral preparations of pancreatic lipase, amylase and protease are readily available. They are rapidly inactivated at low pH so are more effective if taken either in an enteric coated form or preceded by an H2 receptor antagonist. A common mistake is under-prescribing in patients with steatorrhea. With adequate dosage (up to 100,000 units of lipase with each meal), it is usually possible to achieve a reduction in fecal fat excretion of at least 50%. The diet should be high in protein and carbohydrate and low in fat. Diabetes is treated with insulin.

Small Intestinal Bacteria Overgrowth (SIBO)

Natural History and Management

Intestinal stasis is the main factor in the development of clinically important bacterial overgrowth of the small intestine.
- The classic cause of this are surgical blind loops, e.g. the afferent loop of a Polya gastrectomy, small bowel diverticulosis, stricturing, e.g. Crohn's disease and more rarely a motility disorder such as in scleroderma
- It has also been shown that elderly patients without any anatomical blind loop may develop bacterial overgrowth without any clear reason except possibly from overuse of PPIs
- Perhaps up to 20% of patients labeled with IBS-D have SIBO
- Diabetics with autonomic neuropathy and patients with systemic sclerosis have atonic bowel and lead to SIBO.

The two main consequences are B12 deficiency and fat malabsorption. B12 deficiency may be sufficiently severe to cause megaloblastic anemia or neurological defects (subacute combined degeneration of the cord, peripheral neuropathy or dementia). Fat malabsorption may be constant or intermittent and may be complicated by hypoproteinemia and hypocalcemia. Bile salts are deconjugated by anaerobic bacteria and subsequently dehydroxylated by bacteria to secondary bile acids (deoxycholic acid and lithocholic acid). These free acids do not take part in the enterohepatic circulation so are not reabsorbed in the distal ileum and cause impaired absorption of salt and water from the colon thus contributing to the diarrhea. The bile salt pool becomes depleted. Mild-to-moderate inflammatory changes and villous atrophy may occur in the small intestine and also contribute to the malabsorption.

A simple method of testing for bacterial overgrowth is the hydrogen (or methane) breath test. Hydrogen and methane are released by bacteria when given a suitable substrate like glucose or lactulose and the gas can be detected in the breath. An early peak (<90 min) before the substrate reaches the colon suggests a small bowel colonization with bacteria.

Treatment consists of correcting nutritional deficiencies with vitamin B12 and fat-soluble vitamin supplements if necessary. Tetracycline (250 mg qds orally) is the traditional antibiotic of choice and is usually highly effective. Metronidazole should theoretically be as effective since the offending bacteria are almost exclusively anaerobes however long term or recurrent therapy is often necessary and tetracycline is therefore preferable because of its lower risk of side effects in long term use. More recently, the non-absorbable antibiotic rifaximin is increasingly used. If calcium supplements are needed, they should be taken at a different time of day to prevent binding with tetracycline. Surgical correction of the blind loop is not usually necessary or appropriate unless there is stricturing with proximal stasis.

SECRETORY DIARRHEA

Cholera

Cholera is the classic cause of secretory diarrhea and knowledge of its pathophysiology has led to a much fuller understanding of fluid and electrolyte handling by the small intestine. The *Vibrio cholerae* causes no structural damage to the mucosa but its toxin binds irreversibly with a receptor on the epithelial surface and the active component of the toxin then enters the epithelial cell where it stimulates adenylate cyclase. This increases the intracellular concentration of cyclic AMP which stimulates secretion of salt and water from the crypt cells and inhibits absorption by the villous cells. This results in a devastating change in the large fluxes of salt and water that occur normally in the small intestine so that watery diarrhea of up to 25 L/day may result.

This is not solely due to a secretory effect since the healthy small intestine can absorb up to 20 L/day. As with most other examples of secretory diarrhea, there is an absorptive defect as well. If fluid replacement is adequate the diarrhea resolves within a few days and is usually only massive for the first 24 h.

Peptide-secreting Tumors

Other diarrheas usually classed as secretory because of a high stool volume (>300 mL/day) in the fasting state include diarrhea associated with peptide-secreting tumors: vipoma of the pancreas, medullary carcinoma of the thyroid and carcinoid syndrome. In these conditions other mechanisms, particularly altered motility also contribute to the diarrhea.

Vasoactive intestinal peptide (VIP) can be produced in excess by neuroendocrine tumors of the pancreas, neural tissues (ganglioneuroblastoma) or lung (oat cell carcinoma). This results in a syndrome, described by Verner and Morrison in 1958, of watery diarrhea, hypokalemia and achlorhydria. Diarrhea is typically massive (>1 L/day). VIP does not cause sufficient inhibition of adenyl cyclase for this to be its main mechanism of action and it is likely that some other mechanism and possibly also another peptide contributes to the diarrhea.

Diarrhea in medullary carcinoma of the thyroid is usually less massive (300 mL/day or so). Calcitonin levels are greatly increased in the plasma but do not seem to be responsible for the diarrhea which is probably prostaglandin mediated.

Carcinoid syndrome results from excessive release of a wide group of peptides and other factors including 5-hydroxytryptamine (which is probably the cause of the diarrhea), bradykinin, histamine, catecholamines, prostaglandins and other peptide hormones. The syndrome may include flushing attacks, wheezing, abdominal pain, diarrhea and right-sided valvular heart lesions. Pellagra may result from niacin deficiency that results from diversion of tryptophan to serotonin rather than niacin synthesis.

Management of Secretory Diarrhea

Fluid and Electrolyte Replacement: In cholera and all other examples of massive diarrhea, the most essential aspect of treatment is fluid and electrolyte replacement. This may need to be given intravenously but a huge advance has been made in the management of cholera by the realization that sugar/salt solutions, given enterally achieve successful rehydration in most cases. This is because glucose (and neutral amino acids such as glycine) enhances absorption of sodium. The World Health Organization recommends an oral rehydration solution consisting of sodium chloride 4 g/L, sodium acetate 6.5 g/L, potassium chloride 1 g/L and glucose 9 g/L. With adequate rehydration mortality from cholera approaches zero whereas it may otherwise be rapidly fatal.

Management of Peptide-secreting Tumors

Vasoactive intestinal peptide (VIP)-producing tumor can be treated successfully by resection of the tumor in about 50% of cases. If metastases have already developed, symptomatic relief and sometimes tumor shrinkage may be achieved with streptozocin or with radiolabeled octreotide. Symptoms of diarrhea can be controlled with octreotide, sometimes long-term use with depot octreotide is helpful. Corticosteroids are less helpful in controlling the diarrhea.

Carcinoid syndrome invariably implies the presence of hepatic metastases but these are slow growing and if confined to one lobe of the liver a prolonged remission may be achieved by resection. Pharmacological treatment is complicated and not always successful. Octreotide is helpful in controlling the diarrhea and antihistamines occasionally relieve flushing.

If hepatic metastases are too extensive for resection, then palliation may be achieved by hepatic artery radioembolization or transcatheter chemoembolization with doxorubicin or cisplatin. When embolization is unsuccessful or not feasible for liver metastases, percutaneous or intraoperative radiofrequency tumor ablation may be attempted, though it is not ideal for large metastatic tumors. Care must be taken during these maneuvers as release of vasoactive compounds can cause severe symptoms.

Medullary carcinoma of the thyroid occasionally produces diarrhea when metastases have developed but survival is often remarkably good with little progression over several years. Diarrhea may respond to somatostatin or octreotide.

Various forms of chemotherapy have been used for all the peptide-secreting tumors when resection is not possible. Cure is unfortunately very rare but response rates of about 50% have been reported with combinations such as adriamycin and 5-fluorouracil. Occasional impressive tumor regression has also been reported with somatostatin and somatostatin analogs and as these generally case fewer side effects than conventional chemotherapy they probably should be used in preference.

Purgative Abuse

Natural History and Management

Purgative abuse can be notoriously difficult to diagnose. Clinical features in a severe case can include severe malabsorption, clubbing, hypogammaglobulinemia and tetany. Diagnosis requires a high index of suspicion. Although the doctor may feel a great sense of personal triumph when the diagnosis is established, the trouble is usually only just beginning. Direct confrontation of the patient will often produce complete denial or a switch to another self-induced disease which may even lead to a suicide attempt. An air of tolerance and understanding needs to be conveyed rather than victory. Psychiatric help should be sought but there is no clear consensus about the optimal treatment and the prognosis in severe cases is poor.

Bile Acid Diarrhea

Natural History and Management

Bile acid diarrhea most commonly follows resection or irradiation damage to the distal small intestine where 95% of secreted bile acids are normally reabsorbed for recirculation (*see* Fig 3.21). Typically a patient who had a terminal ileal resection for Crohn's disease may present with watery diarrhea. Unabsorbed bile acids stimulate adenyl cyclase in the colonic epithelium resulting in a net loss of salt and water into the lumen. It has been suggested that a small proportion of patients with the IBS particularly those with chronic watery diarrhea (IBS-C), may also suffer from bile salt malabsorption. In some instances of postvagotomy diarrhea, particularly if combined with cholecystectomy, bile salt diarrhea also seems to be an important mechanism. In patients who had a cholecystectomy, there is nowhere to store excess bile and it may leak out unbuffered by food and lead to diarrhea.

A SeHCAT scan can be used to diagnose bile salt malabsorption but a simple therapeutic trial with oral cholestyramine, the ion-exchange resin, is usually dramatically effective and the dose, usually one to two sachets daily, can be adjusted according to the response. Care should be taken to avoid taking other drugs simultaneously as they might be adsorbed by the cholestyramine.

■ FURTHER READING

Inflammatory Bowel Diseases
1. Dignass A, Van Assche G, Lindsay JO, et al. The second European evidence-based consensus on the diagnosis and management of Crohn's disease: current management. J Crohn's Colitis. 2010;4(1):28-62.
2. Dignass A, Eliakim R, Magro F, et al. Second European evidence-based consensus on the diagnosis and management of ulcerative colitis Part 1: definitions and diagnosis. J Crohn's Colitis. 2012;6(10):965-90.
3. Dignass A, Lindsay JO, Sturm A, et al. Second European evidence-based consensus on the diagnosis and management of ulcerative colitis Part 2: current management. J Crohn's Colitis. 2012;6(10):991-1030.
4. Gomollón F, Dignass A, Annese V, et al. Third European evidence-based consensus on the diagnosis and management of Crohn's disease 2016: Part 1: diagnosis and medical management. J Crohn's Colitis. 2017;11(1):3-25.
5. Hodson R. Inflammatory bowel disease. Nature. 2016;540:S97.

Small Intestinal Bacterial Overgrowth/Bile Acid Malabsorption
6. Bures J, Cyrany J, Kohoutova D, et al. Small intestinal bacterial overgrowth syndrome. World J Gastroenterol. 2010;16(24):2978-90.
7. Wilcox C, Turner J, Green J. Systematic review: the management of chronic diarrhea due to bile acid malabsorption. Aliment Pharmacol Ther. 2014;39(9):923-39.

Celiac Disease/Pancreatic Insufficiency
8. Fieker A, Philpott J, Armand M. Enzyme replacement therapy for pancreatic insufficiency: present and future. Clin Exp Gastroenterol. 2011;4:55-73.
9. Green PH, Cellier C. Celiac disease. N Engl J Med. 2007;357(17):1731-43.
10. Struyvenberg MR, Martin CR, Freedman SD. Practical guide to exocrine pancreatic insufficiency—breaking the myths. BMC Med. 2017;15(1):29.

CHAPTER 4

Constipation

Her Hsin Tsai

■ WHAT IS CONSTIPATION?

When patients report having constipation, they may mean a range of different symptoms:
1. Infrequent emptying of bowels, lack of urge to go
2. Painful defecation with hard stools
3. Bloating and abdominal pain with infrequency of defecation
4. Need to strain
5. Feeling of incomplete evacuation
6. Having to sit for long periods in the toilet.

It is remarkably difficult to come to a definition. It is often accepted that less than three spontaneous evacuations a week may be regarded as constipation and this is often the definition used in clinical trials to evaluate laxatives. However, there is little correlation between this definition and patient symptoms. Many may feel very comfortable with fewer than one or two evacuations, while others may be very symptomatic despite spending a considerable amount of time in the toilet. In fact, one definition (Rome III) classifies everyone with at least two of the above symptoms in the past 6 months as having constipation. Of course, this is a completely arbitrary definition. In the final analysis, the physician's task is to alleviate symptoms and exclude important organic disease.

One observation is that the appearance of the stool does correlate very well with symptomatic constipation. This has led to the widespread and helpful use of the Bristol stool chart in evaluating constipation. Patients with hard lumpy stools whether pellet-like or stuck together (Bristol types 1 and 2) can be described as having constipation. There is a reduced content of water in the stool due to its longer transit in the colon and rolled into pill-like shape by the non-propulsive contractions of the lower colon (Fig. 4.1).

If there is any doubt, a whole gut transit study is simple and cheap to perform. This involves swallowing a radiopaque marker and then performing

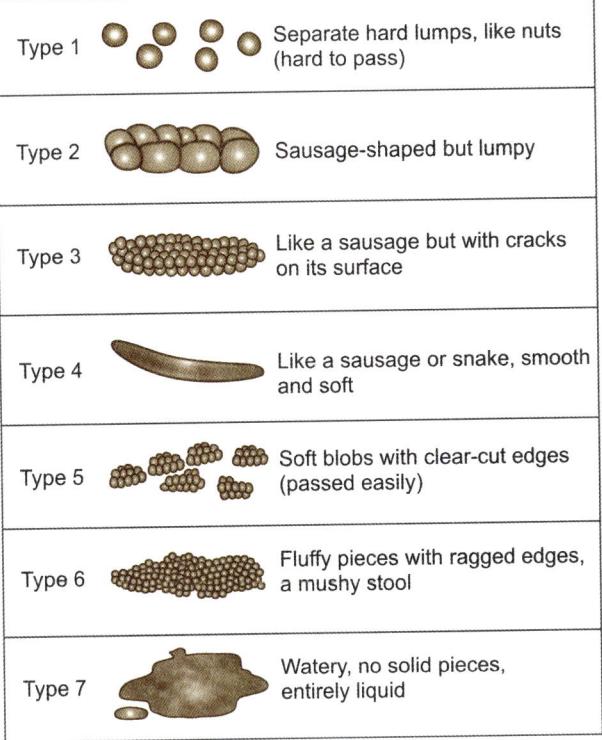

Fig. 4.1: Bristol stool chart.

a plain X-ray 5 days later. Sometimes, two different-shaped markers are used, one swallowed 2 days after the first. This simple test could also show if there is slowing down of the whole colon with markers spread throughout the colon or if the markers are all aggregated in the pelvis when there is obstructed defecation.

Pathophysiology

Constipation may arise from:
- A generalized abnormality of colorectal motility
- Disordered anorectal physiology
- Involuntary overriding of normal response perhaps due to social fear of public toilets or painful anal condition
- Stricture or tumor obstruction
- Inadequate fluid or fiber intake.

The primary function of the gastrointestinal (GI) tract is to digest food and extract nutrients and fluid. Hence, it is not a conveyor belt moving in one direction only. Most of the time, the peristaltic contractions are a to-and-fro activity exposing the food to the absorptive surface. In the colon, about 7–9 times a day, there are coordinated propulsions toward the rectum termed as high-amplitude propagated contractions (HAPC). This is suppressed at night during sleep but increases upon awakening, are much more common during the day, and increases after meals and exercise. They originate in the proximal colon but mostly do not propagate beyond the mid-colon and <5% reach the rectum. When contents reach the rectum, it may lead to internal anal sphincter relaxation stimulating the urge to defecate. HAPCs are reduced in slow-transit constipation and increased in diarrhea predominant irritable bowel syndrome (IBS) and may explain disturbances of colonic transit in these conditions.

When the fecal material reaches the rectum it is held continent by a complex of sphincters and the puborectalis sling that creates an acute angle at the anorectal junction. These are in turn controlled by the sacral and pudendal nerves. Efferent nerves feed into the lower spinal cord where a combination of local reflex and higher control allows for the complex control of continence. In fact, remarkably, the human rectum is capable of distinguishing between solids, liquids and gas and can selectively expel the latter while remaining continent of the former two. At the point of defecation, the anorectal angle straightens up with the relaxation of the puborectalis muscle, the internal and external sphincters relax and defecation takes place. It is worth noting that the angle is at its most straight in the crouching position which is how humans are evolved to defecate and less so (more acute) in the sitting position of Western toilets (Fig. 4.2).

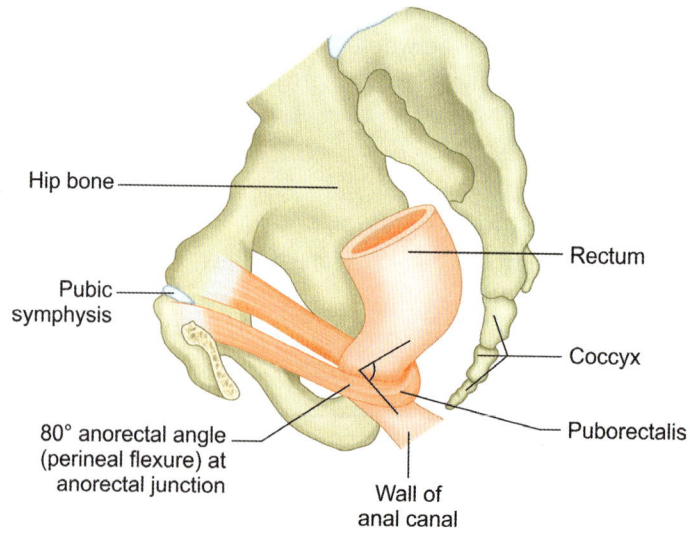

Fig. 4.2: The anorectal angle acts as an effective gatekeeper, relaxation of the puborectalis straightens it up and allows passage of stool.

Approach to the Diagnosis

Taking a good history and taking the patient's age into account helps to make the correct diagnosis and avoids unnecessary unpleasant investigations like a colonoscopy. History of diabetes, cerebrovascular disease and drugs both prescription and over-the-counter remedies gives important clues. The main initial assessment would be to distinguish between primary constipation (also referred to as functional or idiopathic) and secondary causes. In the patient of 45 years or older, where colonic neoplasia needs to be excluded, a colonoscopy should be performed although the pickup for chronic constipation is low. In other patients, abdominal examination may pick up a loaded colon and evidence of bowel spasm or tenderness. Anorectal examination may reveal a prolapsed mucosa or painful fissures or perianal hematomas. A digital examination may reveal abscesses and assess tone of the anal sphincter. A biochemistry profile and thyroid-stimulating hormone could identify metabolic causes of constipation. A flexible sigmoidoscopy is simple and requires only an enema rather than a full bowel prep and may identify rectal conditions like solitary rectal ulcer.

IS IT PRIMARY CONSTIPATION?

Primary constipation can generally be subdivided into the following 3 types, although there may be considerable overlap:
- Irritable bowel syndrome with predominant constipation (IBS-C)
- Slow-transit constipation
- Pelvic floor dysfunction (also referred to as pelvic floor dyssynergia).

IS IT CONSTIPATION-PREDOMINANT IRRITABLE BOWEL SYNDROME?

It is important to try to make a positive diagnosis to avoid unnecessary investigations in this group. Patients are commonly younger women. They often have the classic triad of colicky abdominal pain, bloating and constipation. This meets the criteria for making a diagnosis of IBD-C. In these patients, stool passes through the colon at a normal rate, but they find it difficult to evacuate their bowels. There may be alternating with episodes of diarrhea and pain may be relieved by defecation. The presence of weight loss, rectal bleeding or nocturnal pain requires further investigation. A fuller discussion of IBS may be found in Chapter 1.

Management of IBS-C

Management can be very difficult. An understanding listening sympathetic approach is vital. The doctor is often the best medicine. Occasionally, it is possible to coax the patient to reveal some deep-seated psychological disturbance as a precipitating cause. The physician is then obliged to offer some clinical psychological support. Cognitive behavioral therapy and hypnotherapy wave their advocates. Postinfective IBS tends to lead to diarrhea predominant IBS but may be a long-forgotten trigger. Dietary improvement is also a vital element. In general, patients with constipation should be counseled to eat more fiber. Soluble fibers, which are found in fruits and leafy vegetables, are preferable to non-soluble fibers like bran. They absorb more liquid and produce softer faces. If the predominant symptom is bloating, then advice about FODMAP foods (see Chapter 9) avoidance may be helpful. Gluten sensitivity may cause constipation, even if celiac disease is serologically discounted, hence a trial of gluten or wheat avoidance can be helpful. A referral to a dietitian can be very helpful. Drug therapy may include the use of laxatives or antidepressants. Stimulant laxatives are best avoided for long-term use. Start with a bulking agent in these patients with soluble fibers such as fybogel or methylceluose with encouragement to drink more fluids. However, these may cause more bloating. Osmotic laxatives like macrogol (polyethylene glycol) are effective and safe. Newer agents have been licensed for use if patients fail on the traditional laxatives of which linaclotide and lubiprostone have been licensed specifically for IBS-C. Linaclotide is a peptide that acts on the guanylate cyclase-C receptors in the intestinal neurons leading to increased cyclic guanosine monophosphate, anion secretion, fluid secretion and stimulating intestinal transit. It appears to work topically as it is not absorbed. Lubiprostone is a bicyclic fatty acid derived from prostaglandin E1 that acts by stimulating ClC-2 chloride channels on the apical aspect of GI epithelial cells, producing a chloride-rich fluid secretion. Both these drugs have NICE approval for use if traditional, cheaper laxatives fail. Antidepressants have a role here. Selective serotonin reuptake inhibitors are preferred to tricyclics as the latter is somewhat constipating.

■ IS IT SLOW-TRANSIT CONSTIPATION?

This is characterized by infrequent bowel movements, decreased urgency or straining to defecate. Patients usually have a long history and predominately occur in the young females. Slow-transit constipation as the name implies has impaired phasic colonic motor activity. A 5-day colonic marker test would show considerable retention of markers that may be scattered through the colon. Often there is abdominal distention or palpable stool in the sigmoid colon but pain is unusual. Patients may report alarmingly infrequent bowel movement that can be believed from the amount of marker retention (Fig. 4.3).

Management

This group of patients would normally have gone through the full gamut of drugs mentioned earlier by the time they visit secondary care physician.

Constipation

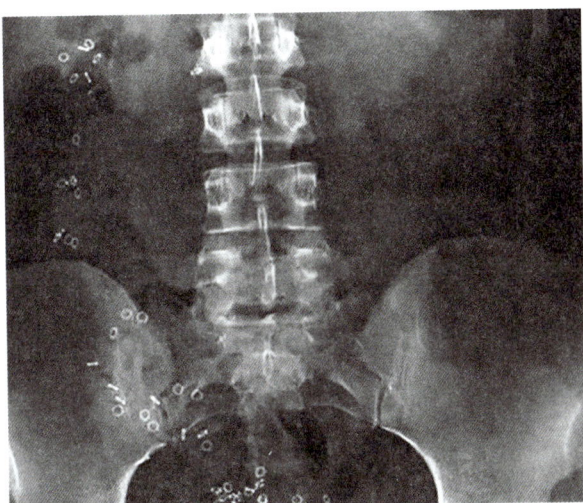

Fig. 4.3: Colonic transit study: these markers have been ingested 5 days earlier and are still in the ascending colon showing marked slow-transit constipation.

Hence, management of the patients at the severe end is very challenging. Psychological factors may play a role. A dietitian consultation is also helpful. Laxatives must be selected with care. Bulking agents generally are best avoided. They may lead to bloating, although soluble fibers could be tried. Stimulant laxatives should be avoided. Osmotic laxatives remain the cornerstone but may quickly lose effect and combination laxatives are often needed. Sometimes, patients may need full doses of macrogol used for bowel preparations for a proper evacuation.

Biofeedback and coaching by an experienced physiologist can be helpful. Provision of a twice weekly irrigation using a self-administered enema pump is helpful to many who are refractory to oral laxatives. Operative procedures include an appendicostomy. Here the appendix is brought to the surface of the abdominal wall and antegrade fluid can be pumped into the colon as a flushing agent at regular intervals. Colectomies should only be reserved for the extreme cases as a last resort. Sacral nerve stimulators have also a role, but long-term results are disappointing.

■ IS IT PELVIC FLOOR DYSFUNCTION?

In pelvic floor dysfunction, patients often report prolonged or excessive straining, a feeling of incomplete evacuation, or they may report digital evacuation of stool with a finger inserted into the rectum or into the vagina pressing posteriorly. Careful history taking usually leads to the diagnosis. Patients may have nerve damage from traumatic virginal deliveries, particularly forceps deliveries.

Here a lower GI physiologist can be very helpful. There is often a failure to coordinate between the relaxation of the puborectalis and the relaxation of the anal sphincters. This is why rectal digitization works. Vaginal pressure posteriorly also straightens the angle allowing passage of feces. Of course, these practices are best discouraged, and patients best find more physiological solutions. Manometry is usually performed and biofeedback is the cornerstone of management. As in the slow-transit constipation, osmotic laxatives are best. Patients should be coached to establish a good bowel habit. Toilet position is helpful, patients could have a child's stool to rest the feet to simulate a more squat position at defecation. Sacral nerve stimulation holds some promise but as a rule in this group, surgery is best avoided.

■ IS IT SECONDARY CONSTIPATION?

By far the commonest cause of constipation is poor diet (or recent change of diet) accompanied by inadequate water intake or inadequate fiber intake or excessive coffee, tea or alcohol. Ignoring the urge to defecate because of phobias of public toilets or during long-distance travel and reduced levels of exercise may play a factor.

Other secondary constipation includes anal fissures, thrombosed hemorrhoids, colonic strictures, obstructing tumors, volvulus and idiopathic megarectum/megacolon (Hirschsprung's disease).

Table 4.1 lists the systemic diseases that may lead to constipation and the list of drugs known to induce constipation is given in Table 4.2.

Table 4.1: Systemic diseases that may cause constipation.
Endocrinological and metabolic disorders
Hypercalcemia and hyperparathyroidism
Hypokalemia
Hypothyroidism
Pregnancy
Diabetes mellitus (constipation is the most common gastrointestinal problem affecting the diabetic population)
Neurological disorders
Hirschsprung's disease
Stroke
Parkinson's disease
Multiple sclerosis
Diabetic autonomic neuropathy
Spinal cord lesion
Head injury
Cerebrovascular accident
Chagas disease

Table 4.2: Drugs that may lead to constipation.
Antidepressants (e.g. cyclic antidepressants and monoamine oxidase inhibitors)
Metals (e.g. iron and bismuth)
Anticholinergics (e.g. benztropine and trihexyphenidyl)
Opioids (e.g. codeine and morphine)
Antacids (e.g. aluminum and calcium compounds)
Calcium channel blockers (e.g. verapamil)
Non-steroidal anti-inflammatory drugs (e.g. ibuprofen and diclofenac)
Sympathomimetics (e.g. pseudoephedrine)
Many psychotropic drugs especially tricyclics
Cholestyramine and stimulant laxatives after prolonged use may lead to the development of a dilated atonic

Management

Treatment of the primary condition usually leads to improved bowel function. If drugs are involved, then selection of the less constipating agent is obvious. However, some patients may need that class of medication. Most commonly encountered situation is patients requiring long-term opioids. Patients on palliative care regiments often include several drugs that constipate. There are now non-absorbable opioid antagonists that prevent opioid drugs from binding onto gut receptors. These are the peripherally acting mu-opioid receptor antagonists, the most widely used of which is naloxegol.

IS THERE HIRSCHSPRUNG'S DISEASE?

This disease is usually identified by the classic toothpaste feces in childhood, but some do go undetected till adulthood. It is a neurological defect with an absence of ganglions in the myenteric plexus. Colon and rectum become pathologically distended. A straight abdominal film will show dilated megacolon. Treatment would involve resection of the aganglionic segment.

SOLITARY RECTAL ULCER SYNDROME

This is a rare curious condition in which ulceration occurs in the rectum in the absence of chronic inflammatory bowel disease like Crohn's. Histologically, there is evidence of ischemia and fibrosis. The name is a misnomer as there may be more than one ulcer. There is often associated history of constipation, straining and rectal prolapse. Patients are often accused of digitally induced trauma but there is little evidence of that. It is more likely that it is due to rectal prolapse and subsequent ischemia. At sigmoidoscopy, the most common site is the posterior wall. Drugs inserted rectally like indomethacin can also cause similar ulceration. Treatment involves correcting

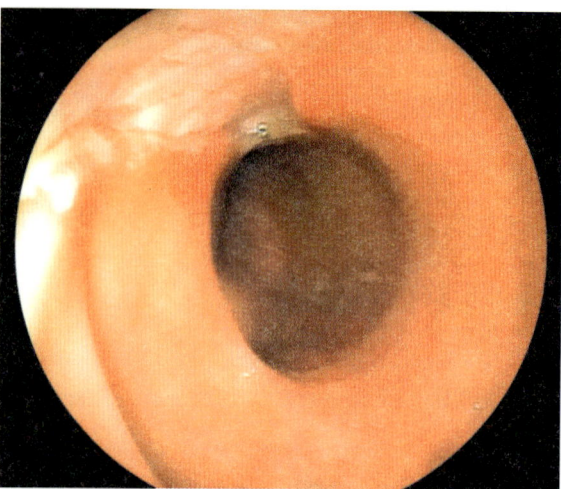

Fig. 4.4: Solitary rectal ulcer.

underlying constipation but can be difficult. Rectal prolapse may need surgical intervention (Fig. 4.4).

FURTHER READING

1. Chatoor D, Emmnauel A. Constipation and evacuation disorders. Best Pract Res Clin Gastroenterol. 2009;23(4):517-30.
2. Thayalasekeran S, Hani A, Tsai HH. Novel therapies for constipation. World J Gastroenterol. 2013;19(45):8247-51. PMC. Web. September 16, 2017.

CHAPTER 5

Anorectal Problems

Her Hsin Tsai

■ DIAGNOSIS

Patients presenting with anorectal problems come with a variety of symptoms; chiefly, bleeding, anal pain, urgency or tenesmus, discharge and incontinence.

Bleeding

It is important to obtain a careful history with the aim of distinguishing (1) blood spotting on toilet paper only (which is almost always due to minor local trauma and occurs in most people at some time), (2) blood in the pan that is separate from feces and (3) blood that is on the surface or mixed in with feces. The diagnostic approach to bleeding and anemia is discussed elsewhere but it is worth repeating that any patient presenting with rectal bleeding as the main problem should at least undergo rigid sigmoidoscopy even if it is just spotting as in (1). At the same occasion, the anal canal should be carefully inspected. Gentle parting of the anal canal will reveal the presence of a fissure and the patient should be asked to strain to allow detection of rectal prolapse or engorgement of the external venous plexus. No further investigation is required if the sigmoidoscopy is normal, if there is never any blood in the pan or on the feces and if there are no other symptoms. Blood in the pan or feces needs more thorough investigation. If the blood is separate from the feces, then flexible sigmoidoscopy is sufficient providing preparation is adequate to allow a clear view. If the nature of bleeding is difficult to establish with certainty from the history or if there is a clear history of blood mixed with feces, then full colonoscopy should be performed.

Blood seen on paper only is usually due either to small hemorrhoids, minor local trauma usually associated with pruritus or anal fissuring. Blood separate from feces is most commonly due to hemorrhoids, but may also be due to a variety of other causes including rectal carcinoma, proctitis (usually associated with passage of mucus per rectum in addition). Blood mixed with feces may be due to carcinoma, vascular abnormalities such as angiodysplasia, inflammatory bowel disease, either ulcerative proctitis or Crohn's disease (more extensive ulcerative colitis that is sufficiently active to cause bleeding will always cause diarrhea so bleeding without diarrhea in a patient with previous extensive ulcerative colitis should always be carefully investigated). Polyps are often found as a chance in finding when bleeding is investigated, but are rarely the cause of bleeding unless very large or frankly malignant. Diverticula can occasionally give rise to brisk arterial bleeding when inflamed but do not usually cause recurrent low-grade blood loss. Very brisk upper gastrointestinal bleeding, e.g. due to duodenal ulceration, may pass through rapidly as bright red blood per rectum but this will invariably be associated with hemodynamic signs of bleeding.

Barium enema is not a very satisfactory examination when rectal bleeding is the only symptom. Vascular lesions will be missed and most patients will not have a cause for the bleeding found and will need to be referred on for colonoscopy. Fecal occult blood testing is also of little help. If positive, it merely confirms the presence of bleeding and if negative just implies that the bleeding is intermittent but in no way reduces the need for further investigation.

Pain

A careful history is needed to determine whether pain is (1) anal, (2) rectal or (3) pelvic. Anal pain is most commonly due either to fissuring or to thrombosed hemorrhoids and careful inspection will usually give an immediate diagnosis. Rectal pain is more difficult. It is only rarely due to organic disease. The commonest form being proctalgia fugax—intermittent severe rectal pain that is not associated with defecation and may even wake the patient. In men, acute prostatitis may be associated with perineal pain and rectal pain that is worse on defecation. Rectal examination will then reveal a tender prostate. Pelvic pain is much commoner in women. Gynecological conditions such as ovarian pathology, endometriosis, uterine or cervical cancer and ectopic pregnancy may all need exclusion but in many patients no obvious cause is found. In many cases, the pain may be a variant of the irritable bowel syndrome. There has been disconcerting evidence that a high proportion of the cases in which no organic cause is found has been subjected to previous sexual abuse. Pelvic abscess, most commonly due to diverticulitis but also due to Crohn's disease, salpingitis or local perforation due to ingestion of animal bones, etc. may present with vague symptoms of malaise and low-grade pyrexia without clear localizing signs. A careful rectal examination is mandatory but a high index of suspicion combined with pelvic ultrasound or computed tomography scanning may be necessary to make a correct diagnosis.

Tenesmus

Tenesmus is a feeling of incomplete evacuation or frequent sensation of the need to evacuate. It is a usual accompaniment of diarrhea whether this has an organic or functional cause but is particularly prominent when there is rectal disease. Any mass lesion in the rectum such as a tumor or large polyp may cause tenesmus and it is often the most unpleasant symptom in ulcerative proctitis. The solitary ulcer syndrome is a cause of tenesmus that is often misdiagnosed. Although it is associated with rectal mucosal prolapse, a clear history of this is often lacking, moreover when the ulcer is seen on sigmoidoscopy, it is sometimes wrongly assumed to indicate some form of inflammatory bowel disease. The ulcer is on the anterior rectal wall in about two-thirds of cases and histology is characteristic, with marked fibromuscular hyperplasia. Carefully performed defecating proctography will usually confirm mucosal prolapse. Tenesmus is usually accompanied by urgency although urgency alone is a common feature of the irritable bowel syndrome and is then not commonly associated with tenesmus.

Discharge

Spontaneous discharge of pus indicates anal or rectal disease. Careful anal inspection should reveal any anal or perianal pathology such as anal tumors or fissuring, perianal fistula or perianal infections such as herpetic ulceration, syphilitic chancre or perianal warts. In the absence of obvious fissuring, sigmoidoscopy should then be performed. If proctitis is present, then a rectal swab should be taken for gonococcal culture in addition to rectal biopsy for routine histology.

Incontinence

Few problems are as unpleasant, as poorly understood, and as poorly treated as fecal incontinence. Incontinence can occur in the presence of a normal sphincter if there is severe diarrhea, but it is more commonly due to poor sphincter function. It is much commoner in women and is then often related to previous obstetric trauma which may have passed unnoticed at the time. This is especially true if there is a history of forceps delivery or episiotomy. Incontinence will also be a feature of neurological disruption like spinal cord injuries or cauda equina lesions. Diagnosis depends on assessment of sphincter function. There are three main components of the sphincter: (1) the puborectalis sling which is the inner component of the levator ani and which maintains an acute angle between the anal canal and rectum, (2) the internal sphincter consisting of involuntary muscle fibers that are a continuation of the circular muscle coat of the rectum and (3) the external sphincter that surrounds the internal sphincter, consists of voluntary muscle fibers and is attached to the coccyx posteriorly and the perineal body anteriorly. The external sphincter can be assessed crudely by voluntary contraction during rectal examination but facilities should now be available in every health region to allow proper objective measurement of sphincter function prior to any consideration of corrective surgery. This assessment should include assessment of (1) resting pressure (normally 60–100 mm Hg until the sixth decade after which it falls progressively) and (2) squeeze pressure (normally 100–220 mm Hg). Barium enema examination could also be performed to allow measurement of the anorectal angle (the angle between the posterior wall of the rectum and the longitudinal axis of the anal canal which should be approximately 80°) (*see* Fig. 4.3).

Anal Lesions

There are two components to the normal anal mucosa; anal skin distal to the dentate line and columnar epithelium between the dentate line and the anorectal junction. Malignant tumors may of course cross the dentate line, but tumors arising above the line are more commonly adenocarcinomas while those below the line are skin tumors and therefore include squamous and basal cell carcinomas and melanomas. Sexually transmitted diseases will need consideration in cases of anal ulceration. Herpetic ulcers usually cause severe pain and tenesmus, whereas syphilitic ulcers are characteristically painless. Anal warts (condylomata acuminata) are usually easily recognized by their papilliferous appearance. Condylomata lata, the mucosal lesions of secondary syphilis, are flatter lesions. Macular, fissured or ulcerated anal lesions should always be biopsied particularly since the malignant conditions Bowen's disease (squamous carcinoma in situ) and Paget's disease (intraepithelial mucous adenocarcinoma) can only be diagnosed with histology.

Perianal Abscess and Fistula

Diagnosis of the lesion itself is usually obvious but there are two main traps: (1) failing to recognize the presence of underlying Crohn's disease and (2) failing to make a correct assessment of the extent of the fistula. The presence of thickened skin tags, usually of a dusky purple color should alert to the possibility of Crohn's disease. This should be excluded not only by assessment of the colon, but also by magnetic resonance enterography to exclude terminal ileal Crohn's disease. It is particularly important not to miss an underlying diagnosis of Crohn's disease since traditional treatment of a fistula or abscess by surgical debridement and laying open will often be disastrous with very poor healing and further fistulation. Magnetic resonance imaging (MRI) of the pelvis is an excellent method of assessing these fistulae, and endoscopic ultrasound can also be helpful prior to surgery. A careful assessment under anesthetic by an experienced surgeon followed by selective draining and seton insertion is the mainstay of treatment.

Pruritus

Pruritus ani is a very common condition which is most commonly associated with poor local hygiene which in turn may be associated with some degree of fecal incontinence. This may not be obvious from the history and if the problem is persistent, then anorectal physiological studies will be indicated. The anal area should be carefully inspected to exclude any local skin conditions such as eczema or Paget's disease and a stool sample should be examined for ova or parasites. Flexible sigmoidoscopy should also be performed to exclude rectal pathology. Pinworm (*Enterobius vermicularis*) infestation is remarkably common especially in the United Kingdom and is a common cause of pruritus ani. Spread is from person to person and family members are often affected. Infection is usually asymptomatic but anal pruritus is a cardinal symptom as the worms migrate out to lay their eggs. A sellotape test should be performed by sticking a piece of sellotape on the anus and sticking it on a microscope slide. The ova of the parasite are readily visible under microscopy.

NATURAL HISTORY AND MANAGEMENT OF ANORECTAL CONDITIONS

Hemorrhoids

Hemorrhoids are usually formed as a result of enlargement of the normal anal cushions which consist of areas of venous dilatation covered by smooth muscle, elastic and fibrous tissue. These venous cushions are found in three characteristic positions: left lateral [3 o'clock, right posterior (7 o'clock) and right anterior (11 o'clock)]. The presence of arteriovenous communications explains the typical bright red color when they bleed and why portal hypertension is associated with rectal varices but not enlarged hemorrhoids. Exclusion of rectal carcinoma is made by flexible sigmoidoscopy. Hemorrhoids are traditionally classified into first degree: bleeding; second degree: prolapse and third degree: prolapse requiring replacement.

Bleeding most commonly occurs at the end of defecation but may occasionally be retained in the rectum to be passed on the next defecation as dark blood. Such a history always necessitates further investigation by flexible sigmoidoscopy or colonoscopy. Uncomplicated hemorrhoids are impalpable but painful thrombosis is a common complication. This may occasionally be extensive, involving the whole circumference but is more commonly localized, typically as a thrombosed venous saccule (previously called perianal hematoma) (Figs. 5.1 and 5.2).

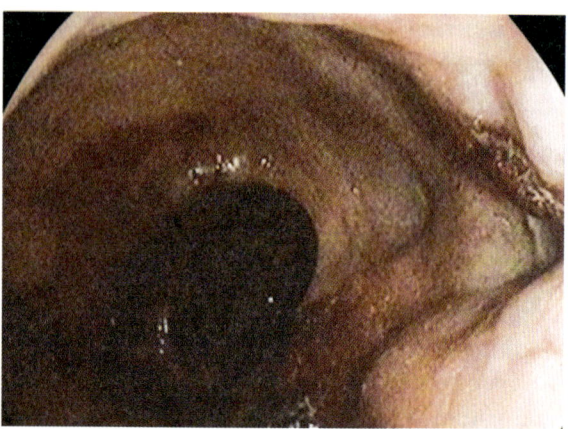

Fig. 5.1: Bleeding hemorrhoids.

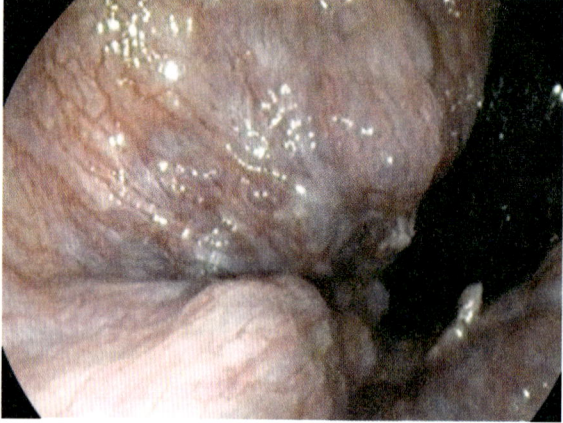

Fig. 5.2: Retroflexing the flexible sigmoidoscope allows for easy visualization of hemorrhoids.

Treatment

Many patients have only minor intermittent bleeding and when other causes of the bleeding have been excluded, they may require no further treatment other than dietary advice or possibly a bulking agent to relieve constipation.

Vigorous anal dilatation under general anesthetic is commonly used to be performed, but is now much less common because of the unpredictable results and appreciable risk of incontinence, particularly in elderly patients. Small hemorrhoids are usually treated by rubber band ligation or if this fails, by excision. Band ligation usually results in pain which persists for about 1 week and secondary hemorrhage may occur in up to 10%. Approximately 10% will require surgical excision. Other techniques in

Anal Fissure

Acute anal fissures consist of a break in the anoderm without surrounding fibrosis. They are usually the result of passage of a large constipated stool. They present with severe pain during defecation associated with bright rectal bleeding. They can usually be treated conservatively with bulking agents. Local anesthetic suppositories or ointment are also commonly used although they are of uncertain benefit. Diagnosis can usually made by direct inspection after parting of the buttocks. Rectal examination is likely to be very painful and should be deferred until symptomatic treatment or spontaneous healing has had a chance to take effect and may then require preliminary administration of local anesthetic ointment. Chronic anal fissures are commonly identifiable by the presence of a classical triad consisting of (1) "sentinel" external tag or "pile," (2) the fissure and (3) a hypertrophied anal papilla at the upper end of the fissure. More than 90% are posterior and midline. There is ulceration down to the transverse muscles of the internal sphincter muscle with associated fibrosis. Medical treatment with 0.3% glyceryl trinitrate (GTN) cream or ointment is helpful in relieving pain and allowing healing. If that fails, then sphincter injection with Botox (Botulinum toxin) under anesthesia can be performed and good results have been reported. Intractable cases may be offered hyperbaric oxygen therapy. Surgical treatment with lateral internal sphincterotomy anal stretching is best avoided as they are associated with a risk for incontinence.

Multiple or lateral fissures should raise the possibility of alternative diagnoses such as traumatic damage, Crohn's disease, leukemia, syphilis or tuberculosis and biopsy should be during an examination under general anesthesia. These "secondary" fissures require treatment of the underlying condition.

Anal Tags

Anal tags do not themselves cause symptoms or require treatment but may be a clue to important underlying conditions. They commonly occur as the end result of a thrombosed external plexus hematoma ("thrombosed external pile") but also mark the external end of chronic anal fissures. Tags associated with Crohn's disease are usually thicker and have a purplish indurated appearance. Biopsy and histology may then be useful as they commonly contain granulomata.

Anal Warts

Anal warts are a contagious sexually transmitted disease caused by some types of human papillomavirus (HPV types 6 and 11). Although the infection is common, <10% develop anal or genital warts. Their presence should therefore alert the clinician to the possible presence of other sexually transmitted disease.

They need to be distinguished from the much rarer mucosal lesions of secondary syphilis (condylomata lata). The latter are more protuberant and moister. Warts are usually treated with topical application of 25% podophyllin or trichloracetic acid but are commonly resistant to treatment. Ablation with cryotherapy (application of liquid nitrogen) and electrocryotherapy is still popular and can be effective without causing scarring.

Anal Tumors

Epidermoid carcinomas of the anus are most commonly squamous but may also be basal cell tumors. They are commoner in homosexuals and may complicate or be mistaken for anal warts. They are also associated with the HPV. Small lesions may be locally excised or ablated with photocoagulation. Surgical excision will result in removal of the sphincters and a permanent colostomy so several sphincter preserving treatment methods are now usually adopted. Chemotherapy (5-FU over 4 days with bolus mitomycin) and radiotherapy are the current mainstay of treatment.

Wide excision is necessary, however, for some of the rare anal tumors including malignant melanoma, mucinous adenocarcinoma occurring in anal canal glands (this causes recurrent anorectal fistulas), Bowen's disease and Paget's disease. Bowen's disease is squamous carcinoma in situ. It often presents with chronic pruritus and may be treated by laser photocoagulation. Paget's disease, quite unlike Paget's disease of the nipple, is an intraepithelial mucinous carcinoma which probably arises in the subepidermal apocrine glands.

Skin Conditions Affecting Perianal Skin

Conditions affecting the anal skin are often difficult to diagnose from appearance alone and are likely to need referral for a dermatological opinion and biopsy if chronic. Differential diagnoses include simple lichenification associated with chronic pruritus ani, the premalignant condition lichen *sclerosus et atrophicus*, leukoplakia, fungal infection, lichen planus or lesions of more generalized diseases such as eczema or psoriasis.

Prolapse and Solitary Rectal Ulcer Syndrome

Prolapse may involve either the full thickness of the rectal wall or prolapse just of the mucosa which may be either external or internal. Mucosal prolapse usually affects the anterior rectal wall. It is commonly internal, i.e. not presented through the anus, and is as a result commonly misdiagnosed. It results in a feeling of incomplete defecation and tenesmus which may be associated with rectal bleeding. Trauma to the mucosa may result in ulceration 6–10 cm above the anal verge, usually a single ulcer, hence "solitary rectal ulcer" but not infrequently there may be more than one ulcer. The ulcer should be biopsied and the histological appearances are characteristic. There is obliteration of the lamina propria by fibromuscular hyperplasia which streams up at right angles to the muscularis mucosae. Glands may be seen in the submucosa ("colitis cystica profunda"). Patients with solitary rectal ulcer are often accused of self-digitating or even of unusual sexual activities and subject should be approached with subtlety. It would appear that the ulcer is probably the result of a combination of local ischemia and trauma directly related to the mucosal prolapse. The perineum should be observed with the patient bearing down but if the prolapse is internal, a defecating proctogram will be necessary to demonstrate the prolapse. Surgical fixation of the posterior rectal wall is usually effective at preventing this prolapse and allowing the ulcer to heal. Medical therapies are usually ineffective although it may be worth a preliminary trial of bulking agents.

Complete prolapse (procidentia) in an adult requires surgical correction as soon as the diagnosis is made. The procedure is usually posterior fixation to the sacrum using some form of synthetic mesh but in frail or very elderly patients, the sphincters may be encircled by a strip of synthetic mesh (Thiersch procedure), a procedure which only requires two very small perineal incisions. These operations are usually effective (>90%) at preventing further prolapse but the sphincters are always weak and incontinence remains a problem in up to 50% (Figs. 5.3 and 5.4).

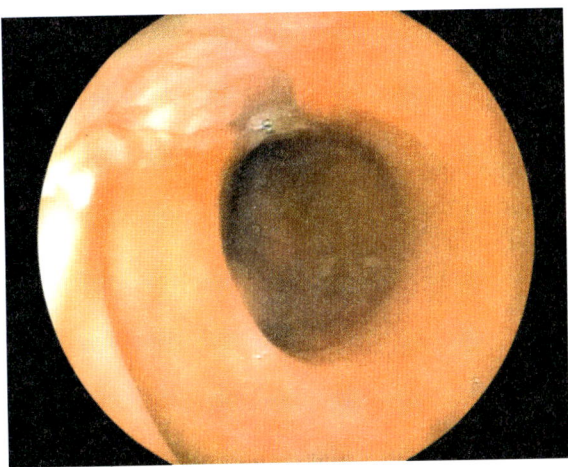

Fig. 5.3: Solitary rectal ulcer.

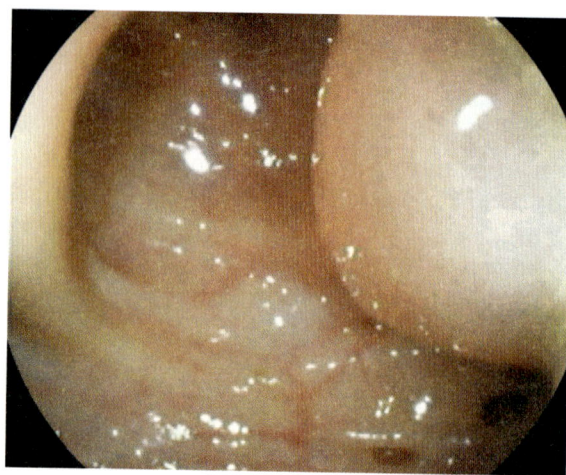

Fig. 5.4: Rectocele presents as a bulge.

Fecal Incontinence

If the feces are liquid, then the first aim should be to establish the cause and treat the diarrhea, remembering that spurious diarrhea due to severe constipation is common in the elderly. Incontinence of formed feces is a distressing condition which is often mismanaged. The obstetric history should be noted since damage to the sphincters is often the result of traumatic childbirth. The cutaneous anal reflex should be checked to exclude a neurological lesion. The anal sphincters should be checked carefully on digital examination, noting the tone, the presence of any obvious defects and the ability to contract. Sigmoidoscopy should be performed to exclude rectal carcinoma and solitary rectal ulcer. If these tests reveal no obvious abnormality, then the patient should be referred to a center specializing in anorectal problems and equipped to perform anorectal manometry and myography. Traumatic sphincter disruption usually needs surgical repair. Other cases may respond to biofeedback but surgical treatment (post-anal repair) may be effective for those with structurally intact sphincters. Electrostimulation of the sacral nerve holds some promise but its effects may not be long-lasting.

Pruritus Ani

In the absence of either local disease of the anal canal or generalized pruritus, pruritus ani is nearly always the result of imperfect local hygiene. Frequent bathing or showering supplemented by the use of impregnated tissues after evacuation will usually allow the condition to settle. Local allergic reactions to topical local anesthetic preparations may compound the problem.

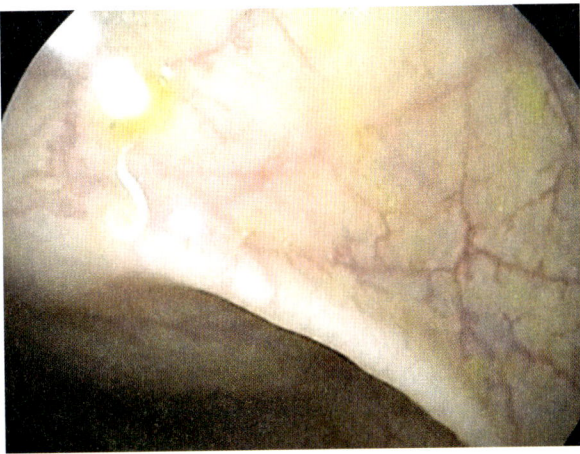

Fig. 5.5: *Enterobius vermicularis* is not uncommonly encountered at colonoscopy.

Infestation with *E. vermicularis* can cause pruritus especially at night when the female worms migrate out to lay their eggs. A sellotape test is helpful. A sticky tape is applied to the anus and put on a slide for the identification of parasite ova. A single dose of mebendazole 100 mg is highly effective but family members should also be treated (Fig. 5.5).

Proctalgia (Rectal Pain)

This is a frustrating condition for both patient and doctor. Seldom is either a cause or an effective treatment found. The solitary rectal ulcer syndrome and associated mucosal prolapse should be excluded but are usually associated with symptoms of incomplete evacuation or tenesmus. The pain is thought usually to result from spasm of the levator ani muscle. Warm baths, simple analgesia and reassurance are usually all that can be offered. In some instances, particularly if there is high anal resting pressure or fissures Botox injection can be effective. GTN ointment applied locally and calcium channel blockers can also be tried.

Coccygodynia, pain in the coccyx is a different but equally perplexing condition. The diagnosis is confirmed by pain on movement of the coccyx. Treatment is usually by injection of local anesthetic although occasionally resection of the coccyx is resorted to with rather mixed results.

Anorectal Abscess

Underlying Crohn's disease, hematological conditions such as leukemia and immune deficiency states may all be predisposing factors although most patients are otherwise healthy but develop infection in an anal crypt which then tracks along the anal ducts through the anal sphincter and then spreads. Abscesses may be (1) perianal, (2) ischiorectal, (3) intersphincteric

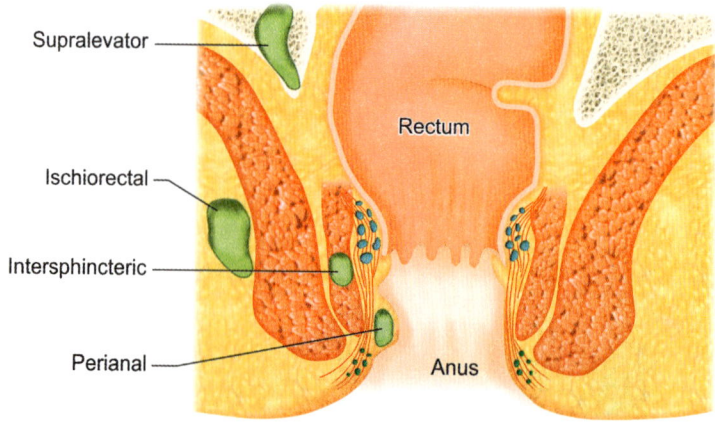

Fig. 5.6: Sites of perianal and ischiorectal abscesses.

or (4) supralevator (Fig. 5.6). Intrasphincteric or supralevator abscesses are diagnosed by digital rectal examination which reveals a tender mass. It is a general rule that all tender masses in the anorectal anatomical spaces contain pus and require drainage whether or not they are fluctuant. Delayed drainage may lead to further extension of the sepsis. It is no longer thought necessary to carry out extensive deroofing and "saucerization" so patients are usually able to return to work with little delay.

Anorectal Fistula

Fistula formation is a common complication of anorectal abscess. Anal crypt infection spreads internally along a track, forming an abscess as described earlier, and when this abscess drains to the exterior, a fistula is inevitable unless the original track from the anal crypt to the abscess has sealed off. The treatment is usually surgical but depends on two factors: (1) the site of the proximal opening and (2) the presence or absence of Crohn's disease.

Magnetic resonance imaging is an invaluable tool in appraising the state of perianal Crohn's disease. This would greatly help the surgeon. An examination under anesthetic will often be necessary to determine the site of the proximal opening although a low track will usually be palpable as a thick cord running toward the anal canal from the internal opening. If there is a fistula, then the surgeon can probe it and insert a loose suture or "seton." This seton keeps the fistula draining and this allows eventual healing. Patients tolerate this remarkably well and may be kept in for many months. Therapy with anti-tumor necrosis factor is indicated. The best evidence for healing of perianal Crohn's is with treatment with infliximab. Nutrition must also be optimized as it will promote healing. Once good healing is achieved, this seton may be removed.

Surgery should be as conservative as possible and damage to anal sphincter is minimized best by specialist surgeons. The standard surgical approach to fistulas can be disastrous in Crohn's disease, resulting in extensive

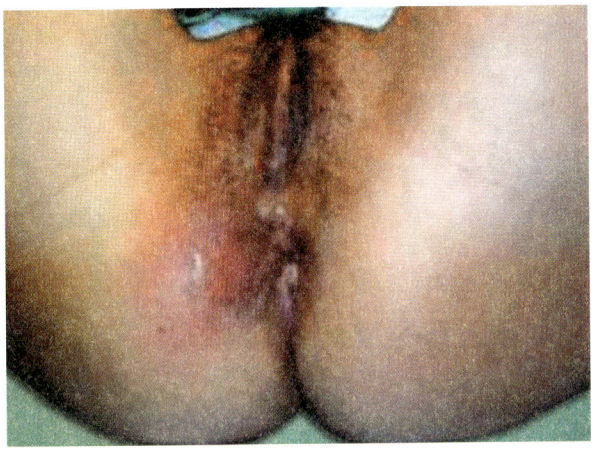

Fig. 5.7: Crohn's disease with scarring from fistulations.

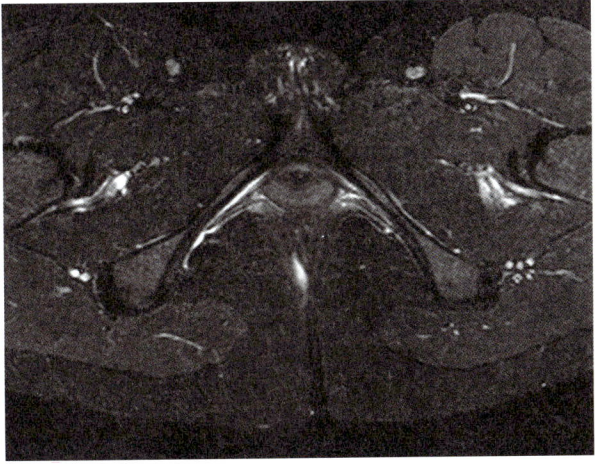

Fig. 5.8: Magnetic resonance imaging is a valuable tool in assessing perianal disease.

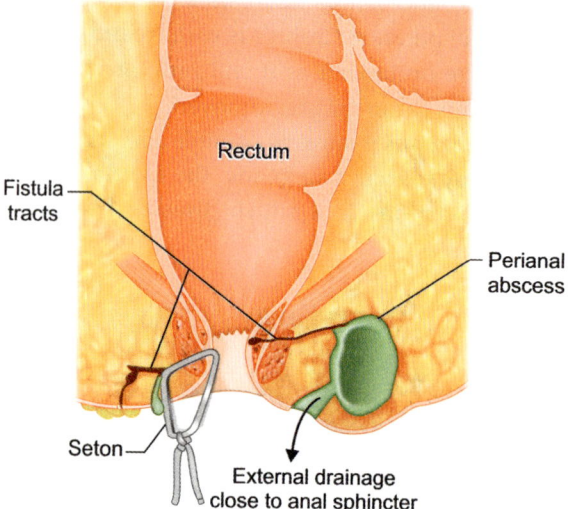

Fig. 5.9: Seton insertion.

perianal infection without granulation or healing. In Crohn's disease, treatment should be as conservative as possible (Figs. 5.7 to 5.9).

■ FURTHER READING

1. Sun Z, Migaly J. Review of hemorrhoid disease: presentation and management. Clin Colon Rectal Surg. 2016;29(1): 22-9.

CHAPTER 6

Gastrointestinal Bleeding and Anemia

Her Hsin Tsai

■ REACHING A DIAGNOSIS AND MANAGEMENT

When a patient appears with acute gastrointestinal (GI) bleeding, it is important to start treatment even before a clear diagnosis has been made. Hence, the general principles and approach to such a patient is one of initial assessments and managements, which has to be performed together. Acute GI bleeding usually occurs from either the upper GI tract presenting as hematemesis and melena or less commonly from the lower GI tract which would present with bright red rectal bleeding. But severe hemorrhage from the upper GI tract can also appear as fresh bleeding per rectum.

The first step in the assessment and management of patients is to ask if there is significant GI bleeding. The patient may present with hematemesis which is vomiting of either bright red blood or altered blood. Altered blood may be described as "coffee grounds". Melena is the passage of black, tarry and sticky stools. Hematochezia is the passage of bright red blood per rectum.

Severe GI bleeding can present with hypotensive shock without external evidence of bleeding or the signs may be delayed. Bleeding from perforated viscus or aortic aneurysm may present with abdominal pain and hypotensive shock. Several caveats should be borne in mind:

- Patients with hemoptysis may be confused with hematemesis. If in doubt it is worth asking the patient to cough up to see whether the bleeding is from genuine hemoptysis rather than hematemesis.
- Swallowed blood from nose bleeding can also cause confusion.
- Patients who vomit from any cause may have small amounts of coffee grounds in the vomitus which may be alarming but is usually harmless.
- Recent ingestion of iron or bismuth compounds, licorice, certain beers like stout and spinach may cause very dark motions and mimic melena.

If it is clear that there is significant evidence of a GI bleed, then clinical assessment can be made quite quickly and efficiently using one of several validated scoring systems. The most widely used scoring systems are the Rockall score and Blatchford score (Table 6.1 and Fig. 6.1).

Table 6.1: Rockall score has two parts, the initial clinical assessment and the endoscopic score. SRH = stigmata of recent hemorrhage.

Variable	Score 0	1	2	3
Age	<60	60–79	>80	
Shock	"No shock," systolic BP ≥100 pulse < 100	"Tachycardia," systolic BP ≥100 pulse ≥100	"Hypotension," systolic BP <100	
Comorbidity	No major comorbidity		Cardiac failure, ischemic heart disease, any major comorbidity	Renal failure, liver failure, disseminated malignancy
Diagnosis	Mallory–Weiss tear, no lesion identified and no SRH	All other diagnoses	Malignancy of upper GI tract	
Major SRH	None or dark spot only		Blood in upper GI tract, adherent clot, visible or spurting vessel	

(SRH: Stigmata of recent hemorrhage; BP: Blood pressure; GI: Gastrointestinal)

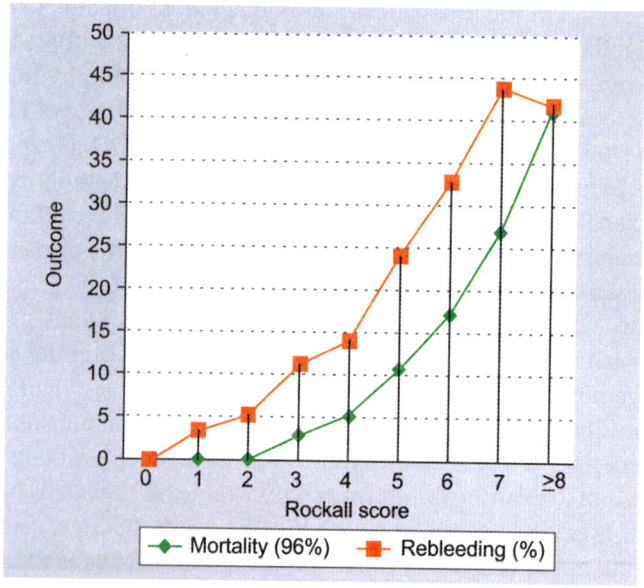

Fig. 6.1: The Rockall score is a good predictor of mortality and rebleeding from upper GI bleeds. (GI: Gastrointestinal.)

Table 6.2: The Blatchford score allows for quick clinical assessment of patients to screen for patients who need urgent endoscopy from those who can be delayed or discharged. Those who have a score of zero have a very low risk and can be discharged.

Admission risk marker	Score
Blood urea mmol/L	
≥6.5–7.9	2
8–9.9	3
10–24.9	4
≥25	6
Hemoglobin g/dL (men)	
≥12–13	1
10–11.9	3
<10	6
Hemoglobin g/dL (women)	
≥10–12	1
<10	6
Systolic blood pressure mm Hg	
100–109	1
90–99	2
<90	3
Other markers	
Pulse ≥100	1
Presentation with melena	1
Presentation with syncope	2
Hepatic disease	2
Cardiac failure	2

The Rockall score has two parts, the first part on clinical parameters and the second part with the addition of endoscopic findings. The Blatchford score is purely a clinical scoring system (Table 6.2).

Both scoring systems depend on measurements of vital signs, systolic blood pressure, pulse and the presence of comorbidity. The Blatchford score has additional laboratory parameters of hemoglobin and urea included as well. No scoring system is perfect and both these scoring systems have their shortcomings. Certainly, the most important skill a physician should acquire is the ability to identify the really ill patients who require immediate resuscitation and stabilization from those who have more trivial symptoms, who may well be suitable for discharge.

The Blatchford score is probably the better score for identifying patients who require urgent endoscopy from those whom endoscopy can be postponed, while the full Rockall score including endoscopic score is valuable for predicting overall severity and likely morbidity and mortality from the GI bleed. Hence, it is best to use the Blatchford score at initial assessment and the Rockall score after endoscopy.

Stabilization

The first priority is to ensure that the patient's hemodynamic status is restored. An intravenous line should be established. The patient's hemoglobin, platelet count and prothrombin times should be checked along with urea and electrolytes. A sample should also be sent for cross-matching of blood.

If the patient is deemed to have significant hypotension and/or significant cardiovascular comorbidity or renal or liver failure, then the risks are high and the patient should be managed in a high dependency or an intensive care unit. Immediate resuscitation with crystalloid fluids like 0.9% sodium chloride or colloids should be started. Patients should also be given supplementary oxygen via a nasal cannula and be kept nil by mouth. If the patient remains hemodynamically unstable despite resuscitation with crystalloids, then blood should be given. Transfusion should be used with caution and a conservative policy should be implemented. Patients who are at high risk should have transfusion if the hemoglobin on admission is <90 g/L (9 g/dL) or <70 g/L (7 g/dL) in patients who are at low risk. It is particularly important to avoid over-transfusion in patients with known gastroesophageal variceal bleeding. Patients with coagulopathy should be corrected with fresh-frozen plasma and patients on warfarin should have consideration for reversal.

Patients should be kept under close monitoring either in a high dependency area or intensive care unit and blood pressure and pulse should be closely monitored.

History and Examination

After stabilization of the patient, a detailed history and examination should be taken. It is important to get a detailed medical history, in particular, history of previous GI hemorrhage, history of previous varices, portal hypertension, peptic ulcer disease, angiodysplasia or malignancy of the GI tract. It is also important to get their history of medication, in particular the use of nonsteroidal drugs, aspirin and antiplatelet agents like clopidogrel. These drugs can cause peptic ulceration and platelet inhibitors would encourage hemorrhage. Anticoagulants like warfarin and directly acting oral anticoagulants (DOACs) increase the severity of GI bleeding. Bismuth products and iron cause black stools which can be confused with melena.

Patients should be examined carefully. Apart from the vital signs, the following signs may help point to a diagnosis:
- Signs of liver disease or portal hypertension (spider nevi, jaundice, ascites and evidence of chronic alcohol use, e.g. parotid swelling)
- Skin lesions like vasculitis, hemangiomas and telangiectasias
- Previous GI surgery: scars in abdomen
- The presence of tender pulsatile aortic aneurysm.

Where is the Bleeding?

Hematemesis is nearly always from a lesion that is proximal to the ligament of Treitz. Melena could occur from lesions beyond that including the small bowel, Meckel's diverticulum or even the colon. Conversely, the passage of bright red rectal bleeding may result from very brisk bleeding from the upper GI tract and not necessarily from a colonic source. Hence, it is important to establish if the bleeding is indeed from the upper GI tract. Passage of a nasogastric tube has been advocated but studies have shown no evidence of its benefit. If a nasogastric tube is already in situ as in many ICU patients, then aspiration can be helpful. However, placing of a nasogastric tube in a patient admitted with possible upper GI bleeding is usually unhelpful. It is far more beneficial for patients to go for early endoscopy if that is available.

Upper GI Endoscopy

Upper GI endoscopy is the diagnostic modality of choice when it comes to GI bleeding. Patients with high-risk scores should go for early endoscopy. This is particularly true for patients with risk factors, the elderly and those who have suspected gastroesophageal varices. Patients with a low-risk score can have the endoscopy at the next available list preferably within 24 h of admission.

Endoscopy should be carried out by experienced endoscopists as it involves not only the ability to perform endoscopy in difficult conditions where visibility can be obscured by clots and blood but also skills are required to perform adequate hemostasis. If the endoscopy is hampered by a great deal of clots and blood, the source of the bleeding may be difficult to find. In this situation, it may be advantageous to give a dose of intravenous erythromycin and re-endoscope the patient at a later time or the next day. Erythromycin helps clear the stomach by its ability to stimulate gastric emptying. Metoclopramide is an alternative.

Very often endoscopy takes place after several days of melena and endoscopy may be entirely normal. Minor lesions like a small Mallory–Weiss tear or a small ulcer may have completely healed and vascular bleeding may no longer be apparent. If the patient is stable and there is no further evidence of bleeding, then a wait and see policy is perfectly acceptable. However, if the bleeding persists and there is still evidence of GI bleeding, then a whole number of possible imaging modalities may be used depending on the circumstances. If the bleeding is quite profuse, then angiography is probably the preferred modality as it can both identify the source and embolize the source of bleeding. Computed tomography (CT) scanning can be helpful. Capsule endoscopy; enteroscopy and colonoscopy virtually covers the entire

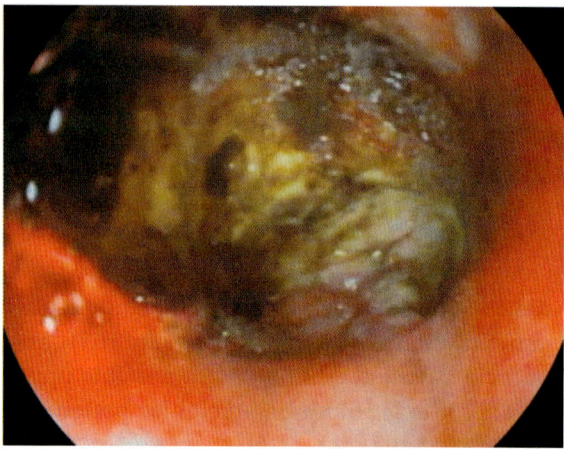

Fig. 6.2: Deep excavated ulcer that is actively bleeding from an eroded vessel at its base.

GI tract for possible causes of bleeding. The choice of test will depend on the clinical suspicion and circumstances (Fig. 6.2).

99mTc Pertechnetate Scanning for Meckel's Diverticulum

In children and young adults with melena, Meckel's diverticulum may be suspected. Meckel's diverticulum may occasionally contain gastric type mucosa which can ulcerate and bleed. Gastric mucosa concentrates the isotope 99mTc pertechnetate. However, bleeding from Meckel's diverticulum is extremely rare in people over the age of 40.

Colonoscopy

In the older patient in whom upper GI bleeding sources have been excluded, a colonoscopy may well be indicated. Colonic cancer, particularly lesions in the cecum and angiodysplasia are important lesions to exclude. A thorough bowel preparation is required if the colonoscopy is to succeed, hence a bowel washout using polyethylene glycol (PEG) solutions usually combine with a stimulant laxative is required to achieve good bowel cleansing. It is best to delay the colonoscopy until the patient is stable as it can be quite invasive. Large lesions like a tumor would easily be picked up on colonoscopy but small lesions like angiodysplasia may be difficult to pick up. Angiodysplastic lesions can be coagulated with argon plasma coagulator (APC) if found and colonic tumors can be biopsied. Colonoscopy is still the investigation of choice if fresh rectal bleeding is the presenting symptom (Fig. 6.3).

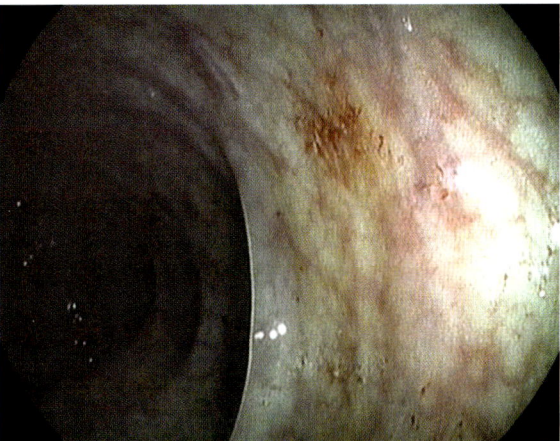

Fig. 6.3: Angiodysplasia in colon can be subtle and best seen on enhanced colonoscopy (i-scan).

Enteroscopy

Enteroscopes are capable of reaching low into the jejunum and some devices like double balloon enteroscopes can achieve deep penetration into the small intestine. However, in an acute setting, they are usually of limited benefit and they are more useful for diagnosing obscure GI bleeds.

Capsule Endoscopy

Capsule endoscopy involves swallowing a pill-shaped capsule which contains a camera and a radio transmitter. The pill is swallowed and the pictures are transmitted out to a radio receiver strapped on the abdomen. Because it may take several hours for the capsule to reach the colon, there is sophisticated software available to highlight possible lesions in the gut. Capsule endoscopy is also not particularly helpful in an acute setting and it is probably better used as a tool for diagnosing an obscure GI bleed in a patient with persistent anemia. It is neither able to precisely define the site of any lesions detected nor is it able to affect any therapy.

Angiography

Interventional vascular radiology is an important contributor to the management of a GI bleed. Not only is it able to identify the source of bleeding; coils which help embolize the vessels can be deployed. It is less invasive than open surgery and therefore particularly helpful in patients with major comorbidities.

Investigating Anemia

The first step in investigating anemia should always be an assessment of a full blood count and blood film. It is also very valuable to check their historical results to look at any patterns in the anemia over the course of time. The full blood count includes the mean corpuscular of volume (MCV) which would inform as to whether the cells are large (macrocytosis) or small (microcytosis).

If there is macrocytosis, then serum folate levels and B12 levels should be measured. A low B12 would indicate probable pernicious anemia and blood checks for an intrinsic factor can be helpful. There are other GI causes for low B12 including previous small bowel surgery of the terminal ileum and bacterial overgrowth.

If the anemia is normocytic, then hematinics including ferritin, iron and iron-binding capacity as well as B12 and folate should all be checked but it is usually due to anemia of chronic disease like renal failure and rheumatological conditions. However, if no clear explanation is found hematological referral may be indicated.

When the anemia is microcytic, it is usually caused by iron deficiency in Northern European patients. In races where there is a high incidence of hemoglobinopathies like thalassemia, it should be checked for. Fecal occult blood testing is of very little value as bleeding is often intermittent and it cannot exclude GI blood loss.

It is important to have a detailed history of drug use. Aspirin, antiplatelet agents in patients who have had recent cardiovascular intervention like angioplasty and stenting often result in a mild chronic anemia. This could be caused by small ulcerations and bleeding from the GI tract caused by these drugs. Another common cause is celiac disease which can affect up to 1% of the population of Northern European extraction. Blood testing of celiac antibodies can be performed. The usual antibody is the anti-TTG (anti-tissue transglutaminase antibody). This is an IgA antibody. Another IgA antibody that is commonly used is the anti-endomysial antibody (EMA). However, up to 10% of celiac patients are IgA deficient. An IgG antibody is available but it is usual to just measure the IgA levels along with the standard antibody assays. If the IgA levels are adequate and the anti-TTG and EMA are negative, then celiac disease is unlikely. If the patient is IgA deficient, then endoscopic biopsies is the only way to exclude celiac disease.

Probably the best investigation for chronic iron deficiency anemia is a combination of upper GI endoscopy and colonoscopy which can be performed at the same sitting. At upper GI endoscopy, duodenal biopsies can be taken if there is a high suspicion of celiac disease. Iron deficiency anemia is often a presenting symptom of colonic cancer, particularly cecal cancer. Hence, it is vital to carry out a full colonoscopy in a well-prepared bowel (Fig. 6.4).

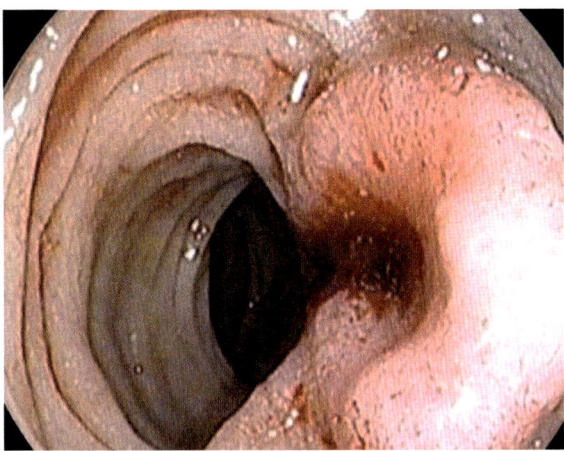

Fig. 6.4: Colon cancer with an ulcerated center that is bleeding. Acute hemorrhage is very unusual and anemia is a common presenting symptom.

Iron deficiency usually signifies significant pathology, and the presence of a hiatus hernia, small duodenal ulcer or diverticular disease cannot be assumed to be the cause of the anemia. Cancers or lymphoma of the GI tract, chronic nonsteroidal use, aspirins, antiplatelet medication, celiac disease, small bowel diverticulosis (leading to intestinal bacterial overgrowth), esophageal varices and inflammatory bowel disease are other possible causes of anemia.

CONDITIONS CAUSING GI BLEEDING: NATURAL HISTORY AND MANAGEMENT

Bleeding Peptic Ulcer

Natural History

The incidence of peptic ulcers of the stomach and duodenum has been decreasing in recent years in developed countries. This is probably related to the reduced incidence of *Helicobacter pylori* infection rates and increased eradication of the bacterium when detected. Although one would expect a similar decrease in the incidence of complications of duodenal ulcer disease, such as bleeding, this fall is relatively modest and does not parallel the fall in the overall incidence of duodenal ulcer disease. This is probably due to the persistent high level of use of nonsteroidal anti-inflammatory agents (NSAIDs), aspirin and other antiplatelet agents. Furthermore, the patients being admitted with bleeding peptic ulcer are increasingly in the older age groups. Of the patients admitted to emergency departments with a GI bleed, some 60% are over the age of 60 years and 20% over the age of 80 years.

Table 6.3: Relative risk of upper GI bleeding in individuals taking NSAIDs.		
NSAIDs	Relative risk (95% CI)	
Celecoxib	1.0 (0.4–2.1)	Low
Diclofenac	3.1 (2.3–4.2)	
Ibuprofen	4.1 (3.1–5.2)	
Naproxen	7.3 (4.7–11.4)	
Ketoprofen	8.6 (2.5–29.2)	
Indomethacin	9.0 (3.9–20.7)	
Meloxicam	9.8 (4.0–23.8)	
Piroxicam	12.6 (7.8–20.3)	High

Source: Adapted from: Lanas A, Garcia-Rodriguez LA, Arroyo MT, et al. Am J Gastroenterol. 2007;102:507–15.
(GI: Gastrointestinal; NSAIDs: Nonsteroidal anti-inflammatory drugs)

The use of nonsteroidal drugs is associated with a higher risk of both bleeding and perforation, and concomitant use of aspirin is associated with an even greater risk. This risk is dose related and drug related (Table 6.3). Furthermore, the risk appears to be highest during the first 30 days of non-steroidal use.

Helicobacter pylori Infection

The causal relationship between peptic ulcer disease and *H. pylori* is now well established. Furthermore, *H. pylori* significantly increase the risk of bleeding from duodenal ulcers but curiously not gastric ulcers. So, in a setting of bleeding duodenal ulcers, it is wise to eradicate the *Helicobacter* when identified.

However, testing for *H. pylori* during an acute bleeding situation can be difficult for several reasons. Biopsies taken during endoscopy using the rapid urease test can be unreliable and patients are often already put on a proton pump inhibitor (PPI) and that may reduce the sensitivity of these tests by inhibiting *H. pylori* urease production. The priority is to stabilize the patient and therefore the patient should be kept on a PPI and should not be withdrawn just purely for *H. pylori* testing. Probably, the best test in this situation is a stool test as it is highly sensitive for detecting *H. pylori* antigen, whether the bacterium is alive or killed.

Aspirin, non-steroidal drugs and *H. pylori* account for the majority of bleeding peptic ulcer diseases. Peptic ulcer disease in the absence of either *H. pylori* or non-steroidal use usually occurs in severely ill patients who have serious comorbidities like renal failure usually in an intensive care setting. Despite modern pharmacological and endoscopic treatment, the mortality from bleeding peptic ulcer disease remains persistently high (9–11%), largely due to increased age and severity of comorbidities of the patient.

Management

The treatment of acutely bleeding duodenal ulcer is a combination of pharmacological and endoscopic treatment largely. When endoscopic treatment fails, then interventional radiology in the form of angiography with/without embolization and surgery may be required.

Endoscopy, Stratification of Severity and Treatment

The initial assessment of patients with bleeding comes from endoscopy. If an ulcer is found on endoscopy, then the Forrest classification of the ulcer is a good predictor of the likelihood of rebleeding from the ulcer. The risk of rebleeding is higher than 50% if any of the following findings are seen on endoscopy: active bleeding (spurting or oozing vessel), adherent blood clot and a visible vessel. Mortality rises considerably up to 20% for patients with a rebleed and the elderly are particularly vulnerable and those with major comorbidities like cancer and renal failure (Table 6.4, Figs. 6.5 and 6.6).

Table 6.4: Risks of rebleeding can be ascertained by the endoscopic appearance of the ulcer.

Forrest classification	Endoscopic finding	Rebleeding rate (%)
Class Ia	Spurting hemorrhage	60
Class Ib	Oozing hemorrhage	30
Class IIa	Non-bleeding visible vessel	30
Class IIb	Adherent clot	20
Class IIc	Flat pigmented spot	<10
Class III	Clean ulcer base	<2

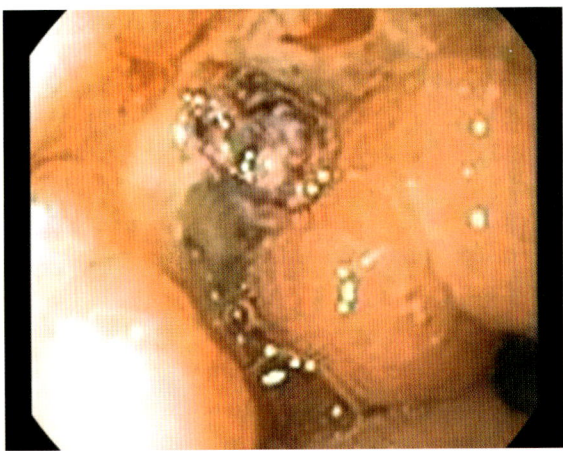

Fig. 6.5: Duodenal ulcer with large aneurysmal vessel has a high risk of rebleeding (30%).

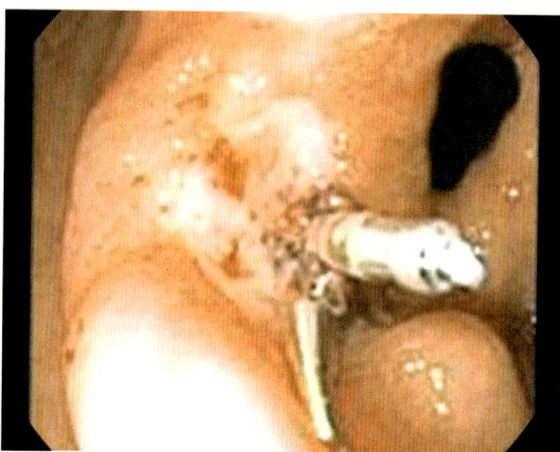

Fig. 6.6: Application of clips can reduce rebleeding risk.

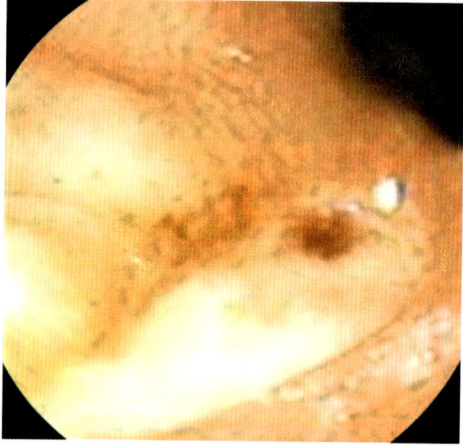

Fig. 6.7: Clean base with a pigmented spot Forrest 2B has a <10% rebleeding tendency.

However, patients with a clean ulcer base with no stigmata or recent hemorrhage at all have a very low risk of rebleeding (Fig. 6.7).

The stratification of the risk using the Rockall score after endoscopy is a good predictor of patients who are safe to be discharged on oral PPIs and those requiring closer supervision. Increasingly, patients presenting with GI bleed from ulcer disease tend to be elderly or have major comorbidities.

Endoscopic Therapy

Various treatment modalities are available to the endoscopist and during the initial endoscopy treatment can be given to those patients with a high risk of rebleeding. This includes patients with active spurting vessels, active oozing or a visible vessel. The methods of treatment include injection usually with adrenaline, application of heat either with a heater probe or diathermy device or the use of hemostatic clips. Usually, a combination of two of these modalities is advised but it depends on the availability and experience of the operator. In general, thermal methods like heat probes or diathermy or clips are better than adrenaline injections alone. However, because adrenaline causes vasoconstriction and stops the bleeding, it can make the field cleaner and blood-free to allow the endoscopist to apply a more definitive therapy like heater probe or hemostatic clips more accurately. Hence, a useful strategy is to inject with adrenaline, wash the area with a water-jet and apply thermal coagulation or clips. Other methods of hemostasis, like "hemospray" which is a fine adhesive powder, are being trialed and may well come into standard practice.

When the patients are identified as high risk or with a risk of rebleeding, treatment with intravenous PPI is indicated. Based on the earlier trials, the current practice is to give intravenous PPIs as a bolus doses rather than an IV infusion for 72 h. Both omeprazole and pantoprazole are available for IV use. Where immediate endoscopy is not available, it may be reasonable to give IV PPIs overnight until endoscopy is available the following day. Recent studies have compared oral with IV dosing and suggest that oral therapy, which is cheaper, may be equally good.

When there is Rebleeding

If despite initial endoscopic therapy and intravenous PPIs, the patient bleeds again, then there is a high risk of mortality. In this situation, it may be worth having another look with endoscope and to attempt further therapy. Posterior duodenal ulcers, very large ulcers and ulcers in the gastric lesser curve are associated with higher risk of rebleeding. Patients with multiple comorbidities or on non-steroidal drugs or anticoagulants have also higher risk and should be managed in a high dependency setting.

Predictors of rebleeding

- Endoscopic findings
- Location of the ulcer (post-DU, high lesser curve)
- Age >60
- Shock/anemia on admission
- Size of the ulcer.

Interventional Radiology

Angiography along with transarterial embolization is an increasingly valuable technique in patients with recurrent peptic ulcer bleeding. This is best done in a setting where endoscopic therapy has failed, and surgery may be considered high risk. Interventional radiology is also valuable for embolizing

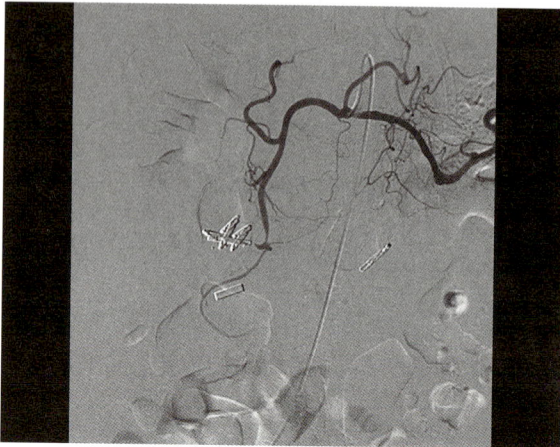

Fig. 6.8: When endoscopy fails to stop the bleeding, angiography can be used. Here, the vessel shows signs of persistent bleeding. Note the clips left by the endoscopist's attempts at arresting the bleed at endoscopy.

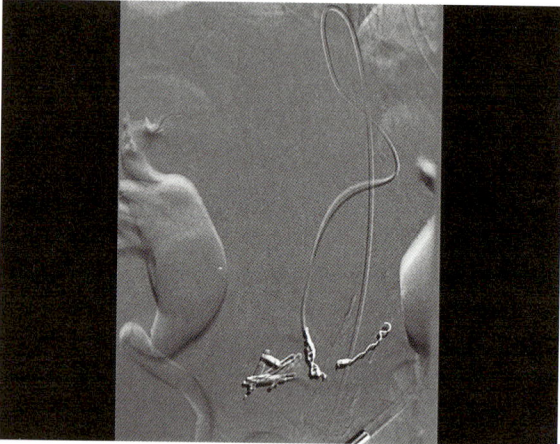

Fig. 6.9: The vascular radiologist then placed several coils to successfully embolize the bleeding vessel.

vessels that are not accessible to the endoscopist like bleeding from biliary tree or pancreatic duct or vessels in the less accessible parts of the GI tract (Figs. 6.8 and 6.9).

Surgery

When endoscopic treatment fails and a patient has further bleeding and in situations where interventional radiology is not easily available, surgery may be the only option available. It is now usually performed when two attempts of endoscopic therapy have failed to stop the bleeding or when angiographic methods are not available or have been unsuccessful. When the decision to perform surgery is made, it is important not to delay and it should be performed as promptly as possible. Usually, surgery involves over-sewing of bleeding vessel but sometimes surgeons can often perform vagotomy and pyloroplasty as well or a partial gastrectomy, but the exact type of surgery will depend on the clinical and surgical findings.

Aftercare

After acute bleed is arrested, patient should be fed as early enteral nutrition is important. If *H. pylori* fecal antigen is detected, then treatment with eradication therapy is indicated as soon as practical. NSAIDs should be avoided and this is usually possible with better rheumatological input. However, it remains true that aspirin and antiplatelet therapy is lifesaving, particularly in the context of recent myocardial event or intervention, such as coronary angioplasty and stenting. In this situation, the early reintroduction of antiplatelet treatment is beneficial as it reduces the overall mortality despite the slight increased risk of rebleeding.

OTHER CAUSES OF NON-VARICEAL UPPER GI BLEEDING

Gastric and Duodenal Erosions

Severe gastric erosions with the development of hemorrhagic lesions with often superficial looking mucosal injury can be either due to drugs like non-steroidal drugs or alcohol or mucosal ischemia and tissue hypoxia seen in trauma, burns and other sepsis. Some chemotherapeutic agents may also cause severe gastric erosion. Curling's ulcers are described in severe burns and these ulcers are also found in patients with severe central nervous system injuries.

Treatment involves the management of their primary medical condition and the withdrawal of erosive agents like alcohol and nonsteroidal drugs or chemotherapeutic agents. Bleeding is often widespread and is not amenable to endoscopic management. Treatment is largely medical and the use of PPIs is usually used though evidence of its benefit is sketchy.

Mallory–Weiss Tear

Mallory–Weiss tears are induced by vomiting. It is particularly associated with alcohol ingestion. It presents with one or more longitudinal tears along the gastric cardia just below the squamocolumnar junction. Sometimes, it extends proximally to the lower esophagus and in severe cases may entirely rupture the esophagus (Boerhaave's syndrome). Similar lacerations of the lower esophagus can occasionally be due to medical instrumentation like endoscopic echosonography. A hiatus hernia is frequently found. In the majority of cases,

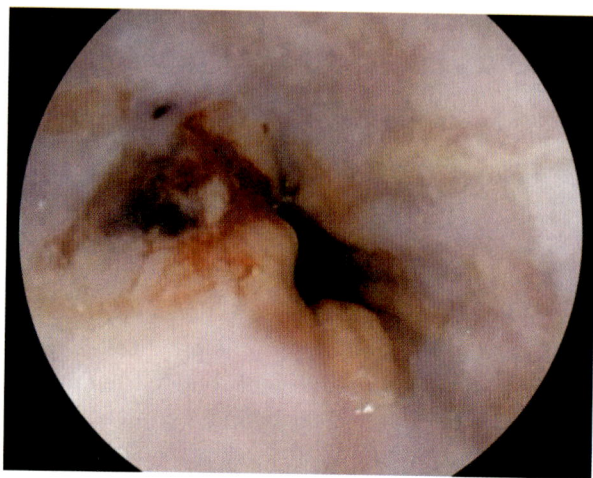

Fig. 6.10: Bleeding from a Mallory–Weiss tear can be severe, although trivial bleeds are more common.

the bleeding is trivial and the lesion heals spontaneously and if endoscopy is carried out after an interval of a few days, it will often be completely healed. A history of prior vomiting of gastric contents initially or retching initially followed by hematemesis can usually be obtained.

The majority of these Mallory-Weiss type bleeds are relatively minor and do not require any active management. If it is found on endoscopy to be actively bleeding, then it can be managed with an injection of adrenaline and if necessary, together with application of a thermal method like heated probe or diathermy. Use of endoscopic clips is also very attractive as it pulls the bleeding edges together. Surgery is very rarely required unless there is a full thickness tear in the lower esophagus (Fig. 6.10).

Dieulafoy's Lesion

This is a rare syndrome where there is unusual prominence of submucosal artery at the fundus of stomach. Angiographically, it looks like a corkscrew that terminates on the mucosa and usually there is a small ulceration at that point and severe bleeding can occur. This is arterial bleeding and thus very brisk and because it is in the fundus, usually underneath a big pool of blood it can be very difficult to locate endoscopically. Endoscopists should be vigilant of a possibility and if a clear bleeding source is not found, a close examination of fundus should be made. When located, the lesion is usually easily treated endoscopically with either hemostatic clips, injection with adrenaline and/or other thermal methods. When an endoscopy fails to locate the bleeding, then angiography is helpful and can locate the bleeding lesion and coils may be deployed to embolize the vessel very effectively (Figs. 6.11 to 6.14).

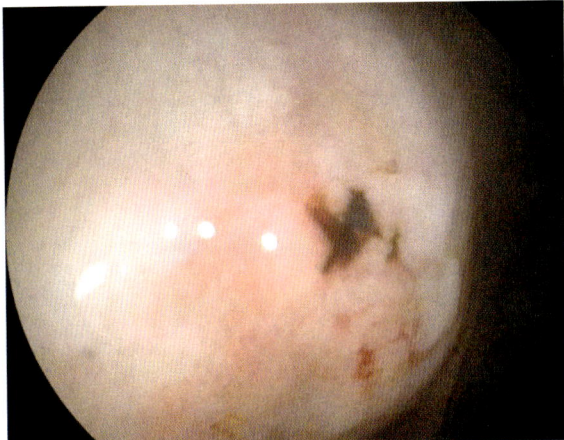

Fig. 6.11: On endoscopy a Dieulafoy lesion can be hard to spot, usually in the body or fundus of the stomach.

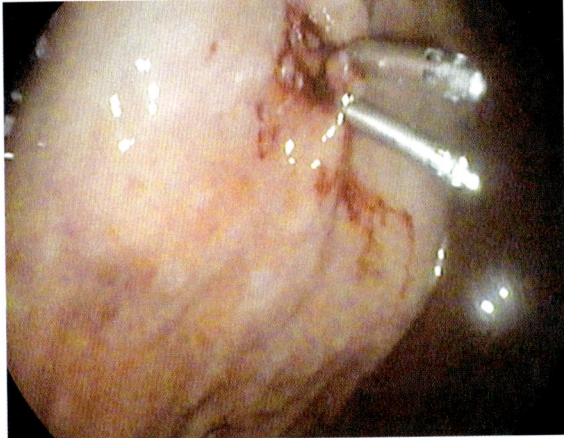

Fig. 6.12: This lesion was treated with hemostatic clips.

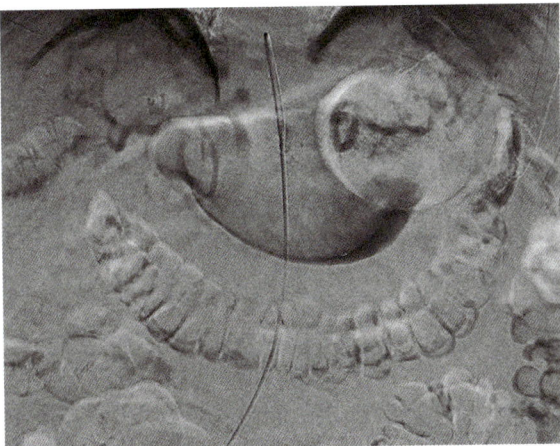

Fig. 6.13: Angiography is often required to identify the lesion.

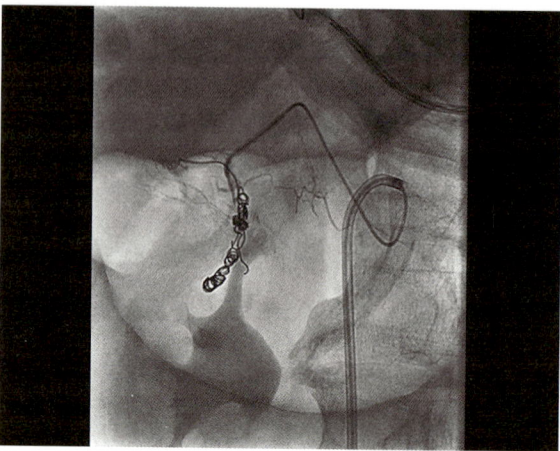

Fig. 6.14: Angiography is often required to identify Dieulafoy lesions and coils placed to achieve hemostasis.

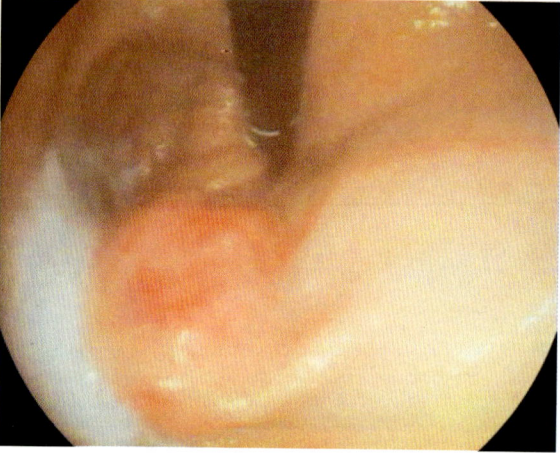

Fig. 6.15: Gastrointestinal stromal tumors in the stomach are often found incidentally but can rarely cause acute GI bleeding. (GI: Gastrointestinal.)

Gastrointestinal Stromal Tumors

Gastrointestinal stromal tumors (GIST) can be found in the stomach along with less common true leiomyomas. GIST in the stomach tend to extend out of the stomach, while leiomyomas tend to extend intraluminally and appear as a bulbous lesion, sometimes within apical crater or ulcer. These lesions can occasionally bleed. When found in the context of an upper GI bleed, it is often treated in the standard fashion for the initial control of bleeding but serious consideration has to be made for surgical resection of these tumors as rebleeding is common and possibility of malignant transformation exists. If found as an incidental finding, small lesions are probably best just observed or endoscopically removed but larger lesions should be assessed for possible malignant transformation (Fig. 6.15).

Gastric Lymphoma

Gastric lymphoma can very rarely present with an acute GI bleed. It is important to recognize that the lesion is malignant and biopsies are carried out. Larger tumors should probably be assessed by endoscopic ultrasound (EUS) and CT scanning. It can sometimes bleed acutely. Treatment depends on the site of bleeding. Often there is bleeding from a wide ulcerated areas, and control of bleeding can be difficult. Hemospray may be helpful in this situation. Treatment is usually by chemoradiotherapy (Figs. 6.16 to 6.18).

Aortoenteric Fistulae

Bleeding into the small intestine from an abdominal aortic aneurysm may occasionally occur without prior surgery but is more commonly a

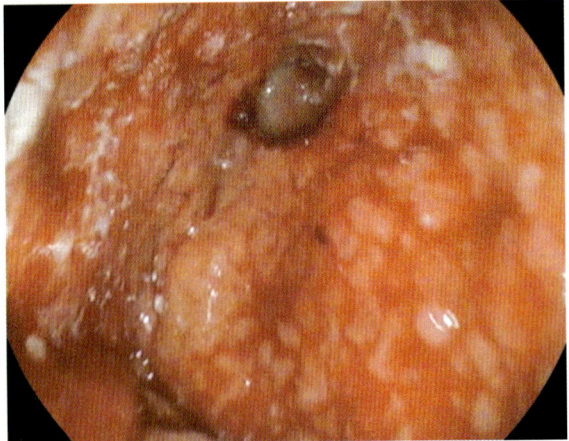

Fig. 6.16: This bulky lesion with bleeding surfaces was a gastric lymphoma.

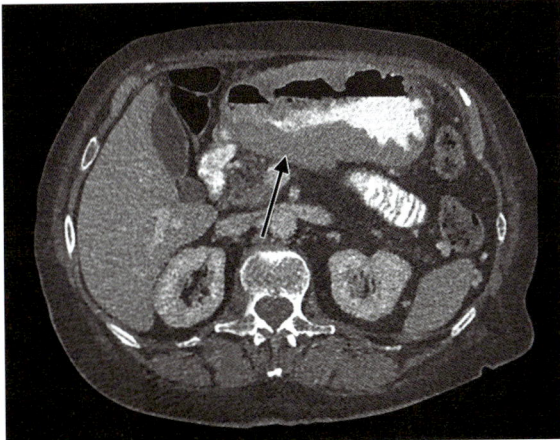

Fig. 6.17: Computed tomography scan shows a grossly thickened gastric body and enlarged lymph nodes of above patient with gastric lymphoma.

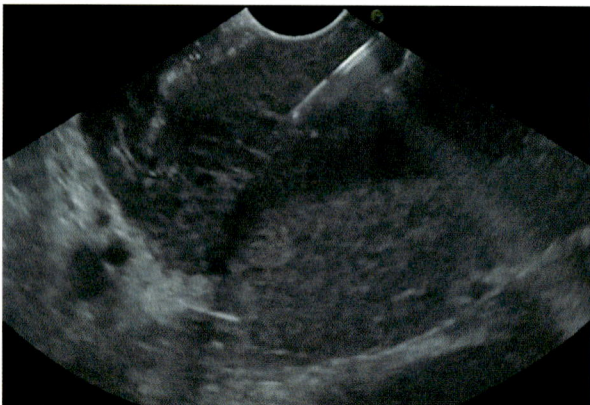

Fig. 6.18: Sampling of deeper layers with EUS is often helpful. (EUS: Endoscopic ultrasound.)

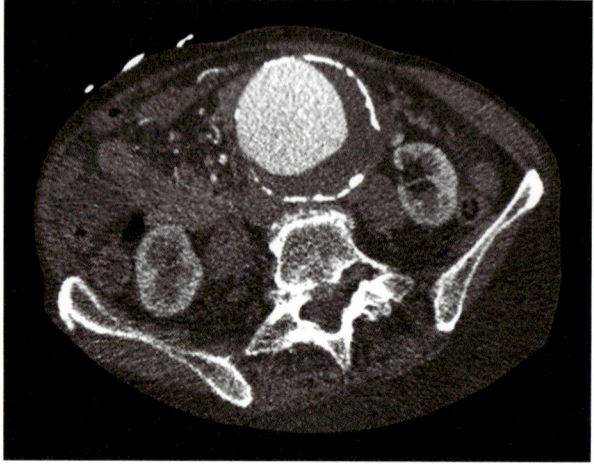

Fig. 6.19: Large abdominal aortic aneurysms can erode into the duodenum.

complication of previous aortic aneurysm repair. There may be back pain from the expanding aneurysm but it is more commonly painless. Bleeding is often massive but may surprisingly be self-limiting. If a patient with a known aortic aneurysm has upper GI hemorrhage and a normal gastroscopy, it should be assumed that the bleeding is coming from the aneurysm. Endoscopy of the distal duodenum may reveal blood but is unlikely to show the actual bleeding site. Angiography may be hazardous and is often unhelpful unless the patient is actively bleeding. CT scanning is the best investigation and may occasionally show gas within the wall of the aortic graft indicating infection by gas-forming organisms which is the usual cause of graft failure. Surgical correction is however a major undertaking and carries a mortality of approximately 50% (Fig. 6.19).

Esophageal Varices

Esophageal varices account for about 10% of admissions with upper GI bleeding but it varies according to prevalence of portal hypertension and in particular alcohol ingestion in the community. It accounts for approximately a third of all deaths from liver cirrhosis.

Etiology and Pathogenesis of Portal Hypertension

Normal portal pressure is about 10 mm Hg but rises to 20–40 mm Hg in portal hypertension. The causes of portal hypertension may be classified as:
- Presinusoidal (i.e. the portal venous side of the liver)
- Sinusoidal
- Postsinusoidal (on the hepatic side of the liver) (Fig. 6.20).

The distinctions of the three different groups can be made using imaging and hepatic vein pressure measurement.

Presinusoidal Portal Hypertension

In this situation where the pressure is raised before the sinusoids, the hepatic vein pressure is low or normal. It may be low because there is reduced flow of blood into the liver. The major causes of presinusoidal portal hypertension include:
- Portal vein thrombosis
- Schistosomiasis
- Primary biliary cirrhosis where the initial injury is to the portal tract within the liver before true cirrhosis occurs.

Portal Vein Thrombosis

Portal vein thrombosis occurs when any part of the portal vein is completely or nearly completely occluded with thrombus. The most common

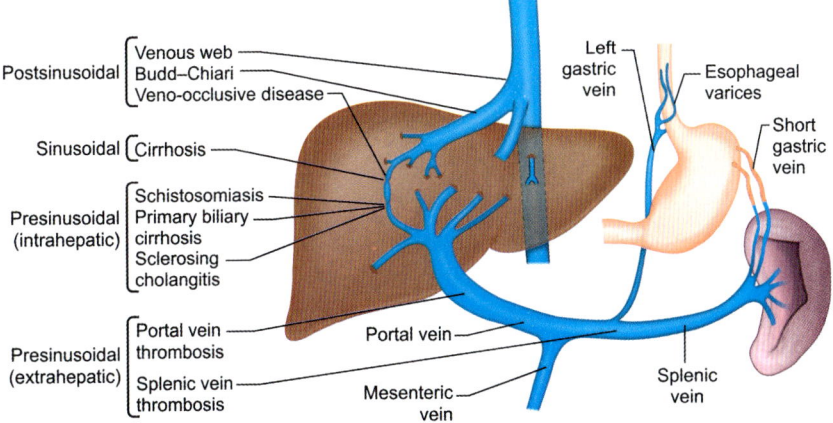

Fig. 6.20: Anatomy of portal hypertension.

cause worldwide would be sepsis, particularly in neonatal umbilical sepsis and appendicitis in children. However, in adult practice in the United Kingdom portal vein thrombosis is often found in patients with known cirrhosis and secondary to reduced portal flow into liver. Pancreatitis can also cause portal vein thrombosis but the commonest non-cirrhotic cause of portal vein thrombosis is malignancy of the pancreas. In this situation where there is portal vein invasion of the pancreatic cancer that results in thrombus formation, the complications of which carries a very grave prognosis. Very occasionally, hypercoagulable states may lead to thrombosis of the portal vein. This includes thrombocytosis and hypercoagulable states like factor V Leiden, prothrombin G20210A mutation, and deficiencies of natural anticoagulants which may be inherited (protein S and C deficiencies) or acquired, or both. The liver receives some oxygen from the portal vein but portal occlusion does not materially compromise the liver function itself and therefore the liver enzymes may not be deranged and coagulation function may actually be normal. Occasionally, a splenic vein thrombosis occurs and this may result in gastric varices caused by increased pressure in the short gastric veins with or without any esophageal varices.

Diagnosis of portal vein thrombosis can be carried out using ultrasound and other imaging like CT scanning. Doppler on ultrasound is very helpful in detecting the flow of the portal venous system, whether the flow is toward liver or away from the liver.

Occasionally, the portal vein may thrombose quite asymptomatically and collaterals would gradually develop to relieve the pressure in the system. This may subsequently be picked up incidentally, especially when investigating asymptomatic patients with a chance of finding esophageal varices. It may sometimes present as an acute abdomen with abdominal pain, shock, splenomegaly and intestinal bleeding from congested mucosa and even extensive infarction of the small bowel. The latter would usually be fatal without immediate surgical intervention.

Sinusoidal Portal Hypertension

Sinusoidal portal hypertension usually is the result of hepatic cirrhosis of any cause. When measured, hepatic wedge pressure is usually raised.

Postsinusoidal Portal Hypertension

Postsinusoidal portal hypertension may be the result of hepatic vein thrombosis. This gives rise to Budd-Chiari's syndrome. There is congestion of the liver with deranged liver function and often significant ascites with high protein content. Because the caudate lobe of the liver drains separately directly into the vena cava it is not affected. It will eventually hypertrophy to compensate. Budd–Chiari can present with an acute form of liver failure or more insidiously over several months. Treatment of the more severe cases would require hepatic transplantation.

Veno-occlusive Disease

Toxic alkaloids like certain bush teas may result in veno-occlusive disease which may also occur as a result of chemotherapy and part of the graft versus host disease, occasionally seen after transplantation.

Clinical Features of Portal Hypertension

The main clinical features of portal hypertension are gastroesophageal varices, splenomegaly, ascites and porto-systemic encephalopathy. Ascites and encephalopathy are discussed elsewhere. Porto-systemic varices may be asymptomatic and may just cause low-grade iron deficiency anemia but may cause dramatic and life-threatening bleeding. Other places where there is portosystemic confluence may develop dilated veins, such as the caput medusae which are the distended veins around umbilicus with blood flow radiating from the umbilicus. This portal system may confluence at the rectum and this may develop into very large rectal varices. There may be an audible venous hum (Cruveilhier-Baumgarten syndrome) between the umbilicus and the xiphisternum due to a collateral flow from a portal system via the umbilical vein.

Management of Variceal Bleeding

The management of esophageal variceal bleeding involves:
1. Prediction of risk of bleeding from esophageal varices
2. Prevention of the first bleed (primary prevention)
3. Acute treatment of an active bleeding
4. Prevention of rebleeding (secondary prophylaxis).

Prediction of Risk of Bleeding from Esophageal Varices

The likelihood of esophageal varices to bleed depends upon three factors: the size of the varices, the presence of red markings (red wale) and the Child's Class of liver disease. The larger the varices, the more likely it is to bleed and the Child's Class C patients are up to 5 times more likely to bleed than the same-sized varices in patients with Class A or B. Calculators and applications on smart devices are available to give an approximate 1-year percentage of probability of bleeding. Patients with known liver cirrhosis should have upper GI endoscopy to look for evidence of varices. In the absence of varices, there is no evidence for any treatment that would delay its development. When varices are noted on endoscopy, even in patients who have never bled from these varices, they should be considered for primary prophylaxis. There are two basic methods of prophylaxis: the use of beta blockers and endoscopic

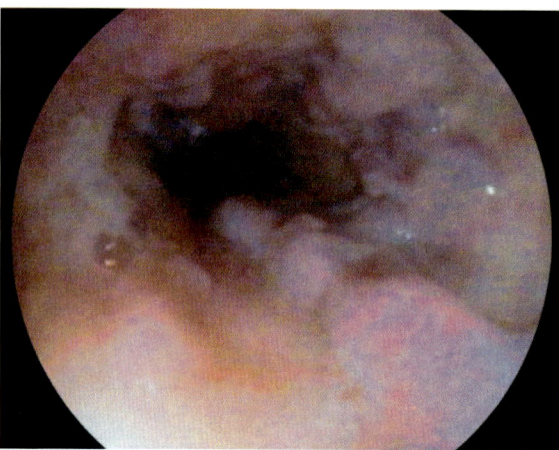

Fig. 6.21: Early varices showing dilated tortuous venous distention.

variceal banding. Because of the low probability of bleeding in patients with small varices and Child's A liver disease, the benefits from primary prophylaxis are relatively minimal and hence not recommended. However, patients who are Child's B or C with medium or large varices with a high risk of bleeding, primary prophylaxis may be justified. Currently, there is no evidence that endoscopic banding is any superior to beta blockers and as beta blockers are low cost and carry low morbidity compared to endoscopic treatment, it is probably the preferred approach. Beta blockers have to be nonselective and propranolol is usually used although nadolol and carvedilol may also be used (Fig. 6.21).

Management of Acute Variceal Bleeding

General Principles: Bleeding from esophageal varices can be dramatic and life-threatening. It is important therefore to achieve stabilization and initial resuscitation followed by methods of reducing and stopping the bleeding and finally to try to reduce the likelihood of complications. Large-bore intravenous lines should be placed immediately and immediate resuscitation with saline and at least four units of blood should be crossmatched and given when available. Coagulopathy is very common in patients with liver disease and a coagulation screen should be carried out and corrected if necessary. Coagulopathy may be corrected with the use of fresh-frozen plasma (Octaplas) between 10 and 20 mL/kg body weight. Platelets may also be lacking in many patients and should be replaced if it is significantly reduced. Blood should be given when initial hemoglobin level is <70 g/dL with aim of no >90 g/dL. A restrictive transfusion policy carries a lower mortality than a liberal one.

Gastrointestinal Bleeding and Anemia

Prevention of hepatic encephalopathy is important and patients should be managed with lactulose and magnesium sulfate enemas. Patients with Child's Pugh Class B and C may succumb from infections and there is now good evidence that antibiotics may reduce mortality. Hence, prophylactic antibiotic therapy at presentation with patients with variceal bleeding is now widely recommended. A broad-spectrum antibiotic like ciprofloxacin or IV tazocin (piperacillin and tazobactam) is usually satisfactory depending on local antibiotic policy.

Drug Therapy

Drugs that lower portal flow may decrease the bleeding rate and may prove very useful in the immediate management of patients with variceal bleeding. These drugs include vasopressin or its synthetic analog terlipressin, somatostatin and its analog octreotide. Vasopressin and terlipressin act by constricting mesenteric arteries and therefore decrease portal venous flow. Terlipressin is given as a 2 mg IV dose every 4 h, while octreotide is usually given as a bolus dose of 50 µg followed by continuous infusion of 50 µg/h.

Vasopressin causes vasoconstriction and may cause vasoconstriction of vessels supplying vital organs like the heart and brain and in patients with known ischemic heart disease it may be wise to combine vasopressin with glyceryl trinitrate (GTN).

Endoscopic Therapy

Suspected variceal bleeding is an emergency that requires immediate endoscopy. This should be carried out by experienced hands and be thorough as bleeding may be from a non-variceal source like a duodenal ulcer. When varices are noted at endoscopy, it should be carefully inspected for recent hemorrhage. Occasionally, blood can be seen spurting out of a bleeding varix. Endoscopic therapy remains the most effective means of stopping esophageal variceal bleeding. The most common method is endoscopic variceal banding (ligation). This is achieved using a ligating device that can apply elastic bands. Bands are best placed in the distal esophagus where the feeding vessels arise. An alternative to esophageal banding is sclerotherapy with sclerosant like ethanolamine but this is associated with a higher complication rate like stricture formation and ulceration. This method is largely obsolete widely replaced by variceal band ligation (Figs. 6.22A and B).

Balloon Tamponade

If bleeding persists despite endoscopic therapy and medical therapy with terlipressin and/or somatostatin, then direct compression of the varices with Sengstaken tube may be necessary. There are various designs of the tube and a disposal, single use version is now widely available. Because of high risk of

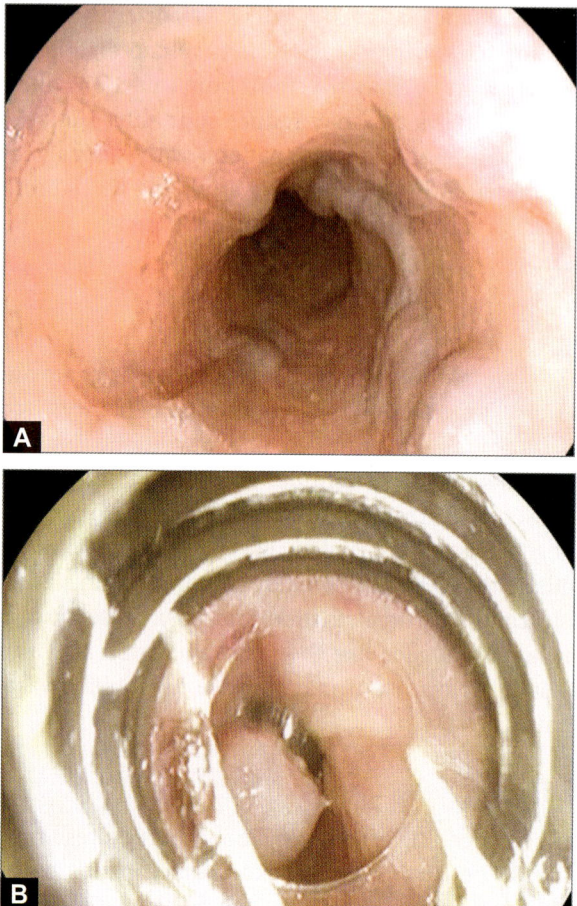

Figs. 6.22A and B: Large varices (A) identified easily on endoscopy and could be banded acutely or prophylactically (B).

aspiration patients who require a balloon tamponade should be intubated in an intensive care setting. The balloon is inserted in the stomach and inflated and traction applied to the fundus of the stomach which would apply pressure on the feeding vessels and stop the bleeding. If necessary an esophageal balloon is also available which can be inflated to further tamponade the bleeding varices. The esophageal balloon is usually inflated to a pressure of about 40 mm Hg. The tube can be left in place for 24–48 h but it is usual to have a second look endoscopy 24 h after placement of the tube to see if any further endoscopic therapy is feasible. Complications of balloon tamponade are very high and usually as a result of misplaced tubes by inexperienced staff. Esophageal rupture is usually fatal in this setting.

A novel device known as Danis stent has been recently made available in which a wide bore expandable metal stent is placed at the gastroesophageal

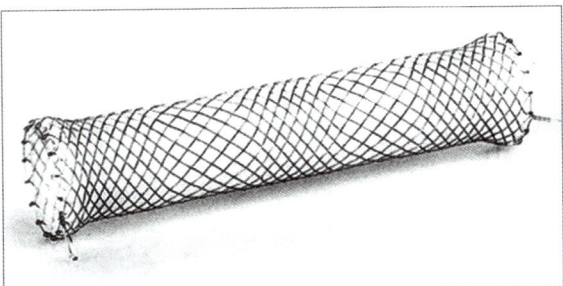

Fig. 6.23: A self-expanding covered nitinol mesh stent can exert adequate lateral pressure to tamponade bleeding esophageal varices.

junction which tamponades the bleeding vessel. It has an additional advantage in which patients may be able to feed normally and there is lower risk of aspiration as a result. These stents can also be placed for a few days until the patient is stabilized and may be removed at a later date (Fig. 6.23).

Transhepatic Portal Systemic Shunting (TIPSS)

The portal pressure may be reduced by placing a stent between the portal vein and the hepatic vein. This can be achieved radiologically by the passage of a catheter through the jugular and passed up the hepatic vein. A fine needle is pushed into the portal vein and a guidewire put through and a track is made. This allows a passage of an expandable stent. To do this successfully, however, a portal vein must be patent and not thrombosed. It is very effective in reducing the portal pressure and therefore stopping the bleeding from esophageal varices. However, it increases the risk of hepatic encephalopathy. This is due to the bypassing of toxic ammonia from the gut to the systemic circulation without being metabolized by liver. The outcome from TIPSS procedure depends on severity of underlying liver disease. Patients with Child's C disease have a high mortality after TIPSS procedures hence should only be used in these patients as an extemporizing procedure to arrest variceal bleeding while awaiting definitive treatment like transplantation (Fig. 6.24).

The overall prognosis of patients who are admitted with a variceal bleed does depend on the stage of liver disease. Patients with Child's C have a poor prognosis. In these situations, patients should be considered as a liver transplant patient. Further discussions of liver failure is found in Chapter 14.

Varices in Other Sites

Gastric varices are not uncommon and its management includes the use of somatostatin or terlipressin IV as primary measure. Endoscopic management is more difficult as banding is technically difficult or impossible and sclerotherapy is associated with a high complication rate. The best technique

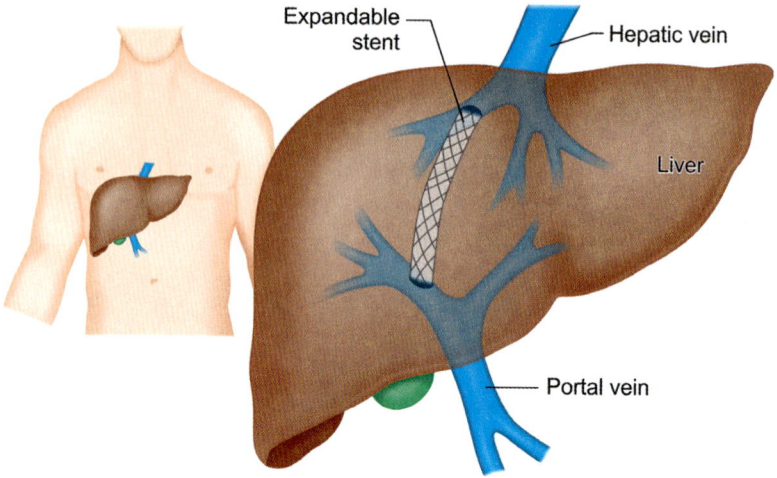

Fig. 6.24: Transhepatic portal systemic shunting.

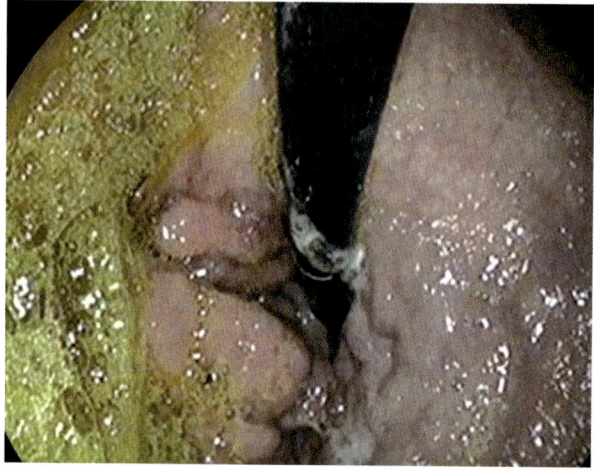

Fig. 6.25: Large gastric varices can be difficult to manage if they bleed.

is injection with cyanoacrylate glue. The technique is quite demanding and is best left to centers where expertise is available. Balloon tamponade can be helpful in difficult situations and TIPSS placement is often required to control bleeding gastric varices.

Very rarely varices can occur in the rectum and sometimes around stomas in patients with previous ileostomy. Rectal varices can be difficult to manage. Sclerotherapy and banding have been used but are difficult and associated with high complication rates. Bleeding from these varices is best managed by a TIPSS procedure (Fig. 6.25).

Portal Hypertensive Gastropathy

Patients with portal hypertension may have a speckled dusky appearance of the gastric mucosa which is often referred to as portal hypertensive gastropathy. It may cause a generalized oozing of blood from the stomach. This often coexists with esophageal varices and in patients who have had a bleed it may be difficult to determine whether the esophageal varices were the source of the bleeding or from the portal hypertensive gastropathy. Treatment is usually with the use of medical measures and if that fails, a TIPSS procedure may be required. Endoscopic management is not possible in this situation.

RARER CAUSES OF SMALL INTESTINAL BLEEDING

Carcinoma of the Small Intestine

Carcinoma of the small intestine is rare but may account for unexplained GI bleeding or anemia. It is found mainly in the duodenum or proximal jejunum so is often accessible to an upper GI endoscope or a longer enteroscope. A lymphoma of the small bowel may ulcerate and present as bleeding but more often as an abdominal mass or small bowel obstruction. CT scan or magnetic resonance imaging (MRI) is usually required to detect small bowel lymphomas. MRI is probably the preferred imaging particularly if combined with enteroclysis (MRE) which involves drinking a solution of PEG as contrast. Crohn's disease may occasionally present as an acute bleed particularly when ulcerating into a vessel (Fig. 6.26).

Peutz–Jeghers' syndrome is an autosomal dominant condition characterized by hamartomatous polyps of the stomach, small and large intestine.

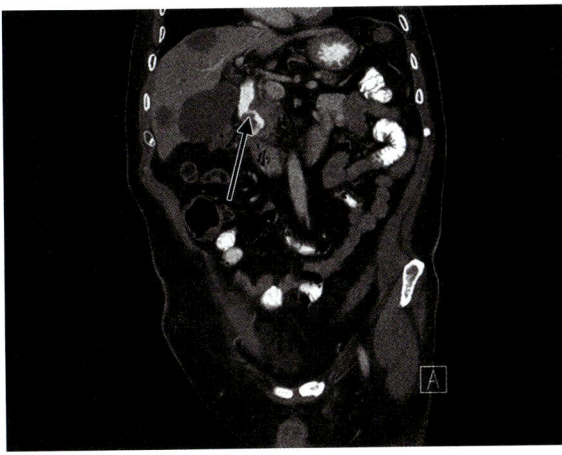

Fig. 6.26: Computed tomography scan showing a duodenal tumor.

It is associated with spotty melanin pigmentation around the mouth, hands and feet and genital areas. In adulthood, all the pigment lesions except those around the mouth usually fade. The polyps themselves are prominent in the small intestine and they can cause obstruction, intussusception or bleeding. They have a very slight malignant potential but not to a degree that requires removal except for complications like bleeding or obstruction. Ovarian and testicular tumors can also occur in greater frequency in this syndrome.

Bleeding from Biliary or Pancreatic Ducts via Ampulla of Vater

Very occasionally, bleeding may occur into the biliary tree and the blood exits through the ampulla of Vater. This is sometimes referred to as hematobilia. It may occasionally spontaneously occur with bleeding from vascular liver lesions or more rarely varices around the portal tracks. Bleeding from pancreatic duct is probably commoner and is usually a result of pancreatitis resulting with erosions into one of the arteries like the splenic artery or its tributaries. This can cause a major bleed through the ampulla. Endoscopy can identify this but usually requires angiography and embolization to stem the hemorrhage which can be quite substantial.

Hemorrhagic Telangiectasia

Hemorrhagic telangiectasia can be an acquired or inherited condition. Lesions may occur anywhere in the GI tract from the mouth to the anus and may present with chronic iron deficiency anemia but occasionally as an acute bleed. Acquired telangiectasia occurs in connection with collagen disorders such as scleroderma and CREST syndrome.

Hereditary hemorrhagic telangiectasia may present as spontaneous and recurrent nosebleeds. Clinical examination under the tongue usually reveals telangiectasia and it can also be found on the hands as well. There is often a family history. In severe forms of the disease, patients may develop massive pulmonary venous malformations which cause shunting which may occasionally rupture particularly in pregnant women. Hepatic arterial venous malformations also exist and may lead to liver failure and cirrhosis in a minority of patients.

Management

Bleeding is managed by standard methods. Patients with repeated GI bleed may be treated with tranexamic acid. Patients with recurrent bleeding problems could also be treated with estrogens. The use of angiogenesis inhibitor, Bevacizumab is very promising and may be the ideal treatment for patients with recurrent bleeding from hereditary hemorrhagic telangiectasia.

COLONIC BLEEDING

Diverticulosis

Diverticular disease is probably the most common cause of colonic bleeding. However, diverticulosis is extremely common and small angiodysplastic lesions may coexist and may be the actual source of the bleeding rather than the diverticular disease itself. The bleeding diverticulum is more likely to be from the right side of the colon as opposed to the left side and patients often have coexisting diverticulitis. This is probably related to the thinner walls of the right colon.

Management

Colonoscopy is the best modality for identifying the site of bleeding. When the bleeding is identified clearly on colonoscopy, attempts at endoscopic therapy can be tried like adrenaline injection and clips or diathermy. It is often technically challenging as the colon has a very thin wall, especially in the right colon. When endoscopy fails to either identify or stop the bleeding, angiography is the best alternative. It would identify bleeding rates of more than half a millimeter per minute but bleeding has often stopped by the time angiography is arranged. Surgical intervention is rarely needed.

Angiodysplasia

Angiodysplastic lesions can occur in any part of the intestine but are most common in the terminal ileum, cecum and ascending colon. They are almost always acquired usually in elderly patients. It is also found in patients where there is a history of valvular heart disease and these patients may be on anticoagulants as well. When it appears in the colon, colonoscopy may show the lesions and application of argon plasma coagulation (APC) to such lesions is efficacious (Figs. 6.27 and 6.28).

Colonic Ulceration

Inflammatory bowel diseases like Crohn's disease and ulcerative colitis often present with rectal bleeding which is usually accompanied by diarrhea and the bleeding is rarely severe. Stool examination often reveals streaks of blood with mucous along with the diarrhea as opposed to frank red bleeding.

Solitary ulcers of the colon may exist and there are three main sites for these ulcers: the rectum, the sigmoid and the cecum. In the rectum, they are often associated with rectal prolapse and in patients with chronic constipation who may digitally evacuate. In sigmoid colon, the ulcers are associated in patients with severe constipation and solitary cecal ulcers also exist, the etiology is uncertain.

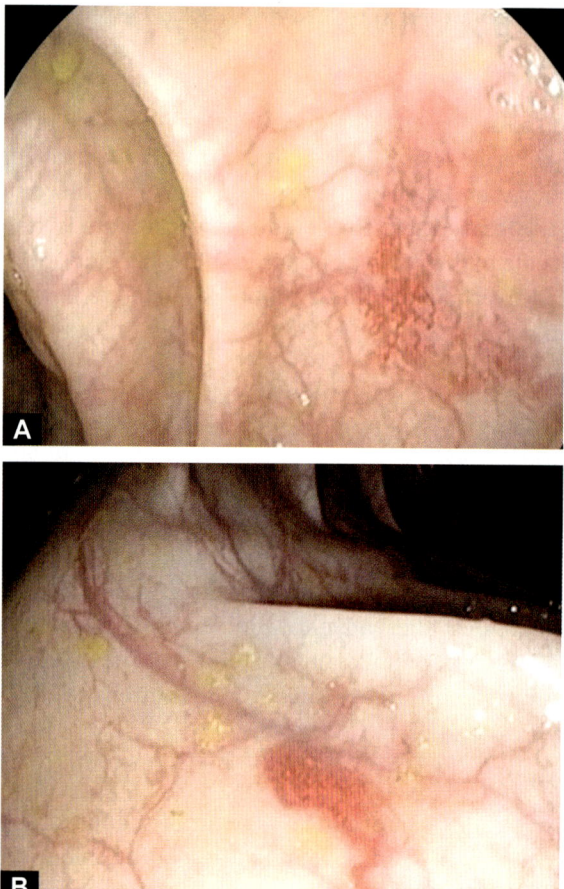

Figs. 6.27A and B: Small angiodysplastic lesions in the colon.

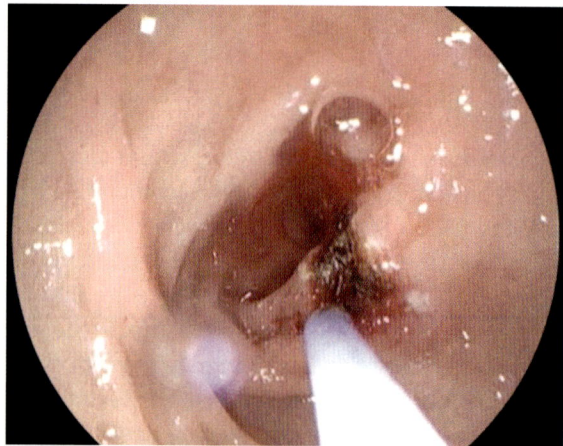

Fig. 6.28: Argon plasma coagulation is an effective method of treatment.

Gastrointestinal Bleeding and Anemia

Pneumatosis coli is a rare condition where there is extensive gas-filled cysts may involve the small intestine as well as the large intestine. It is often associated with chronic obstructive airways disease. These pockets of gas vary in size and may be subserosal or submucosal. They may cause bleeding but more commonly abdominal pain and diarrhea. Large lesions may cause intussusception.

Diagnosis is made through a plain X-ray or a CT scan. Colonoscopy will also display these lesions. They are occasionally picked up incidentally. Management of *pneumatosis coli* involves treating its complications and the use of oxygen, particularly hyperbaric oxygen if this is available (Figs. 6.29 and 6.30).

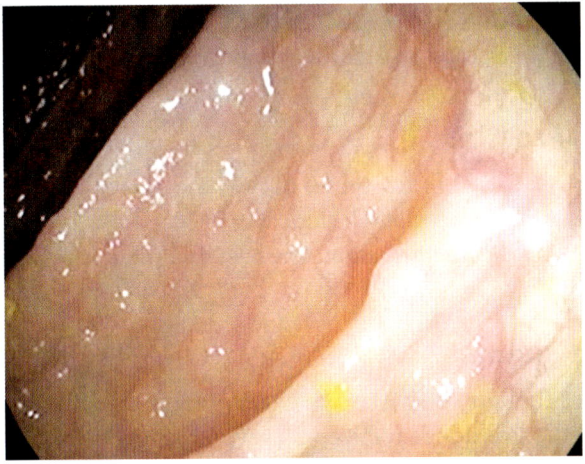

Fig. 6.29: Pneumatosis as seen on colonoscopy.

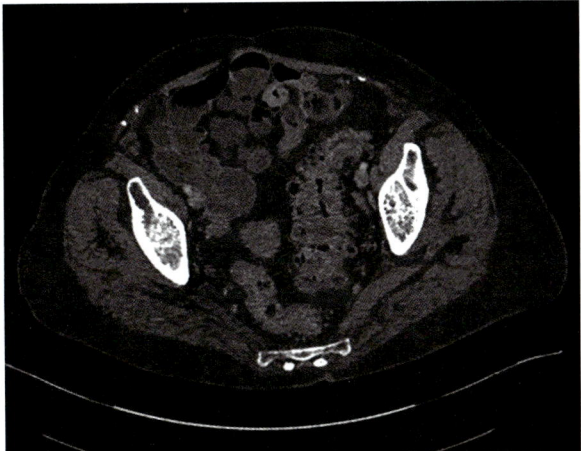

Fig. 6.30: Computed tomography of pneumatosis coli showing the air pockets.

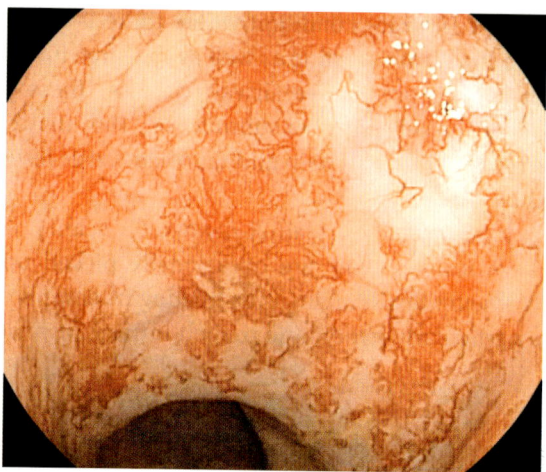

Fig. 6.31: Radiation proctitis: note the fragile superficial capillaries.

Radiation Proctitis

Radiation to rectum from treatment of prostate and gynecological cancers can cause fragile telangiectatic lesions which bleed easily. They are due to ischemia and new vessel formation. The best treatment is hyperbaric oxygen (Fig. 6.31).

Marathon Runners

Long distance runners very rarely can develop rectal bleeding and diarrhea. It is thought that this is due to reduced bowel perfusion and possible ischemia. It is usually self-limiting.

Vasculitis of the Intestine

Vasculitis of the intestine occurs in a number of systemic diseases including:
- Polyarteritis nodosa
- Behçet's syndrome
- Systemic lupus erythematosus
- Rheumatoid arthritis
- Dermatomyositis.

Vasculitis of the intestinal tract results in ischemia or even infarction of the bowel. Abdominal pain is thus the most common symptom and bleeding may occur. Imaging radiologically with CT scan or MRI usually reveals edematous inflamed small bowel. This may be indistinguishable from Crohn's disease. Some conditions like Behçet's syndrome may mimic Crohn's disease and may also have other associated parainflammatory conditions like arteritis, uveitis and mouth ulcers. In Behçet's disease, there are usually genital ulcers as well as uveitis, the former relatively unusual in Crohn's disease. In the acute setting, endoscopic examination can be hazardous as there is a perforation risk associated with endoscopy. The inflamed mucosa can be very friable.

Diagnosis of mesenteric vasculitis should be suspected if there is evidence of vasculitis elsewhere in particular if there is evidence of renal impairment or renal vasculitis or Takayasu's arteritis. Laboratory inflammatory markers are almost invariably raised as is the serum antineutrophil antibodies (P-ANCA). However, this may be unhelpful as P-ANCA may also be found in 60% of ulcerative colitis. However, the P-ANCA found in polyarteritis nodosa is directed toward myeloperoxidase in contrast to P-ANCA in ulcerative colitis which is directed toward other neutrophil granule particularly lactoferrin.

Management of the GI vasculitis involves firstly the treatment of the underlying condition. This is usually some form of immunosuppression, usually a combination of corticosteroids and cyclophosphamide. The other aspect is the acute treatment of complications from the GI tract and may involve surgical resection.

Degos Disease

Degos disease is a rare condition which affects young men and is characterized by the presence of necrotic skin lesions and vasculitis of the duct often resulting in infarction.

Henoch–Schonlein Purpura

Henoch–Schonlein purpura occurs in association with a streptococcal A infection in the throat and consists of a palpable cutaneous purpura, arteritis and abdominal pain. Intestinal bleeding may occur in up to half of these patients and occasionally results in intussusception or even infarction. The purpura is characteristic and occurs in rows in the buttocks and lower abdomen. There may be associated glomerulonephritis. Usually, the disease is self-limiting and carries a good prognosis.

Ehlers–Danlos Syndrome

Ehlers–Danlos syndrome is a relatively rare genetic condition. There are at least six major types identified and they vary in inheritance patterns. The basic defect of these conditions affects collagen and as a result, there is joint laxity, poor wound healing and intermittent intestinal bleeding.

Bleeding and Coagulation Disorders

Hematological disorders of coagulation may result in intestinal bleeding. Coagulopathy may be inherent, acquired, drug induced or therapeutic:
- Hemophiliacs rarely bleed from intestine unless there are additional lesions, in particular, peptic ulceration or esophageal varices. The latter may be from acquired hepatitis C-related cirrhosis.

- In von Willebrand's disease, there is a platelet defect and spontaneous intestinal hemorrhage can be seen. There is an association between von Willebrand's and increased incidence of intestinal angiodysplasia.
- Prolongation of the prothrombin time from warfarin therapy beyond 5 times control may be associated with spontaneous bleeding. Antiplatelet agents may also result in spontaneous bleeding and aspirins have a direct toxic effect on the GI mucosa causing small ulcerations.
- Severely ill patients with disseminated intravascular coagulopathy may bleed spontaneously.
- Severe thrombocytopenia is also associated with spontaneous GI bleeding but this usually occurs in the presence of additional lesions like ulcers or GI malignancy.

Treatment is largely aimed at correcting the underlying coagulopathy usually with hematological advice.

Colon Cancer and Colorectal Polyps

Clinical Features

Patients with colorectal cancer (CRC) may present to health professionals in three possible ways. They may have symptoms suggestive of CRC, they may present as a result of screening in high-risk groups or population screening, or they may present as a result of complications of CRC.

Symptoms of CRC may be from local disease like bleeding per rectum, abdominal pain or discomfort and right-sided tumors may present as an iron deficiency anemia. About half of patients may present with an alteration of bowel habit either constipation or more commonly diarrhea. Patients may also present as a result of metastatic disease like liver metastases with jaundice or palpable tumor. Unfortunately, when these clinical manifestations occur, the malignancy tends to be at a late stage. Other symptoms like weight loss or frank jaundice usually are also grave signs.

Increasingly, patients are picked up on population colorectal screening programs. This may be from fecal occult blood testing or flexible sigmoidoscopy programs. Patients with high risk of developing CRC, such as patients with strong family history or patients with longstanding ulcerative colitis are also usually enrolled on some surveillance program.

About 25% of patients with CRC present as acute emergencies with obstruction, bleeding, paracolic abscess, perforation or jaundice due to secondary deposits. They tend to have late-stage disease.

Epidemiology

Bowel cancer is the third most common cancer worldwide and the second most common cancer in European populations. There is variation in

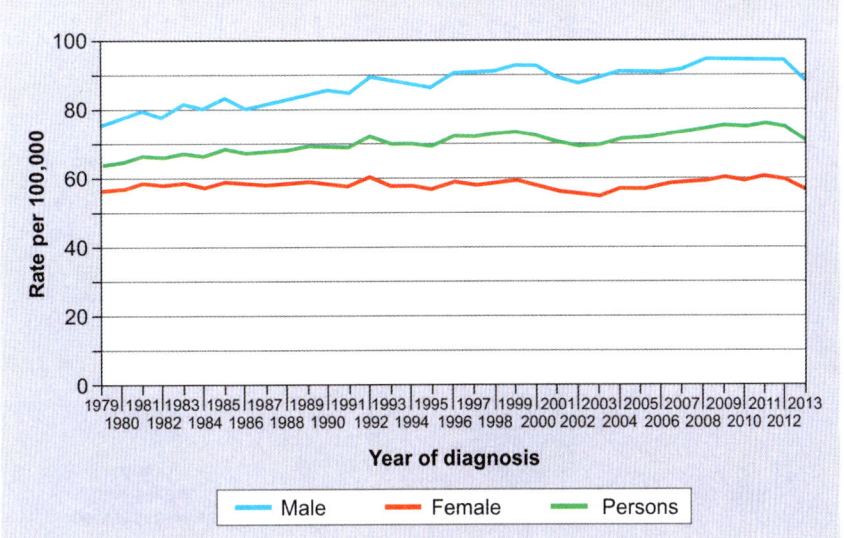

Fig. 6.32: Age-standardized incidence rates per 100,000 population, by sex, United Kingdom.
Source: Cancer Research UK.

incidence rates worldwide with the highest incidents in Australia/New Zealand and the lowest in Western Africa.

In the United Kingdom, based on the latest (2013) data collected by Cancer Research UK, the crude incidence rate in the United Kingdom is 73 per 100,000 males and 56 for every 100,000 females. There are regional differences within the United Kingdom with the incidence highest in Wales.

Bowel cancer incidence rates have increased by 14% in the United Kingdom since the 1970s. This increase is particularly marked in male patients (Fig. 6.32).

Anatomical Distribution of CRC

Colon cancer distribution according to its anatomical site varies between male and female. Proportions of cases of rectum and sigmoid colon cancers are higher in males (32% and 23%, respectively) than females (23% and 20%, respectively). In a cecum and ascending colon, the proportions are higher in females (17% and 10%, respectively) than in males (12% and 7.3%, respectively (Fig. 6.33).

Etiology

There are two main etiological factors contributing to the development of CRC. Patients may have a genetic susceptibility and environmental factors like dietary factors that contribute to development of the cancer.

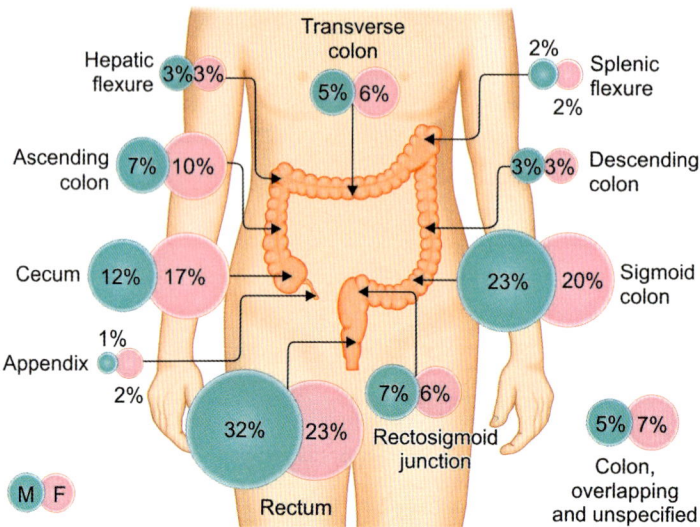

Fig. 6.33: Anatomical distribution of colorectal cancer. *Source*: Cancer Research UK.

Genetic syndromes that lead to CRCs are rare and most cancers encountered would be of the sporadic variety. There are racial differences in rates of CRC, for example, African Americans have the highest rates of CRC in the United States. There are also large studies now suggesting that obesity is associated with a higher incidence as well as type II diabetes and insulin resistance.

There are now large studies on diet which show a high intake of fruit and vegetables protects the individual from the development of colon cancer, whereas intake of high fat, processed meat and red meat is associated with increased risk of colon cancer. Vitamin D deficiencies have been implicated in CRC and higher consumption of omega 3 fatty acids, as found in fish oil, reduces the risk of cancer.

Large trial evidence also suggests that aspirin and other nonsteroidal drugs may be protective against development of colonic polyps and cancers.

Relationship to Adenomatous Polyps

Adenomatous polyps are very common in the colon. The prevalence rises steeply with age. Colonoscopic studies have shown that they are rare in patients in their 20s and 30s and rise to 25–30% in 50-year-old patients and as high as 50% in patients over 70. It is also increased in patients with obesity, particularly correlated to the amount of intra-abdominal visceral fat.

Polyps may be classified according to their morphological appearance or histological type. They may be sessile with a white base or pedunculated having a significant neck. The term "flat lesions" may be used to describe sessile polyps in which the height is perceived to be less than half the diameter of the lesion. Lesions that have a depressed center are likely to harbor malignancy.

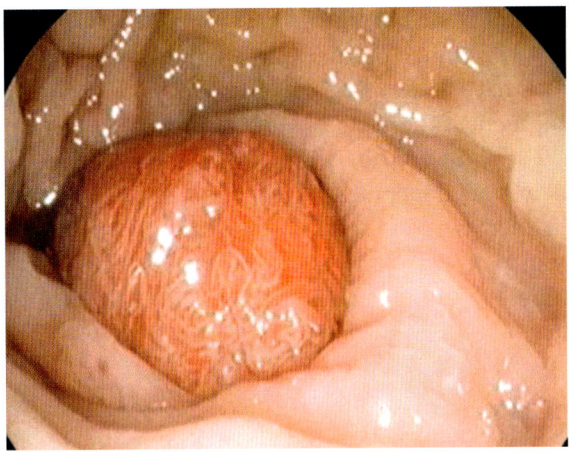

Fig. 6.34: Classic adenomatous polyp in colon.

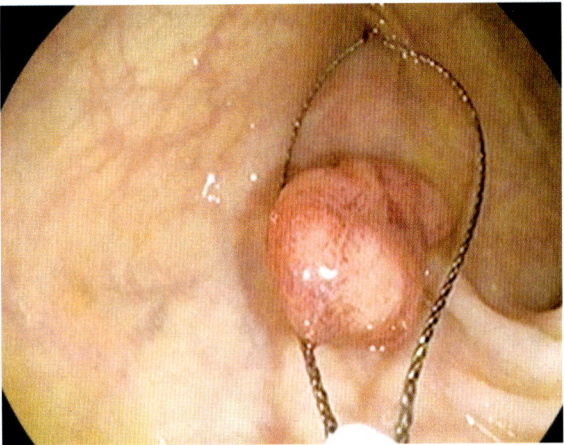

Fig. 6.35: Polyps are easily snared.

Histopathology of these lesions may show glandular architecture suggestive of a tubular lesion or a villous pattern or a mixture of both. All adenomas by definition are dysplastic and histopathologists can classify the degree of dysplasia as low or high grade to intramucosal adenocarcinoma. Frank malignancy is when the muscularis mucosa is invaded by neoplastic cells (Figs. 6.34 and 6.35).

It is widely believed that adenomas grow in variable rates, some may involute spontaneously. The factors that lead to development of cancer include the following:

Polyp size: The larger the polyp, the more likely it is to develop cancers with increased incidence at follow-up of patients with polyps >1 cm in size.

Histology: Polyps with higher grade dysplasia will show more propensities to develop cancers; similarly with patients with more villous type histology is associated with higher risk of cancer.

Number of polyps: It stands to reason that the more polyps a person has, the higher the overall likelihood of cancer developing.

Several trials have shown that polypectomy leads to a decreased likelihood of development of CRCs.

Hyperplastic polyps (polyps which on histology show normal colonic mucosa) have no malignant potential. However, there are lesions, usually flat which are described as sessile serrated adenomas/polyps. These are thought to have potential to develop cancers. It is hoped that better histopathological definitions and the use of molecular markers may help define these lesions more accurately (Figs. 6.36 and 6.37).

Relationship to Inflammatory Bowel Disease

Both idiopathic ulcerative colitis and colonic Crohn's disease are associated with an increased risk of colon cancer. The likelihood of developing colon cancer in patients with ulcerative colitis depends on extent of disease, duration

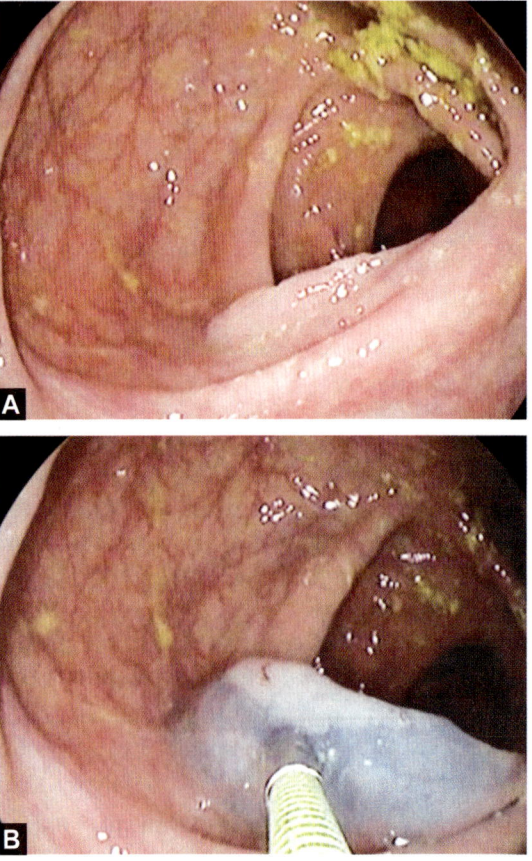

Figs. 6.36A and B

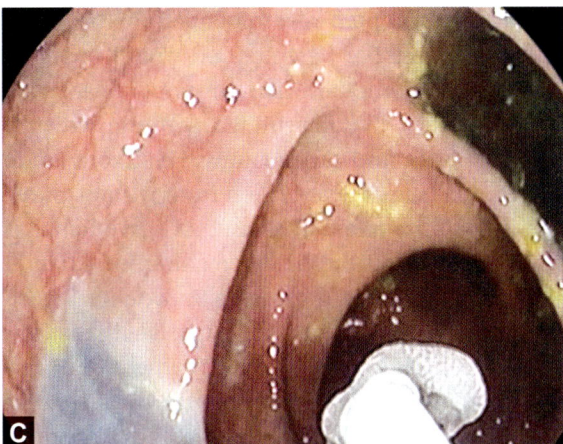

Figs. 6.36A to C: This flat lesion was a serrated adenoma (A). It was lifted by submucosal injection (B) and snared (C).

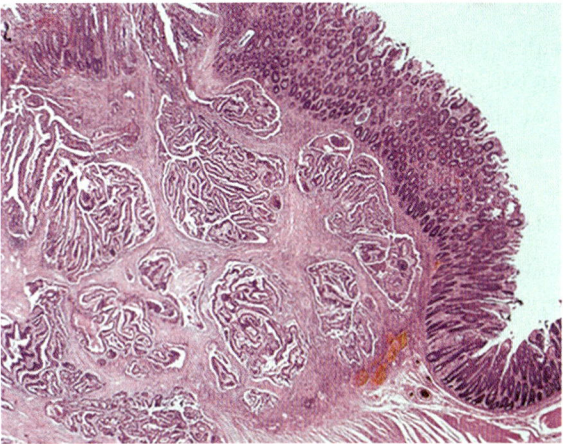

Fig. 6.37: Dysplastic polyp.

of disease and degree activity of inflammation. Patients with proctitis only are probably of little or no increased risk and the highest risk for patients are with extensive disease and pancolitis. It is estimated that patients who have longstanding extensive colitis for >10 years will have an increased risk of about 7 times the normal population for developing colon cancer. Risk for chronic Crohn's disease is probably similar although it may be confounded by the likelihood of smoking in patients with Crohn's disease. The natural history is altered by both medical and treatment and surgery, good control and mucosal healing reduces risk and obviously panproctocolectomy and pouch operations cut the risk dramatically. There may still be a slight risk from any colonic cuff mucosa that remains. There is an additional increased risk in patients who have concomitant primary sclerosing cholangitis.

The increased risk prompted recommendations by various bodies for some form of surveillance. The best method would be colonoscopy, preferably with an enhanced method like chromoendoscopy. This involves spraying the colon with a dye like indigo carmine which enhances the ability to detect dysplasia and target biopsy. If chromoendoscopy is not available, then multiple samples are taken from various parts of the colon. This is largely a hit or miss affair. The value of surveillance is still controversial and it is unclear what the best screening for surveillance strategy is. Clearly, the natural history and progression would suggest that patients should have surveillance only if they have extensive disease and >10 years of disease. Recommendations by national gastroenterology organizations are evolving and current sensible option is to perform a chromoendoscopy at year 10 and stratify risk to those of higher risk requiring yearly inspection and those with low risk who do not.

Hereditary CRC Syndrome

Recent molecular studies have contributed considerably to our understanding of inherited CRC syndrome. Although they are relatively rare and account for about 4% of all CRCs, the understanding of the molecular defects has improved our understanding of the pathogenesis of CRC.

Familial Adenomatous Polyposis

Familial adenomatous polyposis (FAP) accounts for about 1% of colon cancers. It is an autosomal dominant condition and it is caused by mutations of a tumor suppressive gene dubbed adenomatous polyposis coli (*APC*) gene located on chromosome 5q 21–22. There are numerous different mutations described in the literature and they account for the variety of presentations and different penetrations of the gene. Inherited defects are usually termed germline mutations. The same *APC* gene is affected in sporadic CRC as well with somatic as opposed to germline mutations found in as many as 80% of all CRCs.

The location of the mutation on the gene is associated with different severities of colonic polyposis, cancer risk and frequency of extra colonic features. Some mutations are associated with retinal lesions (congenital hypertrophy of the retinal pigment epithelium, CHRPE) sometimes referred to as CHRPE and other mutations associated with desmoid tumors, duodenal polyps or medulloblastomas.

Classic FAP is associated with numerous colonic polyps usually <100 and can be up to a 1000 or more developing in the second or third decade of life. Eventually CRC will develop and usually have an average age of 45 at the diagnosis of cancer. Patients with larger number numbers of polyps are more likely to develop earlier cancer. Other forms of FAP are also described where there is only 10–20 polyps seen and they have older age of onset of colon cancer. Apart from colonic polyps, FAP patients may have other lesions, particularly adenomas in the duodenum and ampulla of Vater. These are more difficult to manage as prophylactic resection is not advocated because of difficulty. Other lesions include gastric polyps usually of the fundic gland variety, osteomas of the skull, mandible and long bones, soft tissue (desmoid) tumors, capillary carcinoma of the thyroid, adrenal adenomas and carcinoma, brain tumors (TURCOT syndrome) and hypertrophy of the retinal pigment epithelium (HRPE). Occasionally, CHRPE's are picked up by ophthalmologists and mandatory colonoscopic screening is recommended.

Management: A total colectomy is mandatory and should be performed in late teens or at initial diagnosis. Usually an ileal pouch procedure is performed but FAP patients tend to tolerate ileal anal pouch procedures less well than ulcerative colitis patients. If patients have duodenal polyps, continuing surveillance is necessary.

Inherited Non-polyposis CRC (Lynch Syndrome)

Lynch's syndrome specifically refers to the hereditary non-polyposis CRC. It is an autosomal dominant disease and accounts for about 3% of all CRCs. It should be suspected in patients with strong family history of CRCs as well as endometrial and other cancers. This group of diseases is associated with defects in DNA mismatch repair gene. These genes, *hMLH1*, *hMSH2*, *hMSH6* or *PMS2*, are involved in repairing DNA whenever there is a defect in the replication of DNA. This will result in a mismatch and these genes repair them. They present predominantly right-sided colon cancers which evolve from flat adenomas. There are many variants with variable associations with other cancers including ovarian, stomach, hepatobiliary and renal tumors.

Identification of families is important and affected families should be offered genetic counseling and screening strategies based on genetic testing, colonoscopic examination and ultrasonic examination of pelvic organs in women.

Pathogenesis of Sporadic Colon Cancer

There is now widespread acceptance of a hypothesis originally put forward by Vogelstein that there is a sequence of events from hyperplasia to dysplasia to malignancy and finally invasion and metastases. During these events, the cells acquire oncogene expression and genetic mutations of tumor suppressor genes that result in the cells becoming malignant. In this process, the normal mucosa develops small adenomas which become large adenomas and eventually, cancer. Evidence of this has been noted from pathologic presence of malignant change within the larger polyps. Further evidence was found when removal of these adenomas reduces cancer risk. There are three important genetic factors that influence CRC formation: oncogenes, onco-suppressor genes and stability genes. The commonest of the oncogenes are *C-MYC* and *C-KiRAS* genes which are involved in cell proliferation. Of the tumor suppressor genes they include a *p53* which is involved in apoptosis (programmed cell death) and help remove cells with damaged DNA. Defect in this gene thus would increase malignant potential. The FAP gene associated with familial adenomatous polyps can undergo spontaneous mutation in somatic cells as well. This is often as the result of chromosome alteration and loss of the 5q arm of the chromosome and a loss of the *APC* gene.

A third genetic alteration is as a result of defects in the stability genes. These help keep genetic alterations to a minimum. They include the genes involved in Lynch's syndromes which are involved in DNA repair (Figs. 6.38 and 6.39).

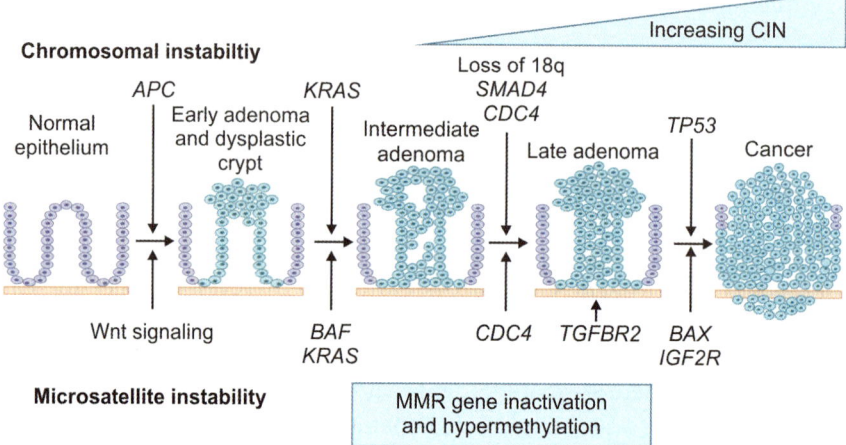

Fig. 6.38: Vogelstein hypothesis is widely accepted as the development majority of left-sided cancers. This pathway accounts for about 80% of sporadic cancers. This is associated with poorer prognosis, more chemoradiosensitive.

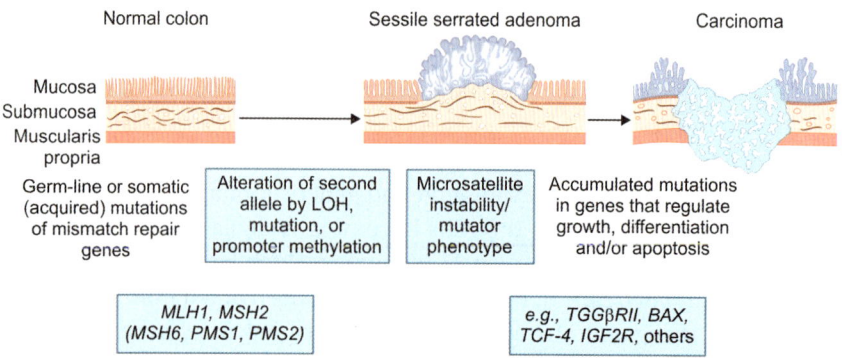

Fig. 6.39: About 20% of sporadic colon cancers occur via mismatch repair defects. They carry a slightly better prognosis but are more chemoradioresistant.

Although all cancers of the colon start as flat lesions, they may become bulky and polypoidal, while others particularly in the left colon become circumferential lesions with an apple core stricturing presentation. This annular growth is probably due to the circular arrangement of lymphatics in the left colon. Histologically, the vast majority are adenocarcinomas. The histological appearances thus carry prognostic value as histopathologists can report the grade of differentiation of the cancer from moderate to undifferentiated in histological appearance (Figs. 6.40 and 6.41).

Tumors in which there is defective DNA miss-match repair will show micro-satellite instability (MSI). MSI testing can be performed on fresh, frozen or paraffin-embedded tumor tissue using a PCR-based assay for detection of instability. The presence or absence of MSI has prognostic and therapeutic implications. Tumors exhibiting MSI are generally found in the proximal colon and in general have a somewhat better overall prognosis. More importantly, tumors with MSI have a poorer response to chemotherapy agents like 5-FU. Hence, it is now widely recommended that histopathologists perform this test.

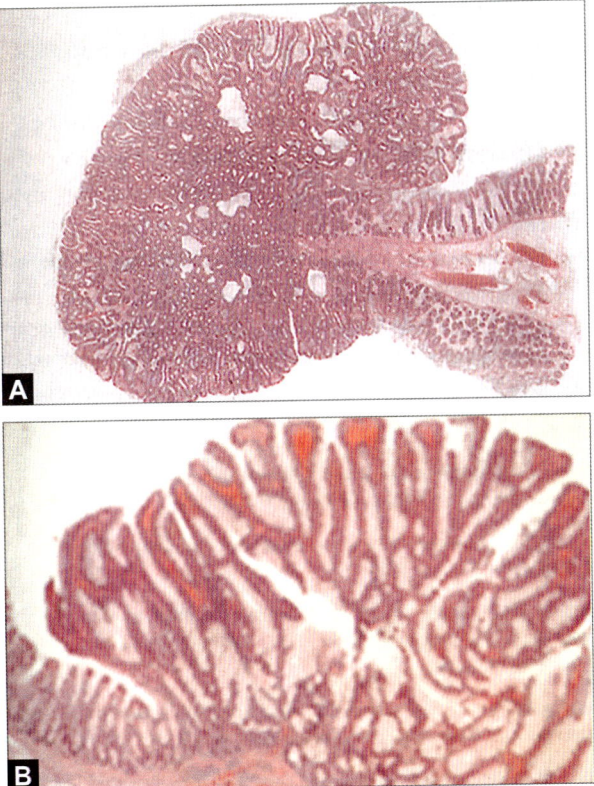

Figs. 6.40A and B

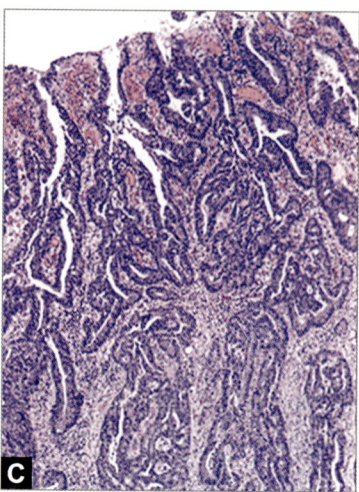

Figs. 6.40A to C: (A) Tubulovillous adenoma; (B) Villous adenoma; (C) Invasive carcinoma.

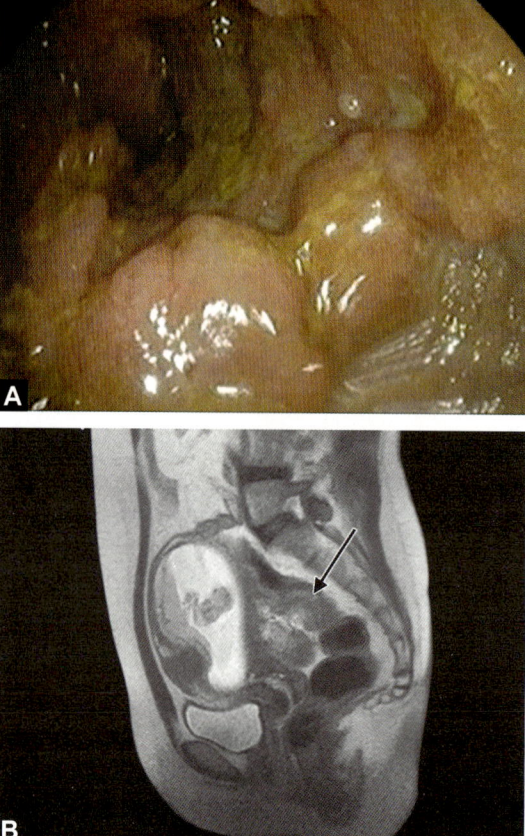

Figs. 6.41A and B: Sigmoid cancer with corresponding CT. (CT: Computed tomography.)

Staging

The staging of colon cancer is a good predictor of prognosis. The original staging system devised by Dukes is now largely replaced by the TNM staging system. This stands for tumor, node and metastases. There have been several versions but the latest version is the 2010 staging system which is now widely adopted. The prognosis and survival figures are given in Figure 6.42.

Clinical evaluation and staging is made by radiological and endoscopic evaluation. CT scan is by far the most commonly used modality and is valuable in assessing tumor extension into the regional lymphatics and distant metastases. MRI, however, is better at assessing liver metastases than CT scanning. Local staging of rectal cancer may be assessed by EUS or pelvic MRI.

Management

Surgical resection is the only curative treatment for CRC. Unfortunately, many patients present late. Survival of advanced cancer of the colon is poor. Furthermore, many patients with CRC have other comorbidities or are elderly. This makes surgery more hazardous. Conversely, early cancers carry a good prognosis.

Cancers found in polyps that are fully resected on endoscopy have a very good prognosis. However, those with poorly differentiated histology and hence invasion into the stalk of the polyp have a higher likelihood of local spread and should be considered for surgical resection.

The use of neoadjuvant chemotherapy (chemotherapy given preoperatively) has not been shown to be effective and the use of adjuvant chemotherapy (chemotherapy given after surgery) remains controversial. However, individual

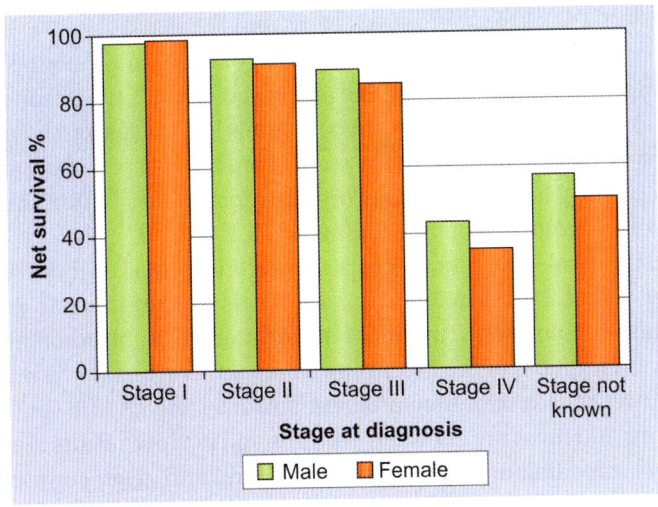

Fig. 6.42: One-year survival by stage of disease at diagnosis.
Source: Cancer Research UK.

cases should be discussed with the relevant surgical and oncological teams on a case-by-case basis.

Surgery is aimed at removing a tumor and at least 5 cm of healthy bowel on either sides plus regional lymph nodes and mesentery.

Hepatic metastases are present at initial presentation in up to 20% of patients. The primary tumor is usually resected and consideration for hepatic resection is made. Resection of the primary tumor prevents subsequent bowel obstruction. Resection of isolated lung metastases is also advocated if surgically feasible.

Follow-up after Colonic Resection

Up to 5% of patients have a second synchronous cancer and up to 35% have one or more adenomatous polyp elsewhere in the colon. Thus, it is reasonable to perform a colonoscopy a few months after surgery if it has not been performed before surgery. Subsequent risk for developing new cancers (metachronous) is about 5%, and about 50% of these will arise within the first 5 years after initial resection. Hence, many surgeons advocate regular colonoscopic screening every 2-5 years thereafter. However, large studies have shown no evidence that regular colonoscopy is a cost-effective method of follow-up. However, it is sensible to consider the risk benefits of regular follow-up and high-risk patients be given the option of surveillance.

Carcinoembryonic antigen (CEA) is a glycoprotein present in low concentration in normal tissues but will rise in concentration in the blood in epithelial malignancies. It has a low sensitivity but a rise in CEA after resection is associated with 60% of recurrences. It is a cheap and effective way of monitoring patients after surgery.

Screening and Prevention

Because colon cancer presents late, detection of early cancers is the best way of reducing mortality from CRCs. The aim of screening is to pick up operable diseases as well as any premalignant conditions like polyps and areas of high grade dysplasia. In many countries some form of CRC screening programs has been publicly funded. This may be in the form of fecal occult blood testing or flexible sigmoidoscopy screening.

The daily fecal blood loss from a normal individual is about 1 mL but the upper end of the normal range 2 mL/day is just sufficient to produce a positive occult blood test. Tumors of the sigmoid colon bleed on average of 2 mL/day and tumors of the ascending colon and cecum up to 9 mL/day. In the UK bowel cancer screening program postal testing kits are sent to target populations and these are analyzed centrally and positive results are fed back to regional screening units. Patients are recalled and given counseling and offered a colonoscopy. In the program for England, there have been about

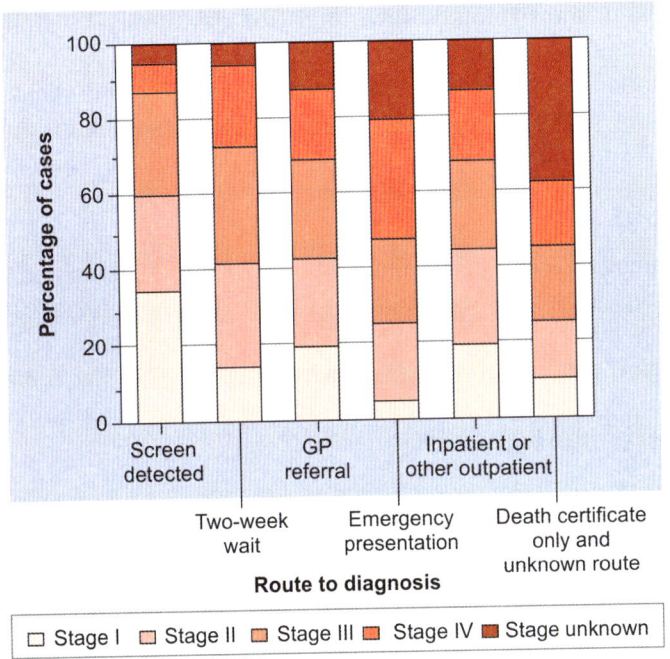

Fig. 6.43: Percentage of cases by stage and route to diagnosis, adults aged 15–99, England.
Source: Cancer Research UK.

a 60% uptake of screening and 2.5% of men and 1.5% of women had positive results. Of those positive individuals, 98% went on to have colonoscopy and cancers were found in 12% of men and 8% of women thus investigated. In addition, 43% of men and 29% of women investigated had high-risk adenomas.

Flexible sigmoidoscopy can be easily performed after a self-administered enema and would be able to pick up left-sided cancers and high risk adenomas. Studies are emerging showing flexible sigmoidoscopy is an effective screening modality for distal CRCs. The cost-effectiveness of public screening programs depends on population incidents of the cancer and uptake of the program. It is remarkably cost-effective in high incidence populations (Fig. 6.43).

OTHER COLONIC MALIGNANCIES

Lymphoma

Primary lymphoma of the colon is rare, accounting for only 0.5% of colonic malignancies and 10–20% of primary GI lymphomas. Lesions may be infiltrative, polypoid or massive and stricturing may occur. Predisposing conditions include ulcerative colitis, long-term immunosuppression, radiation therapy or ureterosigmoidostomy. Increased risk of rectal lymphoma has been reported in homosexual men.

Treatment is usually by a combination of surgery and chemotherapy, sometimes combined with radiotherapy. Cases are too rare for therapeutic trials so the optimal regimen is unclear. The 5-year survival is about 35%.

Carcinoid

Rectal carcinoid accounts for about 10% of carcinoid tumors and for 1% of rectal malignancies. There is a high rate of synchronous rectal carcinoma. About 15% metastasize but carcinoid syndrome is very rare. Treatment is with surgical excision and 5-year survival is about 80%. Carcinoid tumors elsewhere in the colon account for <10% of colonic tumors but behave aggressively with a high rate of metastasis.

Other Colonic Polyps

Hyperplastic (Metaplastic) Polyps

These are the most common polyps found in the colon. Crypts are elongated and the epithelium has a papillary appearance. It has been suggested that they result more from a failure of mature epithelial cells to drop off rather than from an increased rate of proliferation. They are statistically associated with cancer, 90% of patients with rectal cancer have hyperplastic polyps elsewhere in the rectum for example, but it is generally accepted that the polyps themselves have no premalignant potential. They are nearly always small (<5 mm) sessile polyps and can be difficult to differentiate from adenomas on macroscopic appearance. High-definition endoscopes with dye or image enhancement help recognize the surface pit pattern but they are best removed for histological examination. Flat lesions >5 mm should be excised as they may be serrated adenomas.

Juvenile (Hamartomatous) Polyps

These are most common in early childhood and are often familial. They consist of dilated cystic glands and a widened, edematous lamina propria. They are most common in the rectum. They carry a slight increased risk for malignancy because they may contain adenomatous components and should, in any case, be removed, because of the high risk of bleeding.

Peutz–Jeghers (Hamartomatous) Polyps

Hamartomas are benign tumor-like proliferations of normal tissue arranged in an abnormal and disorganized fashion. Peutz–Jeghers polyps differ from juvenile hamartomas in that the lamina propria is normal and the polyp consists of marked smooth muscle hyperplasia. The polyps are always multiple, more common in the small intestine, carry a low but definite risk of malignant change and occur as part of an autosomal dominant syndrome that is characterized also by mucocutaneous pigmentation of the face, perianal area, hands, feet and genitals. Ovarian or testicular (Sertoli cell) tumors may occasionally occur.

Cronkhite–Canada Syndrome

This is an intriguing acquired syndrome that consists of multiple GI polyps from stomach to rectum, dystrophic nails, hair loss, pigmentation, abdominal pain and malabsorption. The polyps are hamartomas with cystic retention similar to that seen in juvenile polyps. The etiology is uncertain and the outlook poor but occasional patients respond to enteral feeding.

■ FURTHER READING

GI Bleeding
1. Acute upper gastrointestinal bleeding in over 16s: management. Clinical guideline [CG141], 2012; NICE.
2. Gralnek IM, Dumonceau JM, Kuipers EJ, et al. Diagnosis and management of nonvariceal upper gastrointestinal hemorrhage: European Society of Gastrointestinal Endoscopy (ESGE) Guideline. Endoscopy. 2015;47(10):a1-a46.

Colon Cancer
3. Colorectal cancer: diagnosis and management. Clinical guideline [CG131], 2011; NICE.
4. Vogelstein B, Papadopoulos N, Velculescu VE, et al. Cancer genome landscapes. Science. 2013;339(6127):1546-58. PMC 3749880 Freely accessible.

CHAPTER 7

Nausea and Vomiting

Her Hsin Tsai

■ NEUROPHYSIOLOGY OF NAUSEA AND VOMITING

The neurological pathway that mediates the sensation of nausea is poorly understood. From an evolutionary survival point of view the vomiting reflex is valuable to expel toxic substances ingested and protection from gastrointestinal (GI) infection. However, the connection with vestibular apparatus is less well argued from a survival point of view. There is clearly also an element of higher conditioning. There may be overlap with the pathway that mediates the sensation of fullness or satiety mediated by largely the vagus nerve. It follows from this that anorexia is an almost universal accompaniment. Vomiting can be induced experimentally by electrical stimulation of the dorsal portion of the tractus solitarius in the medulla. The vomiting center is close to the centers which control respiration and salivation and the process of nausea and retching usually involves activation of both these centers. When retching occurs there is repeated herniation of the abdominal esophagus and cardia into the thorax as a result of a sudden fall in intrathoracic pressure due to inspiratory effort against a closed glottis. This is associated with reflux of gastric contents into the esophagus. The natural antireflux mechanisms of the esophagogastric junction having thus been overcome, vomiting may then follow and is associated with a rise in intrathoracic pressure.

Close to the vomiting center there is a chemoreceptor trigger zone in the floor of the fourth ventricle. Morphine, digoxin, many other drugs and also motion sickness act via stimulation of this center. In addition, sympathetic afferent fibers conduct signals back from the stomach to the vomiting center and are probably responsible for the nausea associated with gastritis and staphylococcal food poisoning. Five principal neurotransmitter receptors mediate vomiting: muscarinic M1, dopamine D2, histamine H1 5-hydroxytryptamine (HT)-3 serotonin, and neurokinin 1 (NK1) and substance P (Fig. 7.1).

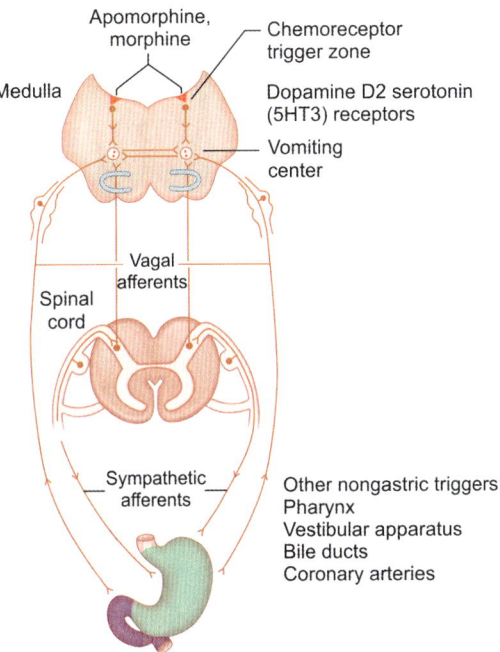

Fig. 7.1: Vomiting reflex is remarkably complex and involves multiple pathways and neurotransmitters.

■ DIAGNOSIS

Causes of Nausea and Vomiting

Abdominal pain is often associated with nausea or vomiting but the diagnosis and management of conditions which cause this combination of symptoms have already been discussed in the section on abdominal pain so will not be dealt with again here in detail. Patients with duodenal ulcer may vomit even in the absence of pyloric stenosis and will often notice relief of the pain after vomiting. Pain associated with biliary colic or pancreatitis will not however be relieved by vomiting. Vomiting is common in acute pancreatitis but uncommon in patients with a perforated viscus and this may be a useful diagnostic clue.

Causes of nausea and vomiting without abdominal pain are listed below:

Causes of Painless Nausea and Vomiting

- Alcoholic gastritis
- Viral gastritis
- Food poisoning

- Gastric carcinoma
- Pyloric stenosis
- Duodenal obstruction
- Biliary reflux following previous gastric surgery
- Diabetic gastroparesis
- Acute hepatitis
- Pregnancy
- Drugs
- Uremia
- Hypercalcemia
- Adrenal insufficiency
- Thyrotoxicosis
- Labyrinthitis
- Meniere's disease
- Psychogenic.

Causes of Vomiting without Nausea

Vomiting without nausea is a characteristic of neurological causes:
- Intracranial tumors
- Raised intracranial pressure
- Encephalitis
- Meningitis
- Migraine
- Cyclical vomiting.

Is the Patient Pregnant?

In a young woman with persistent vomiting this should be the first point to resolve. The vomiting may start shortly after the first missed period so it is not uncommon for patients to be referred up to gastroenterology clinics for investigation of vomiting due to undiagnosed pregnancy. Vomiting in pregnancy usually needs no specific treatment and resolves toward the end of the first trimester. Severe vomiting resulting in electrolyte or fluid depletion (hyperemesis gravidarum) affects about 3.5 per 1000 deliveries and requires hospital admission for fluid and electrolyte replacement and investigation for underlying causes such as twin pregnancy or hydatidiform mole.

Does the Patient Drink Alcohol Excessively?

Patients who habitually drink heavily often seem surprised when they develop alcohol-related gastritis and commonly fail to make any connection between the resulting vomiting and their alcohol intake. Alcoholic gastritis typically causes early morning retching or vomiting, usually of small volumes, the morning after heavy drinking. The vomit often contains flecks of blood.

Is the Patient Taking Drugs which Could be Responsible?

Many drugs will provoke nausea or vomiting by direct stimulation of the chemoreceptor trigger zone. Classical examples include morphine, dopamine agonists and digoxin but it is also a common side effect occurring in a minority of patients with many other drugs. Chemotherapeutic agents are universally emetic and prophylactic antiemetics are used. Sometimes patients receiving chemotherapy become "conditioned" and may develop nausea and vomiting even at the prospect of receiving the treatment.

Is it an Infective Agent?

Epidemics of vomiting are very common especially in winter months. The commonest nonbacterial agent is norovirus. Often dubbed "winter vomiting bug," it is by far the most common cause of infective gastroenteritis in developed countries. Onset is usually sudden and vomiting may be severe and associated with headache, muscle aches, and fever. Non-bloody diarrhea is usual but not always present. Symptoms usually last for 24–48 h and spontaneous recovery is usual. Detection of the infective virus can be made by immune electron microscopy of fecal samples or PCR, serum antibodies can be detected but has low specificity, with cross-reactivity with other homologous viruses. A new strain GII.4 Sydney, first isolated in Australia in 2013, is increasingly reported in the United Kingdom and is associated with higher rates of hospitalization and death in the frail.

Staphylococcus aureus food poisoning may cause a similar explosive onset of vomiting but lasting usually for only 24 h. It has an incubation period of 6–12 h.

Is there Any Evidence of Hepatitis or Hepatic Failure?

Vomiting is a common feature of severe hepatic damage and may be the presenting symptom of fulminant viral hepatitis, hepatic failure due to poisoning (e.g. paracetamol or solvents), fatty liver of pregnancy, Reye's syndrome, idiosyncratic reaction to drugs or acute presentation of Wilson's disease. Blood should be checked for hepatic enzymes and if these are abnormal or there is a strong suspicion of liver failure, the prothrombin time should be checked.

Is the Patient Diabetic?

It has been reported that up to 30% of diabetic patients suffer from intermittent nausea or vomiting. In many cases, this is due to vagal autonomic neuropathy resulting in "diabetic gastroparesis". Patients with this condition typically have longstanding insulin-dependent diabetes and frequently peripheral neuropathy and other signs of autonomic neuropathy such as postural hypotension, impotence, sweating and bladder dysfunction. There is marked delay in gastric emptying which may be seen on barium meal but is

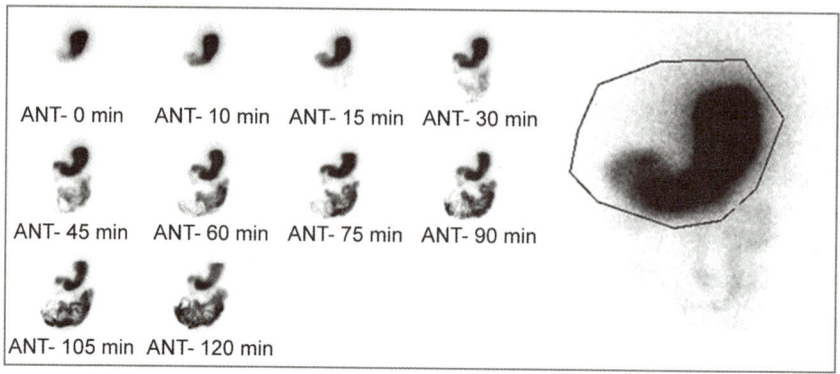

Fig. 7.2: A radiolabeled solid meal is given and the gastric emptying rate can be measured.

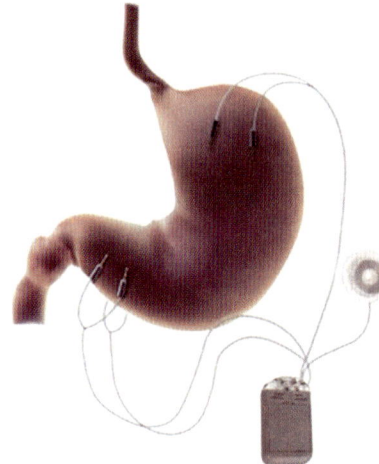

Fig. 7.3: Implantable gastric stimulators are promising treatments for diabetic gastroparesis.

best demonstrated by gastric scanning after ingestion of a radiolabeled meal (Fig. 7.2) (gastric emptying study). Treatment can be difficult. Prokinetics like metoclopramide can be used but carries a risk of tardive dyskinesia. Erythromycin has powerful prokinetic effects but it is short-lived and its effects are temporary. Implantable electric stimulation devices hold some promise (Fig. 7.3). A trial set of temporary electrodes are inserted into the stomach muscles endoscopically and if patients show response, then a permanent device can be inserted.

Could there be a Metabolic Problem?

Addison's disease is a particularly important condition to consider. Postural hypotension and mucosal pigmentation should be looked for. A high-normal or raised plasma potassium is highly suggestive since vomiting will usually result in a fall in plasma potassium. A short Synacthen test should be performed (plasma cortisol measurements before and 1 h after intravenous injection of adrenocorticotropic hormone). Hypercalcemia and hyperthyroidism should also be considered.

Has a Neurological Cause been Excluded?

The absence of nausea is not invariable in neurological vomiting and a neurological cause can easily be missed when vomiting is the only symptom. A careful neurological examination is required checking particularly for nystagmus, hearing loss, normality of gait, incoordination and signs of raised intracranial pressure including fundoscopy for identification of papilledema. If headache is a prominent symptom, intracranial tumor should be suspected. If it is recurrent, migraine should be considered. Magnetic resonance imaging or computed tomography (CT) of the head should be performed if there is a suspicion of intracranial malignancy.

Could there be a Gastric Cause?

Not all gastric lesions which cause vomiting are associated with pain so it is important to exclude gastric pathology. Gastric causes can include carcinoma, which commonly presents with vague symptoms of bloating, belching and nausea without definite pain. Tumors at the gastric outlet (Fig. 7.4) may present with gastric outlet obstruction with vomiting and weight loss. Tumors of the lower esophagus and cardia may present with regurgitation. Infiltrative tumors like linitis plastica are associated with a small shrunken stomach presenting with early satiety and vomiting (Fig. 7.5).

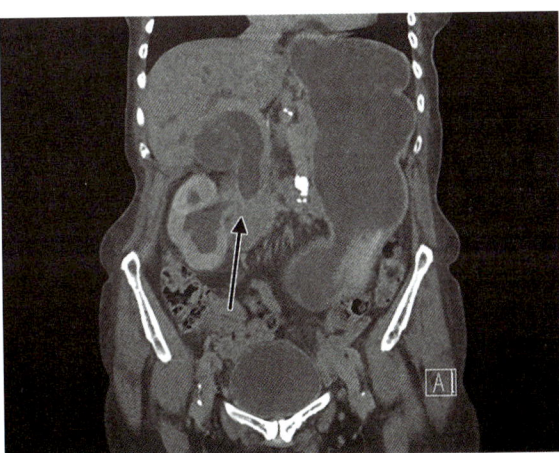

Fig. 7.4: Tumor in duodenum obstructing the gastric outlet and biliary tree.

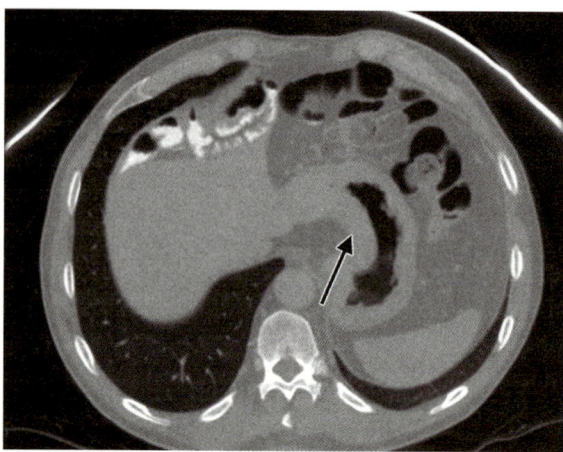

Fig. 7.5: Infiltrative gastric cancer of linitis plastica on computed tomography.

Other possibilities include gastritis (including rare conditions, such as Menetrier's hypertrophic gastritis or gastric Crohn's disease) and benign gastric ulceration. Duodenal stenosis can also be the result of previous benign duodenal ulcers that heal with stricturing.

Bile reflux gastritis is common in patients who have had a previous gastroenterostomy or partial gastrectomy. Endoscopically the mucosa looks diffusely reddened but there may be diagnostic changes of foveolar hyperplasia on histology. Treatment is often unsatisfactory. Bile acid binding agents such as aluminum hydroxide and cholestyramine are worth trying.

A hair bezoar may be an unexpected finding on endoscopy in patients with trichophagia (hair eating) which is the compulsive eating of hair associated with trichotillomania (hair pulling). It can often be broken up endoscopically thus preventing the need for laparotomy.

Is there Intestinal Obstruction?

If there is persistent vomiting associated with abdominal pain, distention and constipation, then intestinal obstruction should be suspected. It may present acutely or subacutely and may be intermittent. A plain abdominal film is very instructive and a CT scan often reveals the cause of the obstruction. This may be any part of the intestine from duodenum to lower colon with the higher lesions causing more vomiting and the lower lesions more bowel changes. Lesions that obstruct the intestine include intrinsic bowel strictures, Crohn's disease, tumors, intussusception or extrinsic lesions like pancreatic head cancers and adhesions.

Is the Vomiting Cyclical?

Cyclical vomiting, usually occurring approximately in 2-month cycles, most commonly present in childhood but may present in teenagers or

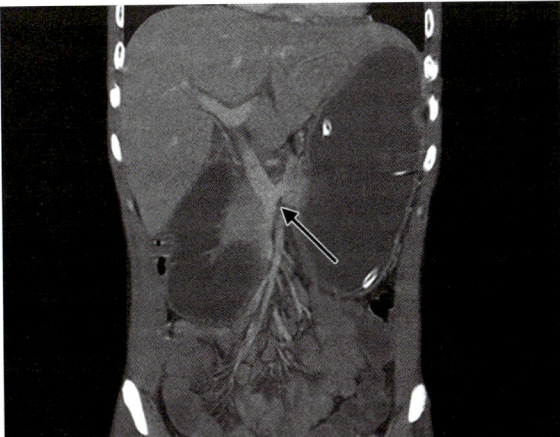

Fig. 7.6: Wilkie's syndrome: note the dilated proximal duodenum and stomach caused by superior mesenteric artery obstructing the distal duodenum.

young adults. It often seems to be a variant of migraine and may be associated with headache or abdominal pain. The condition may respond to propranolol. Care must be taken to exclude alternative GI or neurological causes.

Is it Superior Mesenteric Artery Syndrome (Wilkie's Syndrome)?

Sometimes a barium-meal examination performed in a patient with vomiting will show a dilated proximal duodenum with an apparent obstruction just to the right of the midline. Angiography will show the superior mesenteric artery crossing over the duodenum at this point. CT after non-contrast fluid (PEG solution) ingestion is often the best imaging modality (Fig. 7.6). The patients are usually thin, often female, and have been reported to benefit from duodeno- or gastrojejunostomy. A few cases have been reported after bariatric gastric bypass surgery. The rare possibility of a distal duodenal carcinoma should be considered in this situation.

Is the Vomiting Psychogenic?

Patients with psychogenic vomiting are typically young women with stressful home situations. They usually freely admit to the vomiting, as opposed to patients with bulimia who typically conceal the vomiting.
Features which suggest psychogenic vomiting include:
- Vomiting occurring during meals (organic causes usually result in vomiting after or between meals)
- Lack of preceding nausea
- The ability to delay vomiting until the toilet has been reached
- Apparent lack of concern about the vomiting.

Treatment is generally very difficult. Response to conventional antiemetics is usually poor. The underlying causes need to be addressed. Resolution usually takes place slowly over 1 or 2 years, particularly if the patient is no longer in the situation that he or she finds stressful.

DRUG THERAPY OF VOMITING

Diagnosing the cause of vomiting and instituting appropriate therapy will solve the problem. However, when the cause cannot be removed or treated then symptomatic relief of the unpleasant symptom may be necessary until the condition resolves. Unfortunately many drugs used may have severe extrapyramidal and other adverse reaction after prolonged use.

Prochlorperazine and chlorpromazine have antiemetic effects and may be useful in vestibular problems but both drugs, particularly the latter may cause extrapyramidal problems.

Dopaminergic antagonists like metoclopramide and domperidone can also be effective as they have central action on the vomiting centers as well as peripheral effects on the GI tract by encouraging gastric emptying by its prokinetic effects. However, prolonged use of these drugs may have neurological side effects and possible cardiac effects as well. These drugs too should be used for the short-term only.

5-HT3 receptor antagonists such as ondansetron block serotonin receptors both in the central nervous system and GI tract. They are helpful in postoperative and cytotoxic drug nausea and vomiting. Diarrhea and dry mouth are common side effects. For severe chemotherapy-induced nausea, some of the novel antiemetics like mirtazapine and cannabinoids may be tried.

Histamine receptor (H1) blockers like cyclizine are also helpful in motion sickness.

FURTHER READING

1. Furyk JS, Meek RA, Egerton-Warburton D. Drugs for the treatment of nausea and vomiting in adults in the emergency department setting. Cochrane Database Syst Rev. 2015;9:CD010106.

CHAPTER 8

Eating Disorders and Weight Loss

Her Hsin Tsai

PHYSIOLOGY OF APPETITE

There is a complex physiological mechanism that balances energy intake and expenditure, comprising afferent signals that stimulate appetite and eating and efferent feedback effectors to trigger satiety. The hypothalamus is the main regulatory center for appetite control through a complex neurohormonal mechanism that has recently been elucidated (Fig. 8.1). Hunger leads to initiation of eating and when a meal is ingested, satiety hormones initiate digestion and lead to a feeling of fullness and satiety. Excess energy is stored as adipose tissue, which secretes a hormone leptin that acts as a negative feedback on the hypothalamus. When food reaches the gut, it modulates the production of hormones like ghrelin, PYY 3-36, orexin and cholecystokinin all of which modify the hypothalamic response. Ghrelin is secreted when the stomach is empty. When the stomach is stretched, secretion stops. It acts on hypothalamic brain cells both to increase hunger, and to increase gastric acid secretion and gastrointestinal (GI) motility to prepare the body for food intake. The peptide PYY 3-36 is released from the ileum and colon in response to feeding. PYY acts to reduce appetite (anorexigenic). Other peripheral hormones that signals satiety include glucagon-like peptide-1 (GLP-1) and pancreatic polypeptide (PP). They are both suppressed in obesity and Prader–Willi syndrome, a genetic obesity syndrome. Systemic mediators released in cancer or inflammation and infection, such as tumor necrosis factor-alpha (TNFα), interleukins 1 and 6 and corticotropin-releasing hormone (CRH), suppress appetite and explain why ill people often eat less. Finally, insulin also acts to suppress appetite when glucose levels are elevated.

These peripheral hormonal signals are sensed by the arcuate nucleus of the hypothalamus and it in turn releases stimulatory peptides agouti-related peptide and neuropeptide Y or suppressive signals released in the form of the cocaine and amphetamine-regulated transcript and pro-opiomelanocortin,

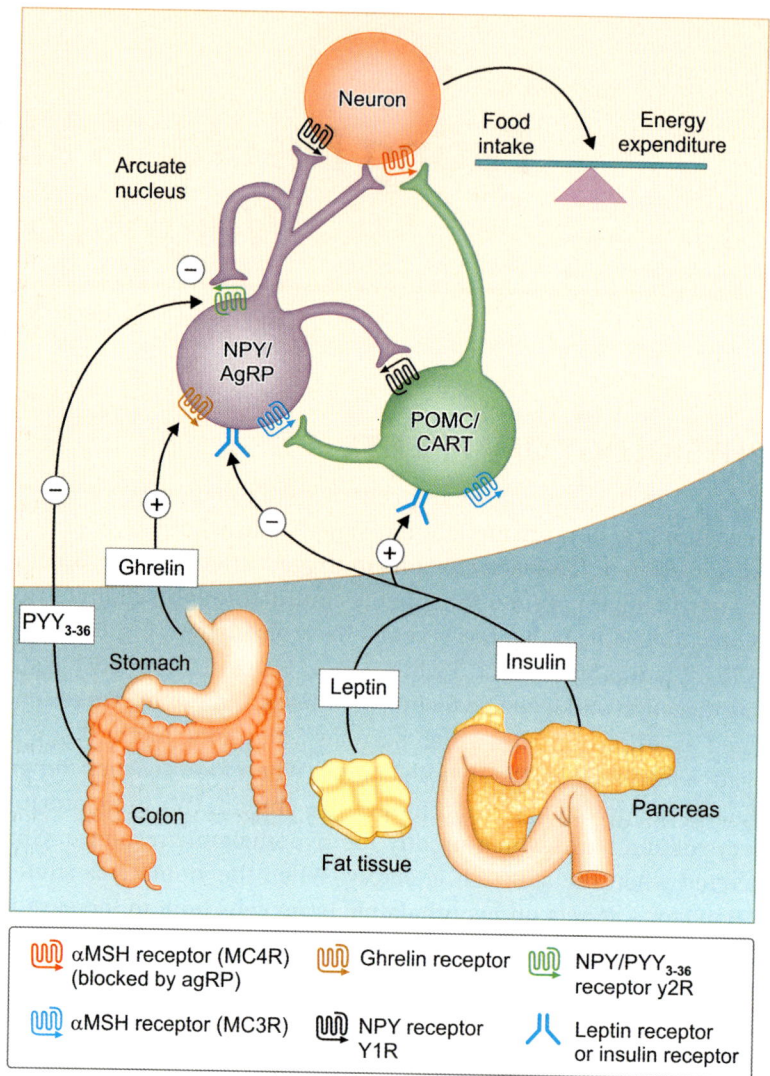

Fig. 8.1: Complex neurohormonal control of appetite.

to the paraventricular nucleus. Close to the hypothalamus are the sensory organs of smell and taste and the higher centers which integrates the signals that lead to eating behavior. Another important hormone in appetite control is orexin which is secreted by the hypothalamus and it promotes wakefulness and stimulates appetite. It is inhibited by leptin (through the leptin receptor pathway) and by hyperglycemia, but are activated by ghrelin. Apart from appetite control orexin has many other important roles in mood control and temperature control.

ANOREXIA AND WEIGHT LOSS

Exclusion of Malignant Disease

Malignant disease can be difficult to exclude in the absence of any localizing symptoms. Family history of cancer and the age of the patient are important considerations in assessing the likely risk. Direct questioning should be used to check for any change in bowel habit, any abdominal discomfort, any recent cough or hemoptysis, gynecological or neurological symptoms. Alcohol consumption should be noted since many patients are unaware of the high-calorific content of alcoholic drinks and are surprised when they lose weight if they cut their alcohol intake.

A careful clinical examination is extremely important with particular attention to lymph nodes. Rectal examination and fecal occult blood testing should be performed.

In the older patient (e.g. over 40) a reasonable program of screening tests would then include full blood count and erythrocyte sedimentation rate, liver biochemistry, chest X-ray, ultrasound scan of liver, pancreas, kidneys and pelvis. Because difficulty in visualizing the whole pancreas is common, it is also reasonable to check for the presence of one of the available pancreas cancer serological markers such as CA19.9. A good quality ultrasound is usually adequate but pancreas may be obscured by gas, and computed tomography (CT) (Figs. 8.2 and 8.3) scanning is probably the best modality. Modern machines produce superb images very quickly with little movement artifact. In the more obese patient, it is preferable to ultrasound. Upper GI endoscopy should be performed since gastric cancer may present as anorexia

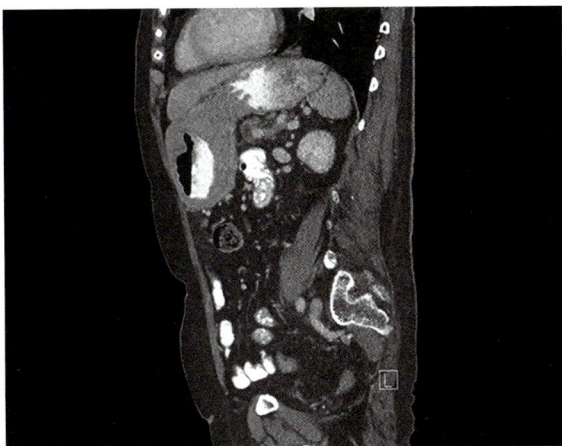

Fig. 8.2: Computed tomography showing thickened stomach with infiltrative disease with prominent lymph nodes; this turned out to be a lymphoma.

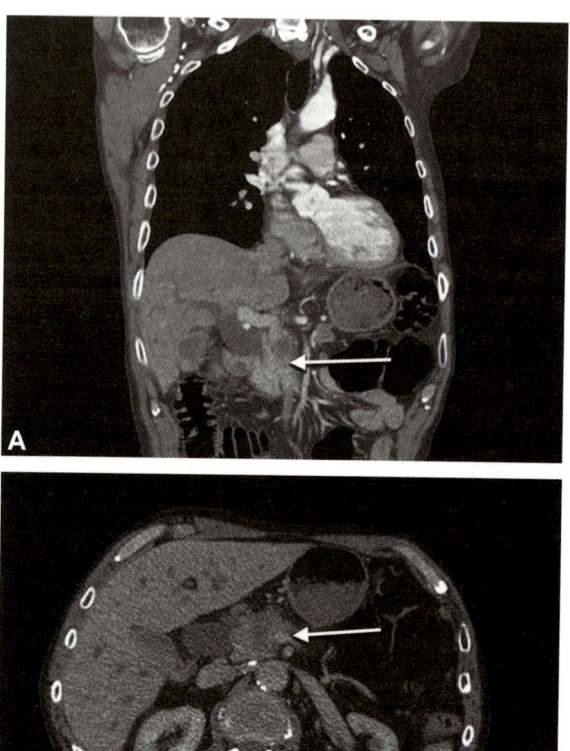

Figs. 8.3A and B: Tumor in the pancreatic head usually is advanced by the time; weight loss is evident. This CT shows a tumor invading vascular structure (A) and blocking the bile duct (B). (CT: Computed tomography)

without pain. Distal duodenal biopsy can be taken at the same time to exclude celiac disease.

If all these tests prove negative a reasonable approach is to review the patient again after a period of about 2 months and reweigh when the patient will often be found to have regained weight. It is particularly important to reexamine the patient thoroughly on subsequent review to check for lymph nodes or other masses that may have become apparent since the first examination.

Exclusion of Metabolic Disease

Tests should include serum calcium, creatinine, glucose, thyroid function tests and plasma electrophoresis. If there is postural hypotension, a short Synacthen test should be performed to exclude Addison's disease.

ANOREXIA NERVOSA

Anorexia nervosa has a male to female ratio of approximately 1:15 which presumably reflects the greater pressure on females to correspond to the socially imposed perception that slimness is desirable. Surveys have shown that it probably affects 4% of females at some time. It is increasingly realized that there are many patients who do not fit all of the previously required diagnostic criteria but who nevertheless have a significant eating disorder. Characteristic features therefore may include some but not necessarily all of the following:

- Loss of 25% of original body weight
- Onset before 25 years
- Distorted body image
- Hoarding of food
- Amenorrhea
- Lanugo hair
- Bradycardia (<60)
- Low luteinizing hormone and follicle-stimulating hormone
- Low T4 and normal thyroid-stimulating hormone
- Low temperature.

Other psychiatric illnesses such as depression or schizophrenia should be excluded.

Management

The patient is often defensive or manipulative. Secretive vomiting or hoarding of food is usual. Purgative and/or diuretic abuses are common. Any patient who has lost >40% of their ideal body weight or >25% within 3 months should be admitted to hospital. A target weight should be agreed with the patient. Meals should be taken at regular times and the patient should be sat with during and for 1 h after each meal.

If the patient does not cooperate with this approach management can be very difficult. A wide range of approaches has been tried reflecting not only the different training but often the different philosophical approach to life of the healthcare personnel involved. There is a need to have a team approach to management. Patients need to their rights protected as well. Psychotherapy and gentle encouragement and agreed objectives must be clear to all healthcare workers. The mortality is at least 5% however and many healthcare professionals find it unacceptable to watch a patient starving to death without attempting some form of assisted feeding.

Enteral feeding, usually with a fine bore nasogastric feeding is quite unobtrusive and is often accepted by patient. Feeding must be done carefully as there is a high risk of refeeding syndrome (*see* Chapter 16). Bloods electrolytes including magnesium should be carefully monitored. There is also a risk of gastric dilatation, vomiting and aspiration and also a risk of pancreatitis. Caloric intake should be increased gradually up to 3000 cal/day over a 2-week period.

If treatment is successful the patient may develop better insight into the problem as her weight approaches normal. At this time careful discussions should be held with the patient and family members to attempt to resolve the underlying conflicts or anxieties which are often present. Between one third and 50% make a complete recovery but persistence of some form of eating disorder (often intermittent bulimia) into later adult life is common and may even persist into old age.

Bulimia (binging and self-induced vomiting) often complicates anorexia but in less severe cases may be the main feature. There is then often a greater insight and the prognosis is generally better. In the short term however severe electrolyte disturbances may occur and can even be fatal. The combination of dehydration and hypokalemia may result in urinary calculi and life-threatening renal failure.

OBESITY

Epidemiology and Morbidity

People are generally considered obese when their body mass index (BMI), a measurement obtained by dividing a person's weight by the square of the person's height, is over 30 kg/m^2, with the range 25–30 kg/m^2 defined as overweight. A recent worldwide survey has shown that the proportion of adults with a BMI of 25 kg/m^2 or greater increased between 1980 and 2013 from 28.8% (95% CI 28.4–29.3) to 36.9% (36.3–37.4) in men, and from 29.8% (29.3–30.2) to 38.0% (37.5–38.5) in women. Prevalence has increased substantially in children and adolescents in developed countries; 23.8% (22.9–24.7) of boys and 22.6% (21.7–23.6) of girls were overweight or obese in 2013. The prevalence of obesity has also increased in children and adolescents in developing countries, from 8.1% (7.7–8.6) to 12.9% (12.3–13.5) in 2013 for boys, and from 8.4% (8.1–8.8) to 13.4% (13.0–13.9) in girls (Fig. 8.4).

Mortality rates compared with those of optimal weight are 28% higher with body weight 120–129% above ideal, 46% higher with 130–139% and 88% higher for those >140% of ideal weight. Mortality is increased from coronary artery disease, diabetes and there is a considerable increase in relative risk for a range of intestinal cancers: in those 140% ideal weight relative risks are for colorectal cancer: 1.73 for males, 1.22 females; for stomach cancer: 1.88 for males, 1.03 females; pancreatic cancer: 1.62 for males, 0.61 for females. In 2010, overweight and obesity were estimated to cause 3.4 million deaths, 4% of years of life lost, and 4% of disability-adjusted life-years worldwide.

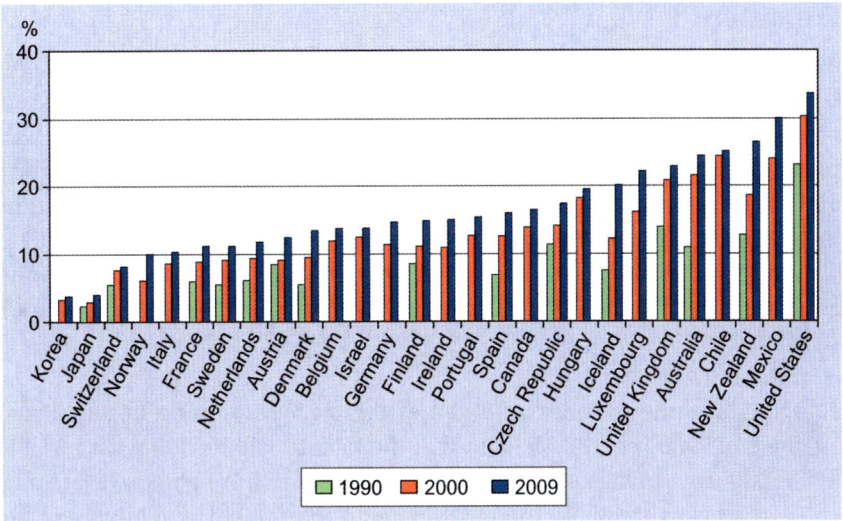

Fig. 8.4: Obesity rates around the world.

Etiology

Underlying genetic defects are very rare and invariably present in childhood. They may be divided into four groups: (1) syndromes with primary hypogonadism and no polydactyly such as Prader–Willi, these children have hypotonia, mental retardation, short stature and hypogenitalism; (2) syndromes with secondary hypogonadism with polydactyly such as Laurence-Moon (+ retinal degeneration, mental deficiency) and (3) without polydactyly such as Bardet–Biedl (also + retinal degeneration and mental deficiency) and (4) obesity without hypogonadism such as triglyceride storage disease (extremely rare). These syndromes have autosomal recessive inheritance and are usually readily recognized by the combination of short stature and mental retardation.

Hypothalamic damage due to trauma or neoplasia is a very rare cause of obesity (which may also be associated with disordered temperature regulation).

There is considerable argument as to whether "simple" obesity is inherited. Fat children usually have fat parents but this might reflect environmental influence. However, children adopted at a young age by overweight foster parents are often of normal weight suggesting that environmental factors may be less important than genetic factors. Children of obese parents have been shown to have lower basal metabolic rates than children of normal-sized parents.

Treatment

A common course of events is for the patient to go on a "crash" diet that is devoid of carbohydrate. Muscle and liver glycogen will start to be broken down and as this is stored with four times its own weight of water there will be rapid weight loss for the first 2–3 weeks. This process will then slow down and ingestion of a relatively small amount of carbohydrate will rapidly undo the weight loss, the patient will become disheartened and give up.

Even more drastic diets such as protein only diets are dangerous, probably because of their low potassium intake, and may be associated with sudden death.

A reasonable course is to:

1. Explain to the patient that a loss of 1 kg of fat requires a negative balance of 7700 kcal (32 MJ) and that the patient will be doing very well if he/she eats 1000 kcal/day less than is consumed. Weight loss averaging 1 kg/week is therefore the most that can reasonably be maintained for any reasonable period.
2. Explain that successful dieting cannot be achieved without feeling hungry, at least for the first 2–3 weeks and that considerable willpower will be needed.
3. Explain that fat has about 9 kcal/g and alcohol has 7 kcal/g compared with carbohydrate of only 4 kcal/g. Reduction in alcohol and fat intake may therefore have a much more dramatic effect than carbohydrate restriction and will also result in a much healthier diet.
4. Ask the patient to keep a diary of what he/she eats. This may highlight indulgencies that the patient may have thought were less frequent than they are and also allows the doctor or dietitian to advise on which items have the highest calorific content.
5. The basic aim is a permanent reduction in intake of sugar, fat and alcohol with maintenance of starch and protein intake.

Commercial slimming organizations may benefit some patients but their success rates are generally only of the order of 15–20%.

Energy expenditure through exercise should be encouraged, water-based activity allows for buoyancy and reduction of load on weight bearing joints.

The most effective treatment for obesity is bariatric surgery. The types of procedures include laparoscopic adjustable gastric banding, Roux-en-Y gastric bypass, vertical-sleeve gastrectomy and biliopancreatic diversion. Gastric restriction surgery alone is often ineffective and addition of a bypass to reduce absorptive surface is necessary. Surgery for severe obesity is associated with long-term weight loss, improvement in obesity-related conditions and decreased overall mortality. However, complications occur in about 17% of cases and reoperation is needed in 7% of cases (*see* Chapter 10). Moreover, bariatric surgery is expensive and may seem excessive.

Drugs are of limited value. Several drugs have been developed for long-term use in obesity. Orlistat is potent natural inhibitor of pancreatic lipases and hence reduced digestion of fats leads to steatorrhea. There is some concern about it causing renal impairment. Liraglutide is a derivative of human incretin (metabolic hormone) glucagon-like peptide-1 (GLP-1) and is an injectable drug which is used in diabetics and suppresses appetite. Bupropion/naltrexone is a combination drug used for weight loss. It combines low doses of bupropion which is an opiate and thus has appetite suppressing effects, and naltrexone, an opiate antagonist. The combination appears to have synergistic effects in reducing appetite and effective as a weight loss agent. Another drug is phentermine/topiramate. Phentermine is a sympathomimetic amine which acts as an appetite suppressant and stimulant, and topiramate is an anticonvulsant which has weight loss side effects. The combination pill is used as a weight reducing drug. However, it is associated with cardiovascular adverse effects. Drug therapy is highly dependent on patient compliance and its many adverse effects limit its use. When dietary treatment alone has failed, drug could be used in combination with a controlled diet.

■ FURTHER READING

1. Attia E. Anorexia nervosa: current status and future directions. Annu Rev Med. 2010;61(1):425-35.

CHAPTER 9

Wind

Her Hsin Tsai

■ BELCHING

Belching, particularly in association with satiety and nausea, may occasionally be a symptom of significant gastric disease, either benign or malignant. Endoscopy is therefore indicated if it occurs as a new symptom in a patient over 40.

In most patients however there is no underlying gastric pathology. Drinking of carbonated drinks naturally can result in burping and the repeated belching results from repeated air swallowing (aerophagia). The air often does not enter the stomach, being noisily regurgitated shortly after it has been swallowed. This usually occurs as a response to stress. The patient is often unaware of the air swallowing but if reassurance is combined with an explanation of the mechanism the problem is usually considerably improved.

■ FLATUS

Much of what we know about flatus has been learnt as a result of meticulous studies by the American researchers, Bond and Levitt. They have shown that the composition of flatus varies widely: nitrogen 11–92%; oxygen 0–11%; carbon dioxide 3–54%; hydrogen 0–69%; methane 0–56%. Hydrogen production is the result of bacterial fermentation of unabsorbed carbohydrate. Methane production varies considerably between individuals and seems to be due to the presence or absence of methane-forming bacteria. The methane-producing status of most individuals seems to remain constant for life and it is presumed that these organisms are established in the colon early in life. Interestingly the feces of methane producers can be recognized by their tendency to float. The main gases are odorless, odor is caused by sulfurous gases like hydrogen sulfide and volatile aromatic compounds like short-chain fatty acids.

Although excessive air swallowing may result in air reaching the anus within 20 min of being swallowed, air swallowing is very rarely the cause of excessive flatus. Some intriguing experiments have shown that the normal range of flatus excretion varies between 200 and 2000 mL/day resulting in an average of about 40 separate passages of gas in young adult male controls. Excessive flatus (although very rarely meticulously documented) is almost always the result of increased production of hydrogen and carbon dioxide as a result of bacterial fermentation of carbohydrate. This usually results from either:

1. The ingestion of high quantities of poorly absorbed dietary fiber or fermentable oligosaccharide, disaccharide, monosaccharide and polyols (FODMAP) foods.
2. Malabsorption of carbohydrate either due to hypolactasia or more generalized malabsorptive syndromes.
3. Small intestinal bacterial overgrowth, perhaps due to previous surgery, duodenal diverticulum or diabetes.

Patients who complain of excessive flatus should generally be reassured and advised that it is entirely normal and do not require invasive investigations. If hypolactasia is suspected, a lactose hydrogen (or methane) breath test could be performed. A glucose (or lactulose) hydrogen breath test is a simple test to exclude intestinal bacterial overgrowth.

Treatment of hypolactasia is simply to avoid dairy products. Supplementation with oral lactase can also be effective. Bacterial overgrowth treatment is dealt with in Chapter 3.

In all other patients, strategies to reduce intestinal gas include:
1. Dietary reduction in FODMAP foods (Table 9.1).
2. Use of surfactants (e.g. Infacol).

Table 9.1: Foods high in FODMAP to avoid.				
High fructose	**Lactose**	**Fructans**	**Galactans**	**Polyols**
Fruits	*Milk*	*Vegetables*	*Legumes*	*Sweeteners*
Apples, applesauce, apricots, dates, canned fruit, cherries, dried fruits, figs, guava, lychee, mango, nectarines, pears, papaya, peaches, plums, prunes, persimmon, watermelon	Cow, goat or sheep milk and products like yoghurt, ice cream	Avocado, artichokes, asparagus, beets, leeks, broccoli, Brussel sprouts, cabbage, cauliflower, fennel, green beans, mushrooms, okra, snow peas, summer squash	Baked bean, chick peas, kidney beans, lentils	Sorbitol, isomalt, maltitol, xylitol, mannitol
Sweeteners	*Cheeses*	*Grain*		*Vegetables*
Fructose	Soft unripened cheeses, cottage, cream, mascarpone, ricotta	Wheat and rye in large amounts as bread or cereal		Peppers, cauliflower, mushroom
Fruit juice from concentrates				
Honey, corn syrup				

3. Probiotics.
4. Nonabsorbable antibiotics like rifaximin.

BLOATING

Bloating is a complaint of abdominal distension usually accompanied by pain or discomfort. It may occasionally be a postprandial fullness resulting from important gastric pathology but more commonly is used to describe the generalized abdominal distension that is commonly a symptom in patients who have other features of the irritable bowel syndrome (IBS) such as alternating constipation with diarrhea and colicky abdominal pain. Patients often have a flat abdomen in the morning and gets bloated as the day progresses (Fig. 9.1). The cause of this is multifactorial. Magnetic resonance imaging studies have shown only a modest increase in abdominal gas volume. This may be due to impaired carbohydrate handling. There is some element of dysmotility allowing gas reflux into the stomach and certainly visceral hypersensitivity. The most important contributor to the distention is phrenic nerve stimulation and a subconscious contraction of the diaphragm with corresponding relaxation of anterior abdominal muscles (Figs. 9.1A to C). This is probably a reflex action to visceral hypersensitivity (abdominophrenic reflex).

It is important to differentiate bloating from IBS from that of ovarian cysts and tumors. In the latter the distension is permanent and the distention occurs while lying down and all day and not intermittent. A simple ultrasound scan should resolve the difference.

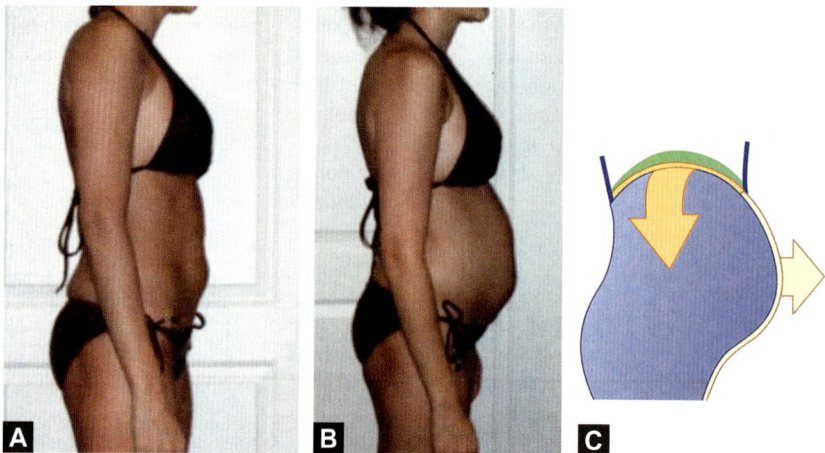

Figs. 9.1A to C: Phrenic dyssynergia: a subconscious contraction of the diaphragm and relaxation of abdominal muscles results in the protrusion of abdomen seen as bloating.

Treatment of IBS-associated bloating can be difficult. The general principles are laid out in Chapter 1. It would involve treatment of underlying psychopathology, dietary and pharmacological therapy. Diets and other measures to reduce gas production as described earlier may be helpful, pain management with the use of small doses of tricyclics and the use of smooth muscle relaxants such as mebeverine or hyoscine or peppermint oil preparations may be effective therapy. In patients with a predominant constipation (IBS-C), lubiprostone and linaclotide have shown to reduce bloating symptom scores in clinical trials.

Teaching Points

Belching
- May indicate significant gastric pathology
- Usually results from excessive air swallowing.

Bloating
- Usually reflects disordered motility rather than increased gas
- Diaphragmatic (phrenic) contraction and abdominal wall relaxation is the main contributor.

Excessive Flatus
- Is not usually due to air swallowing
- Results from increased fermentation of carbohydrate by colonic bacteria
- May be due to carbohydrate malabsorption or excessive intake of fiber.

FODMAP Foods (to Avoid)

The FODMAPs in the diet include:
- Fructose (fruits, honey, high-fructose corn syrup, etc.)
- Lactose (dairy)
- Fructans (wheat, garlic, onion, inulin, etc.)
- Galactans (legumes such as beans, lentils, soybeans, etc.)
- Polyols (sweeteners containing isomaltose, mannitol, sorbitol, xylitol, stone fruits, such as avocado, apricots, cherries, nectarines, peaches, plums, etc.).

FODMAPs may be poorly absorbed and could be fermented by bacteria in the intestinal tract when eaten in excess, releasing gases. Gases like methane are poorly absorbed and remain in the intestine contributing to bloatedness.

FURTHER READING

1. Di Stefano M, Strocchi A, Malservisi S, et al. Non-absorbable antibiotics for managing intestinal gas production and gas-related symptoms. Alimentary Pharmacol Ther. 2000;14(8):1001-8.

2. King TS, Elia M, Hunter JO. Abnormal colonic fermentation in irritable bowel syndrome. Lancet. 1998;352(9135):1187-9.
3. Levitt MD, Bond JH. Volume, composition and source of intestinal gas. Gastroenterology. 1970;59:921.
4. Tangerman A. Measurement and biological significance of the volatile sulfur compounds hydrogen sulfide, methanethiol and dimethyl sulfide in various biological matrices. J Chromatogr B Analyt Technol Biomed Life Sci. 2009;877(28):3366-77.

CHAPTER 10

Gastrointestinal Complications of Obesity Surgery and Other Gastric Operations

Her Hsin Tsai

■ INTRODUCTION

In the past 20 years, there has been a major shift in the practice of gastric surgery. The old procedures for duodenal ulcer surgery such as vagotomy and drainage procedures are largely obsolete and rarely performed. There has however been a great increase in numbers of gastric operations for obesity also known as bariatric surgery. This takes the form of restrictive and bypass procedures of the stomach and may result in gastrointestinal (GI) complications. Some complications are specific for weight reduction surgery, while others occur with gastric surgery for any reason such as cancer surgery or as a result of emergency surgery.

Obesity, as defined by a body mass index of 30 and over, has in many countries reached epidemic proportions. UK figures in 2014 show that 25% of adults are obese. Obesity is associated with risk of major medical problems like hypertension, cardiac, chest problems, diabetes, embolic disease and some cancers. There is the associated increased morbidity and mortality. Calorie restriction through behavioral change is often unsuccessful and weight reduction surgery (bariatric surgery) is increasingly performed. As a consequence, gastroenterologists are increasing faced with GI complications in patients with previous bariatric surgery. Some of the complications are specific to bariatric surgery but others are in common with other types of gastric surgery as may be encountered for malignant gastric disease or in lesser frequency for benign gastric and duodenal ulcers as a result of complications like perforation.

Bariatric surgery involves some form of volume restriction of the stomach to solid foods with or without some enteric diversion to reduce absorptive surface. They can be performed laparoscopically or by open surgery. There are many variations but can be generalized as four types (Figs. 10.1A to D):

1. **Gastric Band Placement**: A silastic band is placed just below the gastroesophageal junction that simply restricts food passage. Adjustable bands are preferred which are laparoscopically placed around the upper stomach to create a restrictive pouch. The balloon in the band is

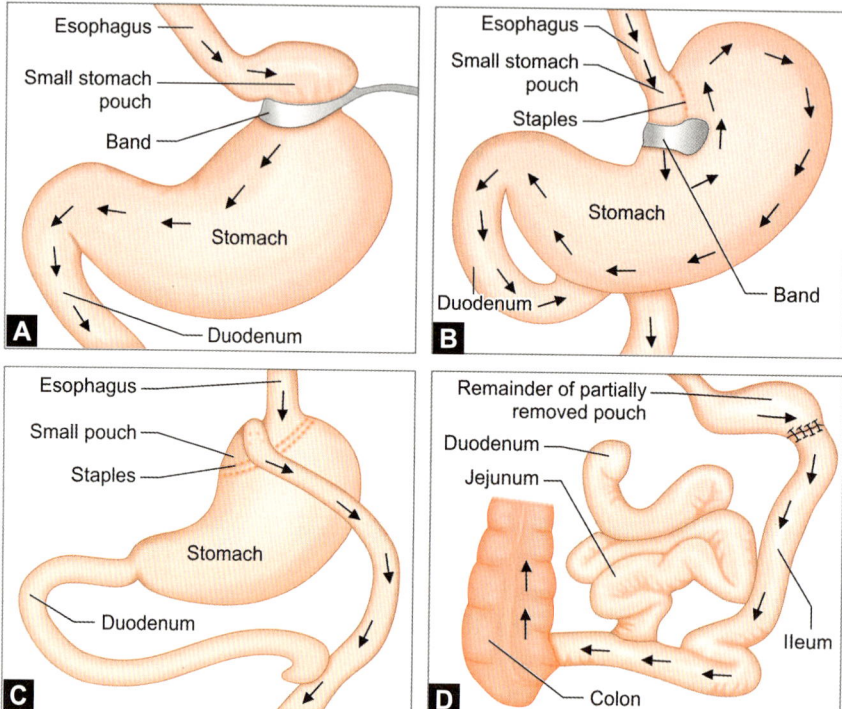

Figs. 10.1A to D: Four main types of bariatric surgery. (A) Laparoscopic adjustable gastric band; (B) Vertical banded gastroplasty; (C) Roux-en-Y gastric bypass; (D) Biliopancreatic diversion.

connected to a port that is placed subcutaneously and can be accessed to inflate or deflate the balloon, consequently changing the size of the band circumference.

2. **Vertical Band Gastropexy**: This involves stapling of the stomach from the fundus and placement of a band in order that gastric volume is restricted to a small pouch.
3. **Gastric Bypass (Roux-en-Y Gastric Bypass)**: Roux-en-Y gastric bypass is mainly a gastric-restrictive procedure, but there is an element of diversion, bypassing of some absorptive jejunum that contributes to weight loss by causing malabsorption of calories and inducing dumping syndrome. A small pouch is constructed by stapling or transecting the proximal stomach and the length of the limb can be varied depending on the size of the patient and can be anything from 50 to 100 cm in length.
4. **Biliopancreatic Diversion**: This is a more radical approach in which a very long Roux-en-Y is created along with a limited gastrectomy. A long segment of jejunum and ileum is thus bypassed by the operation. This can lead to drastic reduction in absorptive surface and lead to substantial weight loss but also risks of malnutrition especially of micronutrients.

There are two ways of fashioning the reconstruction: a classic (Polya style) or by preserving the pylorus with a sleeve gastrectomy. The latter reduces the frequency of dumping syndrome.

ABDOMINAL PAIN

Abdominal pain is not uncommon after bariatric surgery. There can be many causes and include:
- Acute gastric distention/anastomotic leaks
- Stomal ulceration
- Internal herniation
- Gallstones
- Afferent loop syndrome.

Is it a Perioperative Complication?

In the days immediately after bariatric surgery patients may complain of acute abdominal pain. Anastomotic leaks should be suspected. It may be obvious signs of peritonitis but may be subtle with mild abdominal pain, shoulder pain, back pain, unexplained tachycardia or increased urinary and bowel frequency. A high degree of vigilance coupled with water-soluble contrasts are helpful in demonstrating leaks. Treatment is surgical exploration. Gastrocolic fistulae can also be a complication of sleeve gastrectomy leaks and present with pain and diarrhea. Acute gastric distention is another major complication of surgery and presents abdominal pain, distention and has picked up clinical examination and X-ray. If left untreated, it could lead to staple-line dehiscence which can be catastrophic in consequence with sepsis and mortality. It is usually caused by edema at the enteroenteric anastomosis. Treatment is a radiologically inserted gastrostomy to decompress the stomach.

Is it Stomal Ulceration?

In patients who had surgery involving a gastroenterostomy, stomal ulceration is notoriously common affecting up to 50% of all Roux-en-Y type operations. Usually the remnant of the stomach still possesses acid-secreting cells and the ulcers are acid related. It is worth checking the *Helicobacter* status as it may be a contributory factor and smoking and nonsteroidal anti-inflationary drugs (NSAIDs) are other etiological factors. Majority of stomal ulcers are asymptomatic but when pain is present it tends to resemble duodenal ulcer pain. Occasionally it may present with upper GI bleeding without a history of pain. Large stomal ulcers may perforate and fistulation into the colon has been described. If left untreated, stomal ulcers may lead to stricture formation.

Diagnosis is by endoscopy. Treatment is usually medical with PPI's at full or enhanced doses and eradiation of *Helicobacter pylori* if found.

Addition of oral sucralfate is necessary if ulcers do not heal on proton pump inhibitors (PPIs) alone. Smoking must be discouraged. Prevention of stomal ulcers is advocated for all patients after bariatric surgery with PPIs given for up to 6 months postoperatively.

Is it an Internal Hernia?

Patients who complain of abdominal pain with signs of bowel obstruction may have an internal hernia. It can occur at any time after bariatric surgery but most often occur between 6 and 24 months after operation. It is more common in laparoscopic surgery compared to open operations. This is probably due to greater adhesion formation after open surgery, thus preventing small bowel mobility. The reorganization of the alimentary tract results in defects in mesentery leading to possible internal herniation. The defect is dependent on the exact operation, with an antecolic approach leading to two possible defects in the mesocolon. Weight loss itself is a contributory factor in the creation of these spaces. Pregnancy is also seen as another factor. A high index of clinical suspicion is important. Computed tomography (CT) scans are the imaging modality of choice but the findings can be very subtle. Signs of small bowel obstruction, twisting or swirling may be present. It is important to have a radiological conference with an experienced GI radiologist to reach a diagnosis. Treatment is surgery, usually managed laparoscopically. If clinical suspicion is strong, exploratory laparoscopy with intention to proceed to surgical therapy should be performed.

Is it Gallstones?

Obesity and rapid weight loss are independent risk factors for gallstone formation. Hence, patients having bariatric surgery may develop gallstone diseases (Fig. 10.2). If gallstones are present prior to weight reduction surgery,

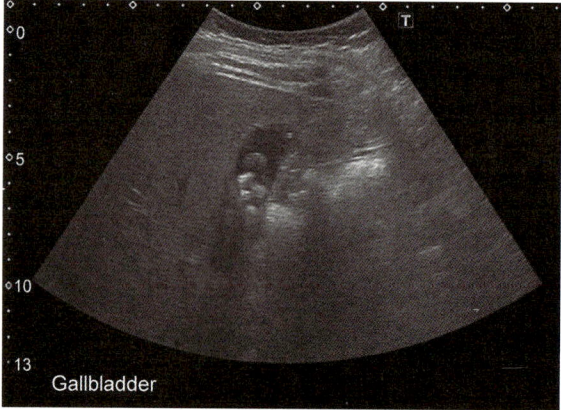

Fig. 10.2: Gallstones are common after obesity surgery and rapid weight loss.

some surgeons advocate cholecystectomy at the same time whether or not they are symptomatic. New gallstone development is common in the first year after surgery and about 15% of all patients are symptomatic enough to warrant cholecystectomy. Symptoms are not different from other non-bariatric patients (*see* Chapter 1). Due to the relatively high incidence of gallstone formation, prophylactic treatment with ursodeoxycholic acid has been advocated. Trials have shown a remarkable reduction in gallstone formation if the drug is given for 6 months after surgery.

Is it Afferent Loop Obstruction Syndrome?

Afferent loop obstruction syndrome is relatively rare complication where there is a sizable biliopancreatic loop (afferent loop). Obstruction may occur as a result of internal herniation, stricture of anastomosis or adhesions. Symptoms include severe abdominal pain and distention. In patients with Polya gastrectomy, partial obstruction may occur where pain and distention occurs after meals and is relieved by vomiting of bile. Classic plain abdominal film of loop dilatation is uncommon. Diagnosis is best reached by CT abdomen. Surgical intervention is usually necessary.

■ VOMITING

Vomiting is a common symptom after bariatric surgery. The most common reason is not adhering to a postgastroplasty advice. Patients should take very small meals, chew well, eat undisturbed and not to drink for at least 2 hours after food. Understandably, old habits are tenacious. Specific coaching, usually with dietetic input usually resolves the problem.

Vomiting accompanied by abdominal pain is discussed earlier. Gastroparesis is not uncommon after gastric surgery and patients who have diabetes can have diabetic autonomic neuropathy leading to gastric emptying issues, which can be exacerbated by surgery.

Stenosis of the stoma may occur as a result of edema from stomal ulcers or its fibrotic sequelae. Vomiting may or may not be associated with abdominal pain. Endoscopy is helpful, but contrast meal is also helpful. Strictures may be dilated endoscopically. Patients with restrictive procedures, such as vertical band gastroplasty, may also develop nausea and vomiting secondary to stomal stenosis, erosion of the restrictive band or ring (Fig. 10.3).

■ DYSPHAGIA

Dysphagia may occur after bariatric surgery. There is often an increased tendency to have gastroesophageal reflux after restrictive surgery to the stomach which may lead to esophagitis. Postoperative use of PPIs prophylactically may reduce its frequency.

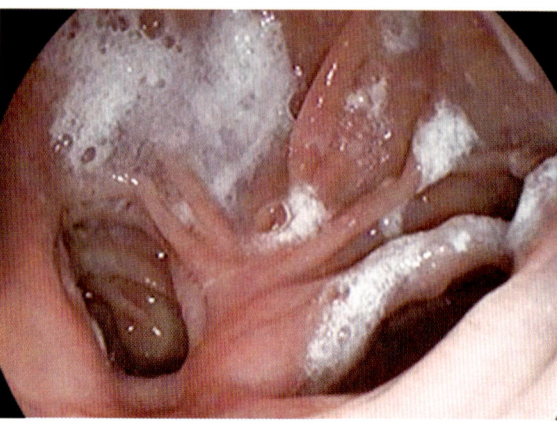

Fig. 10.3: Endoscopic appearance of obesity surgery varies according to the type of operation.

The restrictive nature of the operation, particularly with the use of a gastric band also lends itself to food bolus obstruction. Poorly masticated piece of meat can easily get lodged. Patients will complain of a sudden often painful dysphagia after eating. Occasionally, with a gastric pouch the anastomosis may become strictured, although it is rarely severe enough to cause significant dysphagia, but may lend itself to food bolus impaction.

DIARRHEA

Diarrhea is usually a direct consequence of bariatric surgery due to reduction of absorptive surface and biliopancreatic diversion. However, other causes of diarrhea should be considered:
- Dumping syndrome
- Bile salt diarrhea (also *see* Chapter 3)
- Small bowel bacterial overgrowth (also *see* Chapter 3).

Dumping Syndrome

Dumping syndrome can be a problem after some forms of bariatric operations where there is a gastroenterostomy involved. A pylorus preserving procedure such as the switch operation reduces the possibility of dumping occurring. When it occurs, the symptoms can be crippling to the patient. There are two manifestations: early and late dumping.

Early Dumping

Early dumping manifests within 10–20 min after a meal with symptoms of faintness and abdominal discomfort. Systemic symptoms include palpitations, fatigue, headaches, flushing and syncope. Abdominal discomfort is associated with nausea and diarrhea with abdominal cramps. The pathophysiology of early dumping is multifactorial. There is rapid gastric emptying resulting in rapid intestinal juice sequestration with consequent in hypovolemia and hypotension. There is resultant bloating and diarrhea as a result of inappropriate gut hormone release.

It is possible to set up a dumping provocation test by monitoring the pulse, blood pressure and serum potassium and monitor symptoms during a test meal (typically a drink containing 50 g of glucose). A fall of blood pressure and potassium levels is indicative of early dumping. If still in doubt a gastric emptying study could document early emptying, and a glucose breath hydrogen test will be (falsely) positive due to the early arrival of glucose into the large bowel.

Late Dumping

This occurs 2–3 h after a meal with faintness, perspiration, shakiness, hunger pains and drowsiness. The mechanism is often attributed to insulin release as a result of a glucose load delivered to the small bowel. The dumping of glucose in the jejunum results in enhanced hyperinsulinemia, more so than for equivalent intravenous glucose; the so-called incretin effect. This effect is thought to involve two incretin peptides glucagon-like peptide 1 (GLP-1) and glucose-dependent insulinotropic peptide (also known as gastric inhibitory polypeptide). These are released by the K cells of the small bowel in response to arrival of carbohydrate in the lumen. This effect is enhanced after gastric surgery with the early arrival of a carbohydrate meal. These peptides induce enhanced insulin secretion resulting in the hyperinsulinemia observed. The result is hypoglycemia, and the reflex adrenaline response resulting in the symptoms.

Treatment

Treatment can be difficult. Both early and late dumping is managed in a similar fashion. This can be dietary, medical or surgical interventions.

Diet is important. Taking smaller more frequent meals will limit dumping. Simple sugars like sucrose should be limited and carbohydrates replaced by protein and fat for calorific equivalents. Generally dairy products are poorly tolerated. Increasing soluble fiber content would also flatten out the glucose peaks after meals.

Acarbose: Acarbose is an alpha-glycoside hydrolase inhibitor which is used in type 2 diabetes. It interferes with carbohydrate absorption by inhibiting alpha-glucosidases associated with the brush border of the intestine and thus delays the insulin peak. It also acts by reducing GLP-1 secretion and hence reduces the hyperinsulinemia. Doses of 100 mg with every meal can significantly blunt both early and late dumping symptoms.

Octreotide: Somatostatin and its synthetic analogs have been used in the treatment of dumping syndrome with good efficacy demonstrated in both early and late dumping. It is a hormone with wide-ranging effects on the gut, including inhibition of excessive release of insulin of late dumping. It delays gastric emptying and small bowel transit, reducing the diarrhea and has many vascular effects like splanchnic vasoconstriction and thus counteracting the unpleasant symptoms endured by these patients. It is highly effective when often other medical interventions fail. A long acting version of octreotide and lanreotide is available which only require monthly injections. Long-term use is often necessary to continue management of dumping symptoms and patients are often grateful and happy to continue the injection despite possible long-term adverse effects of weight gain and gallstone formation.

Surgery: As a final resort, surgery may be required. However, no surgical interventions have been shown to be effective in the longer term. Depending on the original surgery, some form of correction or revision may be attempted.

Anemia

Anemia is common after all forms of gastric surgery. It occurs late, after many years and can be very insidious.

Iron deficiency is the most common, occurring because of poor iron absorption. Gastric acid helps to make dietary iron to be more soluble and thus more easily absorbed. The lack of acid after partial gastrectomy thus reduces iron absorption. After total or subtotal gastrectomy dumping can also lead to iron and folate deficiency and small bowel bacterial overgrowth can follow Polya and Roux-en-Y reconstructions with stasis being good reservoirs for bacteria. B12 absorption is also compromised due to lack of intrinsic factor or bacterial overgrowth.

When a patient presents with iron deficiency, it cannot be assumed that gastric surgery is the cause and lower GI malignancy may have to be excluded with a colonoscopy first.

Management

Simple iron replacement therapy may suffice but addition of vitamin C is sensible and helps iron absorption. Oral iron can be poorly tolerated and parenteral iron is a consideration. It is routine to check B12 and folate levels as well and they can be replaced. B12 deficiency will require intramuscular B12 injections (hydrocyanocobalamin) for life.

Other Micronutrient Deficiencies

After weight loss surgery, particularly the versions that involve a bypass, deficiencies of various vitamins and minerals have been reported. Apart from iron and B12 deficiencies already described earlier, there have been reports of vitamin D and calcium deficiency leading to osteoporosis, zinc and copper deficiencies and thiamine deficiency leading to beriberi and Wernicke's encephalopathy. Adequate vitamin and mineral replacement should be prophylactically given to prevent these complications.

FURTHER READING

1. Welbourn R. Why the NHS should do more bariatric surgery; how much should we do? BMJ. 2016;353:i1472.

CHAPTER 11

Esophageal Pain and Difficulty with Swallowing

Her Hsin Tsai

■ DIAGNOSIS

Esophageal Pain

A carefully taken history is particularly important in the diagnosis of esophageal pain. There are three main types of esophageal pain: (1) heartburn, a retrosternal burning discomfort that is often made worse by bending, stooping or lying flat; (2) esophageal colic or spasm, a severe retrosternal discomfort that is similar to and often indistinguishable from cardiac pain and which may radiate to the neck, jaw or arms and (3) odynophagia, a pain which occurs on swallowing.

Heartburn

Heartburn is usually relieved by antacids and may occasionally be accompanied by reflux of bitter or sour fluid into the mouth. Sometimes, "water brash" occurs. This is a reflex outpouring of saliva which is not specific for acid reflux and may occur in many other upper gastrointestinal disorders. Heartburn may be precipitated by relaxation of the lower esophageal sphincter (LES) caused by drinking alcohol, fizzy drinks, coffee or chocolate or smoking.

The pathophysiology of gastroesophageal reflux is complex. The integrity of the gastroesophageal junction in preventing reflux is dependent on the lower esophageal sphincter primarily but also the diaphragmatic sphincter and the angle of the cardia of the stomach to the esophagus (angle of His). The latter two are compromised in the presence of an hiatus hernia. There is a need for the stomach to vent gasses (burping). This is achieved physiologically by transient relaxations of the lower esophageal sphincter (tLESRs). These are relaxations lasting 10–30 s and not associated with food deglutination. It is believed that these transient relaxations allow gastric acid and other contents to temporally access the lower esophagus. Although this is physiological, poor esophageal clearance may be an important factor in causing symptoms and increasing the duration of acid contact with the esophageal mucosa leading to mucosal inflammation. Thus, a degree of dysmotility is another important factor in causing reflux disease. Furthermore, there is often poor gastric emptying contributing to reflux episodes. Going to bed after a full rich meal and alcohol is a recipe for nocturnal reflux.

The lower esophageal sphincter is 2–3 cm long muscle that is contracted with a resting tone of 10–30 mm Hg. This tone may be lowered by alcohol, caffeine, smoking and drugs like nitrates and calcium channel blockers. The esophagus is protected from the caustic effects of gastric juice by buffering with saliva and a mucus layer. Lower salivation during sleep and other causes of decreased salivation (drugs, Sjögren's syndrome) would increase risk of injury to the lower esophagus.

Typically, a patient would have symptoms during episodes of reflux measured on a pH probe. However, patients vary considerably in whether or not they report symptoms. Some patients report symptoms without concomitant pH drop. This suggests that there is a wide range of sensitivities and patients who complain of symptoms may have heightened sensitivity.

Investigation

If patients are over the age of 45 and have new symptoms or sinister "alarm" symptoms like dysphagia and weight loss, then, they should have an endoscopy urgently to exclude sinister pathology. Otherwise, if the symptoms respond well to symptomatic treatment with antacids, there is no need for further investigation. If symptoms cannot be readily controlled by antacids endoscopy should be performed to assess the degree of inflammation endoscopically and histologically. There is little correlation between severity of symptoms and the extent of mucosal damage and more vigorous therapies such as lifelong proton pump inhibitors (PPIs) or antireflux surgery should probably be avoided if endoscopy reveals minimal or no inflammation. Columnar epithelialization of the lower esophagus (Barrett's esophagus) is also important to diagnose because of its associated increased risk for adenocarcinoma (AC) and is another justification for endoscopy in this group of patients. A barium swallow examination will demonstrate the presence of hiatus hernias or strictures but is poor for assessing inflammation or columnar epithelialization and is a largely obsolete investigation of reflux disease. Quantification of acid reflux requires 24 h pH monitoring and can therefore only be performed on selected patients, particularly any patient being considered for antireflux surgery. A probe is inserted to just above the LES and pH is monitored and correlated to symptoms. A scoring system is available, the DeMeeseter score being one of the commonest systems used. Documented evidence of acid reflux should be obtained before recommending antireflux surgery. Manometric measurements are also recommended before surgery to identify those with achalasia or other motility disorders for which antireflux surgery would be detrimental. The older water-perfused equipment is now largely replaced by multichannel solid-state high-resolution probes. These are now linked to sophisticated software to produce a color plot of both anatomical site and time (spatiotemporal) of a swallow with the pressure represented by prismatic color spectrum (blue to red representing low to high pressures, Figs. 11.1 to 11.3).

Esophageal Colic

The distinction between esophageal colic and cardiac pain is one of the most difficult diagnostic problems that confront the general physician. If the pain only occurs on exercise it is much more likely to be cardiac but it has to be

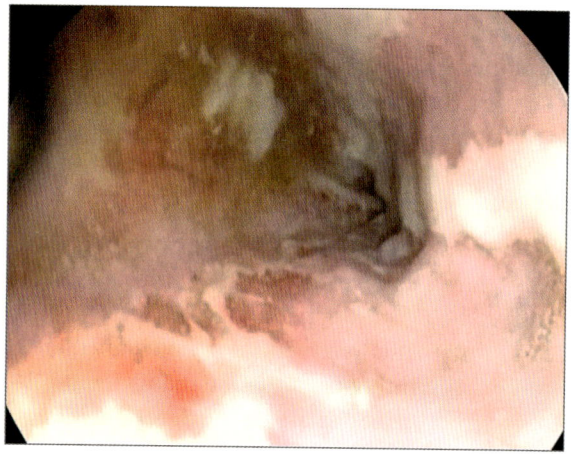

Fig. 11.1: Linear streaks of ulceration are common findings on endoscopy of reflux disease.

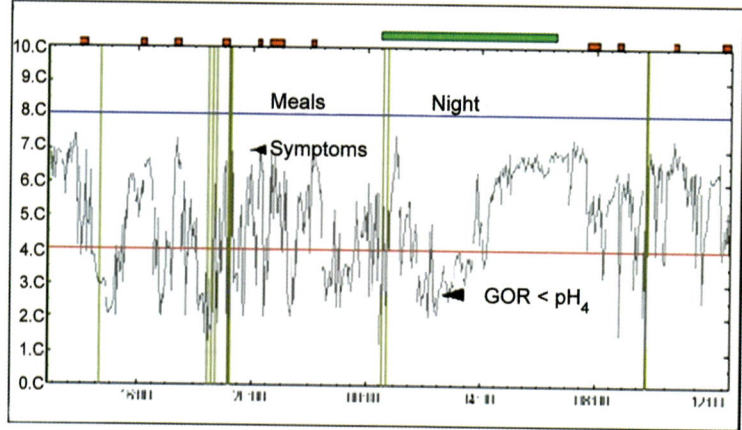

Fig. 11.2: Typical pH monitoring result: the red marks the episodes of heartburn acknowledged by patient and green denotes sleep. Note that some of the episodes of pH drops <4 are symptomatic but not all.

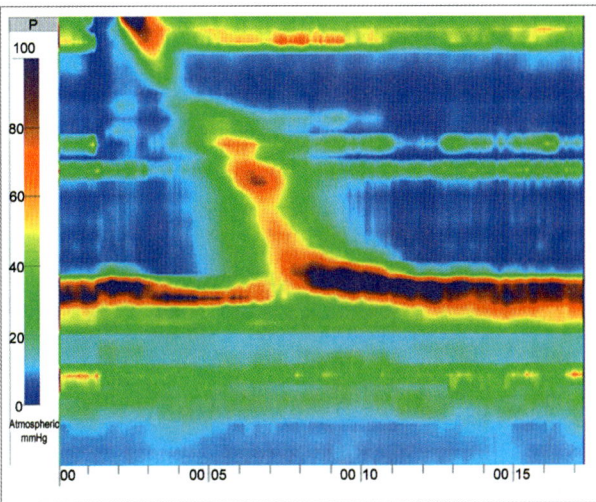

Fig. 11.3: High-resolution manometry: The color indicates esophageal pressure in real time during a swallow.

remembered that esophageal reflux can also be precipitated by exercise. Antacid therapy is not always effective in esophageal spasm and nitrate and calcium antagonists are effective in both conditions so a therapeutic trial does not help to clarify the diagnosis. The Bernstein acid perfusion test is the traditional way of resolving the problem. In total, 0.1N HCl is infused at a rate of 6–8 mL/min via a tube sited in the middle third of the esophagus. Acid is then exchanged for physiological saline without the patient's knowledge. Pain with acid but not with saline is taken as a positive result. Many normal subjects experience discomfort with the acid infusion however and in any case the esophageal pain that mimics cardiac pain is due to spasm rather than acid reflux and the two are often not related. A barium swallow examination may occasionally be helpful if it shows evidence of one of the more extreme forms of esophageal dysmotility such as the "corkscrew" esophagus. The only logical solution at present seems to be to monitor intraesophageal pressure and electrocardiograph for long enough for the patient to have experienced at least one spontaneous attack of pain. Pain that is associated with non-propagating muscular contraction in the esophagus with no ECG change can then be assumed to be esophageal. Such testing is clearly very laborious and is at present only carried out on a minority of patients. It is however clearly more logical and less invasive than turning to coronary angiography early in the patient's diagnostic workup as is commonly done (Fig. 11.4).

Odynophagia

Patients with reflux esophagitis commonly experience some discomfort on swallowing but intense pain on swallowing is a feature of esophagitis due to

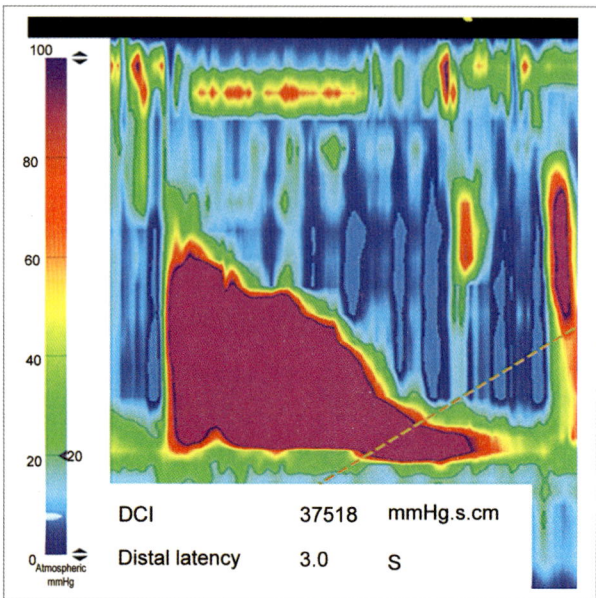

Fig. 11.4: Manometry shows high pressure, non- or poorly propagated swallow of esophageal spasm.

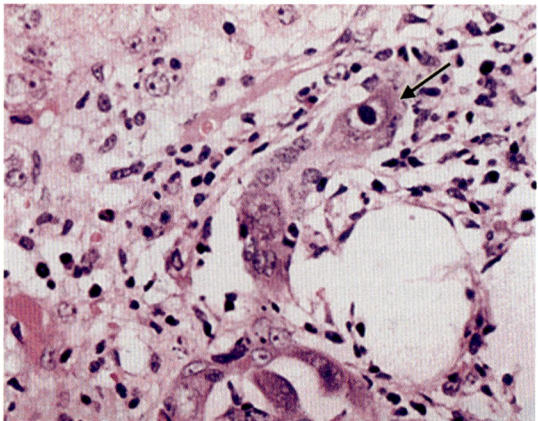

Fig. 11.5: Inclusion bodies (arrow) are seen on cytomegalovirus (CMV) biopsies.

infection with herpes simplex or cytomegalovirus. Endoscopy then reveals small circular or occasionally confluent ulcers and brush cytology shows characteristic inclusions (Fig. 11.5).

Difficulty with Swallowing (Dysphagia)

Globus Hystericus

It is usually possible to distinguish globus hystericus from dysphagia from the history. If a young patient gives a clear description of a constant feeling of a lump in the throat no further investigation is required. In an older patient, it may be more difficult to distinguish this from cricopharyngeal spasm causing difficulty in initiating deglutition. Watching the patient attempt to drink a glass of water may help to make the diagnosis.

Dysphagia

Difficulty with swallowing must always be investigated as it is almost always due to organic disease. The patient's impression of the point where food sticks is a notoriously poor guide to the site of obstruction but it is usually possible to assess whether the patient has difficulty in initiating deglutition or finds that the food sticks after it has been swallowed. This is often distinguishable by taking a history. Dysphagia may therefore be either oropharyngeal or esophageal. The causes of dysphagia may be either mechanical or disruption of motor function or a combination.

Oropharyngeal Dysphagia: The patient is observed to drool with inability to initiate the swallowing reflex. There may be spillage into the larynx causing coughing spells or into the pulmonary passages with resultant aspiration. Assessment by observation of a controlled swallow by a speech therapist is often helpful. A video contrast swallow can be informative if there is uncertainty but not in a frail or uncooperative patient, as it may lead to aspiration. Oropharyngeal dysphagia most commonly occurs in patients after a stroke. It may occur in elderly frail patients without any obvious neurological disease elsewhere but more commonly results from dysfunction of the bulbar muscles due to bulbar or pseudobulbar palsy from cerebrovascular events or primary neuromuscular diseases such as motor neurone disease, myasthenia gravis or polymyositis. Longstanding cricopharyngeal dysmotility is thought to be the major factor in the etiology of pharyngeal pouch. This is a diverticulum arising between the upper border of the cricopharyngeus muscle and the inferior constrictor. If large it may cause dysphagia by compressing the adjacent esophagus. Oral pain from pharyngeal infection with herpes simplex or fungal species may lead to pain, narrowing and swallowing refusal. A check of the pharynx is always helpful (Figs. 11.6 and 11.7).

Esophageal Dysphagia: The history may give valuable clues to the nature of the obstruction. Dysphagia of solids in the absence of a previous history of heartburn is ominous and likely to be due to a malignant stricture while equal difficulty with liquids and solids possibly associated with a lengthy history of regurgitation may suggest achalasia.

It is a very reasonable practice to perform barium swallow as the initial investigation of dysphagia rather than endoscopy. There are two reasons

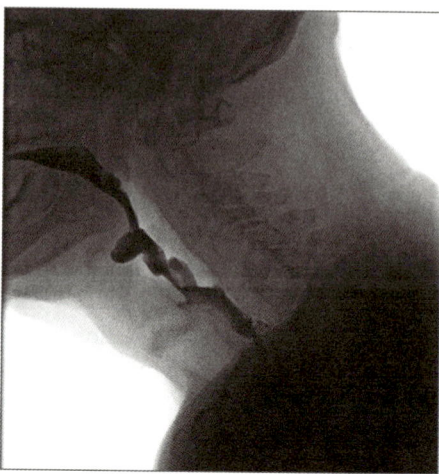

Fig. 11.6: Radiological appearance of a small pharyngeal pouch.

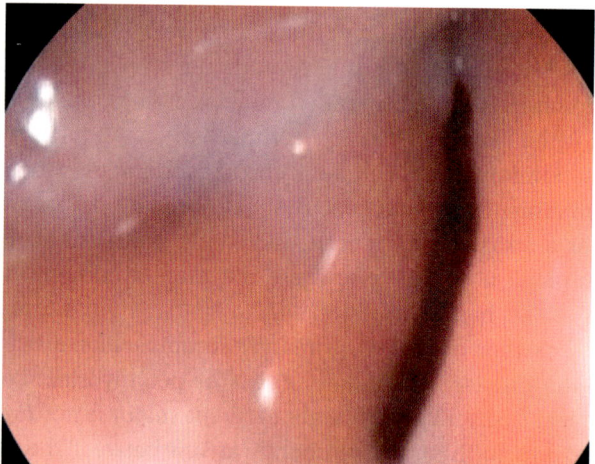

Fig. 11.7: Endoscopic appearance of a small pharyngeal pouch.

for this. First, an upper esophageal pouch may present with dysphagia and there is then a risk of perforation if endoscopy is performed particularly if the endoscope is not introduced under direct vision. Second, motility problems such as achalasia are very difficult to detect endoscopically as the increased tone at the lower esophageal sphincter usually causes surprisingly little resistance to passage of the endoscope. If there is any suggestion of an obstructing lesion on the barium swallow, then endoscopy should then be performed. The endoscope should be introduced into the upper esophagus under direct vision. Many experienced endoscopists would perform endoscopy as the initial investigation, always taking care to introduce the endoscope into the upper esophagus under direct vision.

Lesions that may be seen include:

1. *Upper esophageal web:* Webs are seen more frequently on barium swallow examination than by endoscopy and this discrepancy has not been adequately explained. Presumably localized spasm may account for some of the apparent webs seen on X-ray. Endoscopically, a web appears as a thin fibrous stricture in the upper third of the esophagus which can easily be broken by passage of the endoscope so is often missed if the endoscope is not passed under direct vision.
2. *Caustic stricture:* Strictures resulting from accidental or deliberate ingestion of caustic substances are usually sited in the upper esophagus and may be distinguished from peptic strictures by the presence of squamous mucosa below the stricture.
3. *Peptic strictures* can usually be recognized by the presence of circumferential slough. If they can be passed by the endoscope either with or without prior dilatation, columnar epithelium (which has a deeper color than squamous epithelium) can be recognized below the stricture, usually in association with a hiatus hernia. It must be emphasized though that benign and malignant strictures cannot be reliably distinguished by appearances alone. Biopsy samples should always be taken but it may be difficult reliably to biopsy the relevant site because of the tangential approach. It is therefore particularly important to take multiple biopsies and brush cytology in addition. Cytology is more useful if performed before biopsy to avoid heavy contamination of smears by blood clot (Figs. 11.8 to 11.10).
4. *Malignant strictures* often have a fleshy irregular polypoid appearance with friable mucosa but less slough than is seen in association with peptic strictures. Tumors may occur at any level in the esophagus. Squamous carcinomas arise from the esophageal squamous epithelium and occur above the Z-line, while esophageal adenocarcinomas (ACs) arise from transformed esophageal mucosa (Barrett's mucosa) or invasion of tumors from the cardia. ACs of the esophagus have seen a remarkable increase in the last two decades. Invasion of the esophagus by carcinoma of the left bronchus or from malignant mediastinal nodes is not uncommon (Fig. 11.11).
5. *Benign tumors:* These are very rare and include leiomyomas, lipomas and lymphangiomas (Fig. 11.12).
6. *Achalasia* may produce subtle changes on endoscopy. There is usually only little or no resistance to passage of the endoscope through the cardia and greater difficulty in the absence of any mucosal abnormality should raise the suspicion of external compression by a low mediastinal tumor. Careful examination may show the absence of peristalsis in achalasia. If the achalasia has been longstanding, the esophagus may be grossly

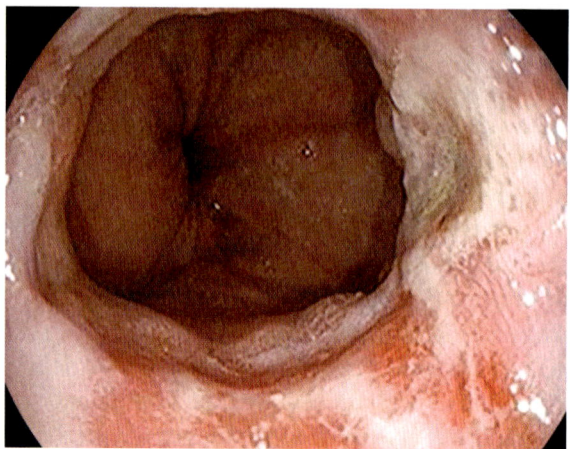

Fig. 11.8: Benign esophageal ulcer: may look benign but should be biopsied.

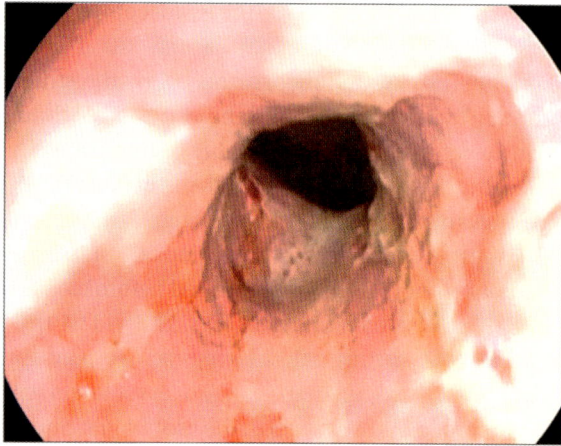

Fig. 11.9: Ulcerated peptic stricture of esophagus.

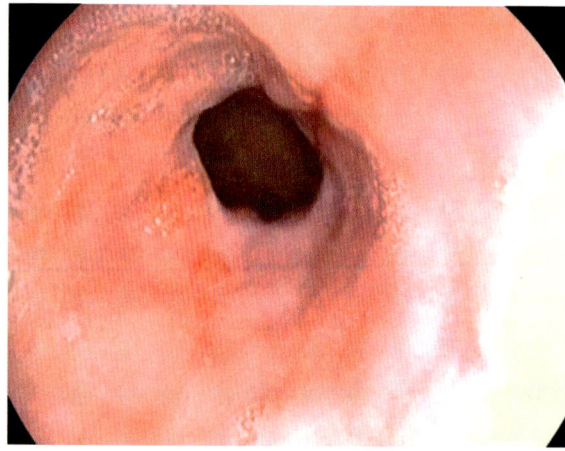

Fig. 11.10: Mild stricture.

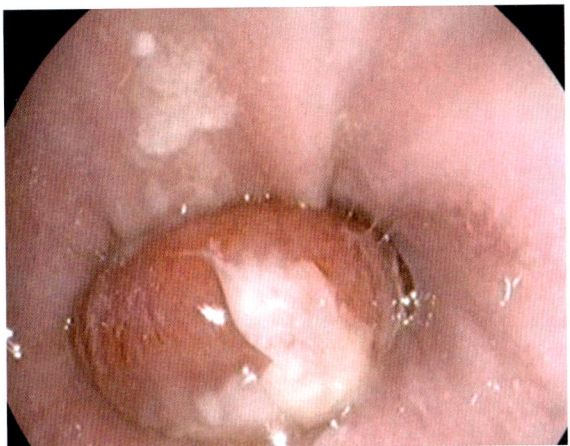

Fig. 11.11: Polypoidal esophageal tumor (malignant).

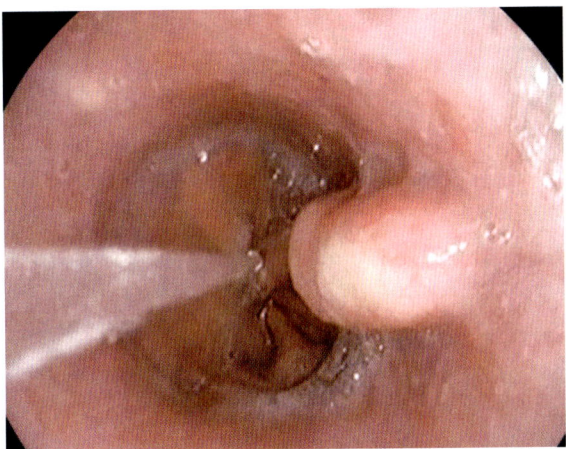

Fig. 11.12: Esophageal lipoma.

dilated and contain a large residue of undigested food. Malignancy of the lower esophagus or cardia may invade the nerves of the lower esophageal sphincter causing a phenomenon of pseudoachalasia and may lead to misdiagnosis. Careful endoscopy with J-maneuver should be performed (Figs. 11.13 and 11.14).

7. A *Schatzki ring* appears similar to an upper esophageal web but is always sited in the lower esophagus. It is a fibromuscular ring occurring at the point where diaphragmatic fibers wrap around the esophagus usually at the upper margin of a small hiatus hernia. It only extends about 2 mm into the lumen but may cause bolus obstruction if the food is not well chewed.

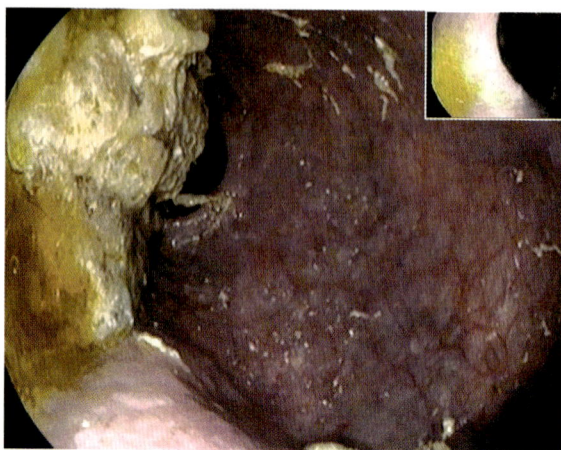

Fig. 11.13: Endoscopy showing food accumulation and grossly dilated esophagus in achalasia.

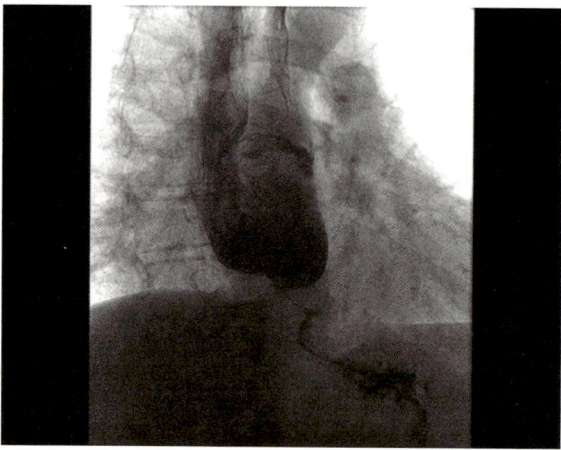

Fig. 11.14: Barium swallow of pseudoachalasia: the dilated esophagus terminates with a classic apple-core appearance of a cancer. Endoscopy confirmed a gastroesophageal tumor.

8. *Eosinophilic esophagitis.* This condition has only been identified recently and encountered not infrequently. Patients report intermittent dysphagia or food impaction. A history of atopy or asthma may be a clue. Endoscopic appearances can vary and may be subtle in the form of concentric rings to edema and stricturing from eosinophilic infiltration of the esophageal mucosa. Diagnosis is made from endoscopic mid-esophageal biopsies and a high degree of suspicion in patients presenting with food impaction without any obvious stricture (Figs. 11.15 and 11.16).

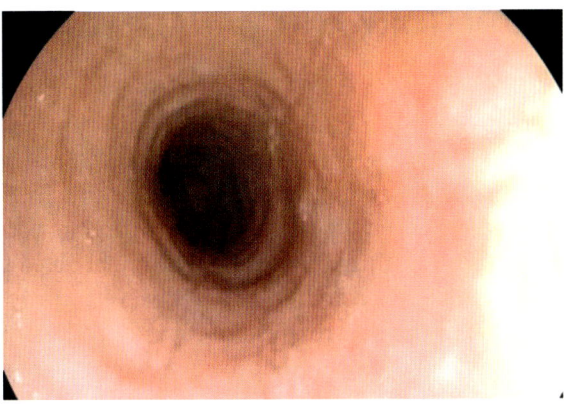

Fig. 11.15: Concentric esophageal rings are seen in eosinophilic esophagitis. Biopsy in this patient was positive.

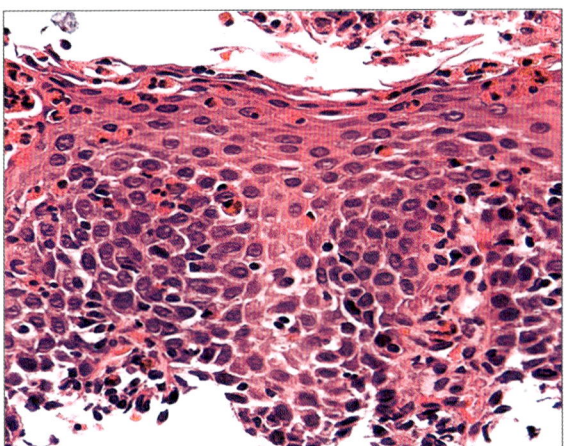

Fig. 11.16: Esophageal biopsy showing eosinophil infiltrates.

Esophageal Rupture

The sudden onset of epigastric pain and shock occurring shortly after vomiting suggests acute rupture of the esophagus, first described by Boerhaave in 1724. The victim is usually a male who has just eaten a heavy meal. Profuse pallor, cyanosis, dyspnea and sweating occur and signs of mediastinal air become apparent within a few hours. These include crepitation over the chest wall and neck and there may be a systolic "crunch" audible on auscultation over the heart. Rapid diagnosis is very important as mediastinitis with an associated high mortality inevitably follows.

Plain chest X-ray will show mediastinal air and a chest computed tomography (CT) can usually reveal the diagnosis. A water soluble contrast agent such as gastrografin is sometimes necessary. Upper GI endoscopy and endoscopic treatment may be feasible in limited cases.

NATURAL HISTORY AND MANAGEMENT

Gastroesophageal Reflux Diseases

Gastroesophageal reflux is common and symptom severity often does not correlate with endoscopic severity. Objective evidence can be sought by 24-h pH monitoring where symptoms may match with falls in esophageal pH. However, it became quite obvious that many patients with reflux have few symptoms and many with symptoms have minimal objective reflux. On one end of the spectrum, there are patients with severe erosive esophagitis on endoscopy and others with normal endoscopy with equally severe symptoms. These are sometimes referred to as non-erosive gastroesophageal reflux disease.

Apart from causing esophagitis, reflux diseases have been implicated in causing a number of respiratory and ENT conditions like asthma exacerbations, cough, laryngeal and sinus issues. Acid may not be the only irritant to the airways as gastric enzymes, bile and other food content could be easily as an irritant. Hence, PPIs alone may not be effective therapy of cough symptoms.

Esophagitis

Natural History

Reflux esophagitis is commonly termed "peptic" although it is unclear if the major damaging factor is acid, bile or pepsin being the other main candidates. Although antacids and even histamine H2 antagonists are relatively ineffective at treating reflux esophagitis, the PPIs, such as omeprazole and lansoprazole, which are extremely potent inhibitors of acid secretion, have been shown to be very effective therapy for esophagitis. This suggests that acid is the major factor although its presence may just be ensuring an optimal pH for peptic activity rather than having a directly damaging effect.

The reasons why some people suffer from excessive reflux and not others are also unclear. Two factors which seem particularly important are a low pressure at the lower esophageal sphincter and the presence of a hiatus hernia but the relative importance of these is uncertain. The frequency of tLESRs and the effectiveness of the lower esophagus to clear the gastric contents are probably the most important factors. In patients who have poor gastric emptying reflux episodes more likely and patients with recurrent vomiting or those who have intubations like a Ryle's tube or feeding tube are also prone to reflux esophagitis.

A small minority of patients have a congenitally short esophagus. This usually occurs in association with an hiatus hernia but there may just be columnar epithelium extending up the lower esophagus without an hiatus hernia. In either case, severe reflux symptoms and even stricturing may occur in early childhood.

Reflux symptoms are extremely common in pregnancy possibly either due to raised intra-abdominal pressure or hormonal effects on lower sphincter pressure. Esophageal involvement by scleroderma causes particularly severe reflux combined with dysmotility resulting in esophageal stricturing and an increased risk for esophageal cancer.

Many drugs reduce lower sphincter pressure and provoke reflux. These include alcohol, tobacco and xanthine derivatives contained in coffee and chocolate as well as theophylline.

Management

Gravity is clearly a major factor in the cause of reflux and some benefit results from following a few simple guidelines. Much of the problem occurs at night and elevation of the head of the bed has been shown to have a beneficial effect. Overweight patients should try to lose weight and not wear tight clothing around the waist. Drugs such as alcohol and tobacco which relax the lower esophageal sphincter should be avoided. Although these methods bring some relief in most patients, some form of drug therapy is required.

Drug Therapy

Antacids: Most patients with intermittent heartburn can be adequately treated with antacids. It may be more convenient to take these in the form of chewable tablets that can be taken whenever symptoms occur. Some preparations combine antacid with the seaweed derivative sodium alginate. This helps to form a poorly soluble "raft" which floats on top of the gastric juice, the principle being that this will result in coating of the esophagus whenever reflux occurs. These preparations are certainly effective and easy to take although there is no good evidence that they work better than antacids alone.

Histamine H2 Antagonists: Although antacids are quite good at relieving heartburn, they have little effect on esophagitis. If patients still have unacceptably frequent symptoms despite antacid therapy endoscopy should be performed. The next step will be to prescribe histamine H2 antagonists but because the course of therapy will probably have to be prolonged it is preferable to assess the extent of inflammation first. Histamine H2 antagonists are relatively much less effective in treating esophagitis than in duodenal ulceration. Higher doses are often necessary, for example ranitidine 300 mg bd or cimetidine 800 mg bd or even qds. Once daily treatment is usually inadequate.

Drugs which Raise Lower Esophageal Sphincter Pressure: Metoclopramide has been tried on the grounds that it raises lower esophageal sphincter pressure but it seems to have no additional therapeutic effect when prescribed with H2 antagonists and has a much poorer side effect profile (particularly extrapyramidal effects of involuntary facial movements which may not always reverse on stopping therapy).

Domperidone is another dopamine antagonist which raises lower esophageal sphincter pressure, stimulates peristalsis and speeds gastric emptying. It does not pass the blood brain barrier and the risk of extrapyramidal side effects is lower but there are concerns about adverse cardiac effects.

Proton Pump Inhibitors: Omeprazole, a substituted benzimidazole, acts as a PPI, i.e. by inhibiting the K+/H+ transporting ATPase in the parietal cells. It causes almost total suppression of acid output and is without doubt the most effective drug for treating reflux esophagitis (in doses of 20–40 mg/day). PPIs can heal up to 70% of reflux esophagitis in 8 weeks. However, relapses are frequent when the drug is stopped, necessitating long-term maintenance treatment. Recent cohort studies suggest of renal impairment and worrying suggestion that dementia risk may be increased in individuals who take long-term PPIs. There must remain some anxiety however about the wisdom of embarking on lifelong therapy in young patients who may need treatment for decades.

Other Medical Therapies: Pyrogastrone, a combination of carbenoxolone (a licorice derivative) and sodium alginate is effective and may help some younger patients who are not responding to H2 antagonists but cannot be used in the elderly because of its side effects of fluid accumulation and hypokalemia due to its mineralocorticoid activity.

Sucralfate, an aluminum hydroxide salt of sucrose-octasulfate is designed to act by coating ulcerated mucosa thus providing an acid buffering layer. It has an efficacy that is roughly similar to H2 antagonists.

Antireflux Surgery: If medical therapy fails to produce satisfactory relief of symptoms or healing of ulceration, then antireflux surgery should be considered. This procedure is now almost always carried out laparoscopically. The pioneer of this operation was Rudolf Nissen and a modified version of his operation is now the norm. The aim is generally to wrap (plicate) the fundus of the stomach around the lower esophagus. Mortality is low and day surgery is possible with patients discharged on the same or following day. Dysphagia may result if the plication is too tight and occurs as a temporary feature. Reported recurrence of reflux symptoms vary considerably from 10% in some series but up to 50% in others followed over a 10-year period.

It follows that the decision to undertake antireflux surgery should not be taken lightly. Suitable patients should be relatively young, have endoscopic evidence of significant mucosal damage and should have failed to respond to a trial of vigorous medical therapy which should include at least 3 months treatment with proton pump blockers. In patients with non-erosive esophageal reflux, evidence from 24 h pH monitoring should be sought before surgery. Manometry is sensible to exclude esophageal dysmotility but there is no evidence that it affects outcome. It is also sensible to assess gastric emptying in diabetics who might have autonomic neuropathy as it would result in poorer outcome.

Barrett's Esophagus

It is thought that prolonged exposure of the lower esophagus to acid and other refluxate results in transformation of the squamous epithelium of the lower esophagus to a columnar or intestinal type of mucosa. Such a transformation (metaplasia) was described by Barrett over 80 years ago. There is good epidemiological evidence association with Barrett's esophagus and the development of AC. However, most patients with Barrett's esophagus will not develop esophageal cancer, with the risk of progression to AC of the esophagus being estimated at approximately 0.5% per year in patients without dysplasia on initial surveillance biopsies. The presence of dysplasia increases the risk considerably.

It is not unreasonable to expect that patients with more extensive Barrett's esophagus will have the higher risk. Indeed patients with circumferential Barrett's extending for >3 cm (called long segment Barrett's esophagus) are 10 times more likely to develop esophageal cancer than those with shorter than 3 cm of transformed mucosa. Thus, it is not unreasonable to undergo regular surveillance endoscopy with multiple biopsies at regular intervals. When low-grade dysplasia is detected, patients should be surveyed more closely for histological signs of progression. If there is high-grade dysplasia, various treatment options are available. If there are visible areas of dysplasia, it can be managed by endoscopic resection. New mucosal ablation therapy such as radio-frequency ablation (RFA) has been demonstrated to improve mortality and prevent cancer progression in controlled trials. One such device is the HALO device. It delivers a controlled thermal ablation to a depth of about 2 mm hence only ablating the mucosa. New mucosal growth of squamous epithelium usually follows. Although stricture formation is a known adverse, it is relatively rare. Using this device for low-grade dysplasia may be justified and currently undergoing long-term evaluation. In some cases, full esophagectomy for high-grade dysplasia may still be the best treatment. The optimal treatment will depend on patient's fitness, histology and extent of disease and thus a multidisciplinary discussion should take place (Figs. 11.17 and 11.18).

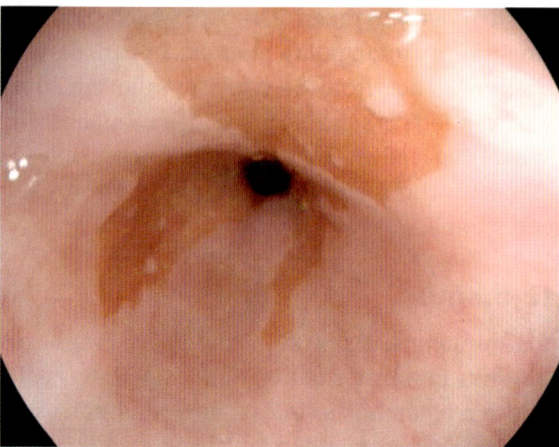

Fig. 11.17: Barrett's esophagus may manifest as tongues of metaplasia.

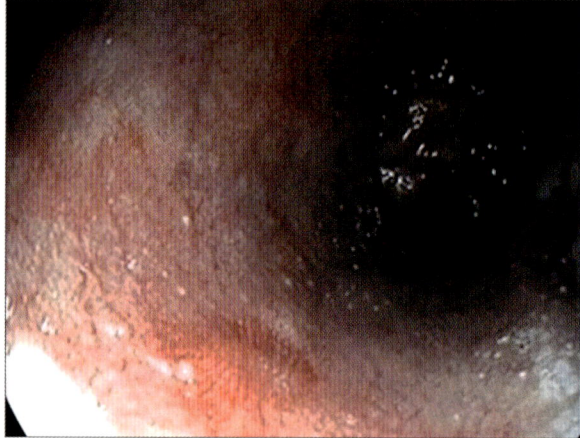

Fig. 11.18: Barrett's visible dysplasia: Endoscopic resection confirms high-grade dysplasia.

Peptic Esophageal Stricture

Endoscopy is the main method of managing benign esophageal stricturing. Dilatation can be carried out under intravenous sedation as an outpatient procedure. A guidewire is passed under endoscopic control through the stricture, the endoscope is removed and a dilator passed over the guidewire. Plastic balloons with graded insufflation diameters are also available and are popular among some endoscopists (Fig. 11.19).

Most patients will eventually develop a recurrence of the stricture but the timing of this is very variable being anything from a few weeks to years. The simplest approach to this is to ask the patient to contact the unit directly when

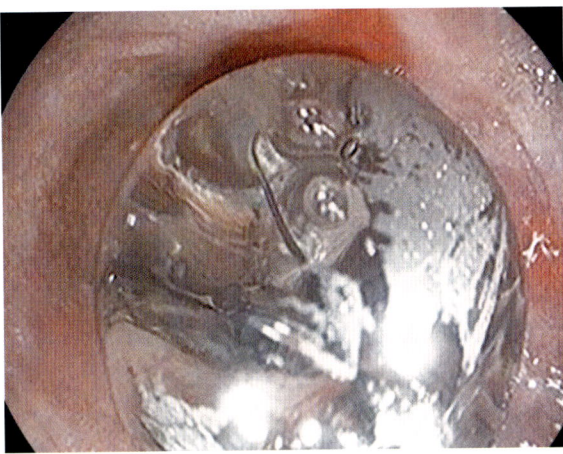

Fig. 11.19: Balloon dilation of esophageal stricture.

symptoms recur so that repeated dilatation can be organized without delay. Use of PPIs after dilation help prevent recurrences. The incidence of esophageal peptic strictures has declined massively after the introduction of PPIs.

Infective Esophagitis

Cytomegalovirus and *Herpes simplex* virus may both cause esophageal ulcers, either separate aphthoid ulcers or confluent ulceration. This may occur either as a result of primary infection or as a result of reactivation in an immunocompromised individual. Very severe pain on swallowing (odynophagia) may result and may prevent an adequate intake of fluids. A cause of immunodeficiency such as HIV infection should be sought and antiviral therapy commenced with intravenous acyclovir. This usually brings about impressive relief of symptoms within 24–48 h (Fig. 11.20).

Extensive *esophageal candidiasis* can be very difficult to eradicate. Oral nystatin or amphotericin should be tried initially. Patients may be immunocompromised or on steroids, either inhaled for asthma or systemic steroids. Alcohol and achalasia are also associated with esophageal candidiasis. Systemic therapy may be needed particularly if there is evidence of candida septicemia; however, this will usually require intravenous amphotericin which is highly nephrotoxic and should only be used when clearly indicated. Fluconazole may be used as a less toxic alternative but is probably less effective in candida septicemia.

Eosinophilic Esophagitis

This is a newly recognized condition and our understanding of the condition is thus evolving. Presence of eosinophilis in the esophageal mucosa may

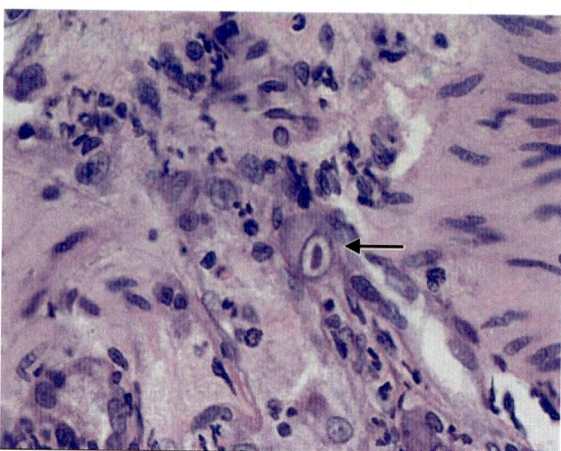

Fig. 11.20: Cytomegalovirus inclusion body.

be found in gastroesophageal reflux disease with or without esophagitis and may be responsive to PPI treatment. Conversely endoscopically eosinophilic esophagitis may resemble classic peptic esophagitis. Hence, it is important to take biopsies at least 5 cm proximal to the gastroesophageal junction.

This condition is now defined as a chronic immune/antigen-mediated esophageal disease characterized clinically by symptoms related to esophageal dysfunction and histologically by eosinophil-predominant inflammation. To make a diagnosis, three criteria had to be fulfilled: (1) symptoms of esophageal dysfunction, (2) a maximum eosinophil count of ≥15 per high magnification field and (3) eosinophilia limited to the esophagus, with exclusion of other possible causes of esophageal eosinophilia especially reflux disease.

The endoscopic appearances and clinical features are not specific hence a high degree of clinical suspicion, with histology in the correct clinical setting allows for a correct diagnosis. A history of atopy like asthma may be a clue but not all patients will have it.

Treatment is often described in as the three Ds: Diet, Drugs and Dilatation. Elimination diets have been shown to be of benefit. Patients are started with elemental diets containing no whole proteins and then foods gradually reintroduced. Such diets are difficult to follow and expensive. Alternatively, some advocate elimination of six common allergenic foods: milk, eggs, wheat, soy, seafood and nuts. Drug therapy primarily relies on topical steroids. This can be easily achieved using steroid inhalers containing fluticasone and budesonide but by swallowing it rather than inhaling it. Preparations containing budesonide in liquid preparation are now available and shown to improve symptoms of the disease. In more recalcitrant disease, systemic steroids are effective. But with risks of adverse effects, long-term use is not practical.

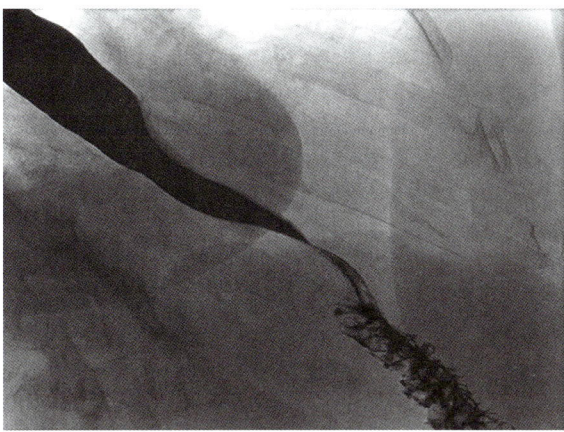

Fig. 11.21: Early achalasia may present with delayed LES opening on barium study. (LES: Lower esophageal sphincter).

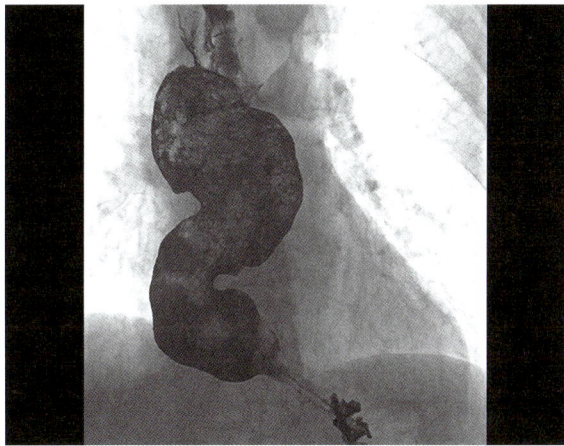

Fig. 11.22: In late achalasia, the esophagus becomes atonic and may dilate considerably.

Treatment with the leukotriene antagonist montelukast showed efficacy but reserved as second-line therapy. Azathioprine may be required in patients as a steroid-sparing agent and the use of biologics such as the anti-IL-5 (mepolizumab) are under evaluation (*see* Figs. 11.15 and 11.16).

Achalasia (Figs. 11.21 and 11.22)

Achalasia is a condition of unknown etiology in which there is a marked reduction in the number of Auerbach's ganglion cells in the lower esophagus. Heightened response to intravenous injection of synthetic acetyl choline (Mecholyl) is supportive evidence of denervation hypersensitivity. A similar end result is seen in Chagas disease, a disease which occurs in Latin

America as a result of infection with *Trypanosoma cruzi*. The two main consequences are disordered peristalsis and lack of the normal relaxation of the LES. High-resolution manometry of the esophagus can make the diagnosis is most cases. Barium meal may show a classic bird's beak appearance of a dilated esophagus with a tapered lower sphincter. It is important to perform an endoscopy to exclude malignancy (pseudoachalasia) and where there is still doubt endoscopic ultrasound (EUS) can be helpful.

Manometry, especially high-resolution manometry, classifies achalasia into three types: the classic achalasia has low or no esophageal pressure and no lower esophageal sphincter relaxation. Type 2 has normal esophageal pressure but poor propagation and type 3 is associated with high pressure spasms.

Dysphagia for both liquids and solids results and in some patients, there may have episodes of severe pain due to spasm, "vigorous achalasia" as the esophagus contracts against a non-relaxing sphincter. The esophagus may gradually dilate to a very marked degree ("classical") and regurgitation is a common feature and may result in recurrent inhalational pneumonia (Fig. 11.23).

Treatment is aimed at reducing the lower esophageal sphincter pressure. Drug therapy with calcium antagonists, e.g. sublingual nifedipine 20 mg before meals, is sometimes effective in milder cases but dilatation is usually required. This is performed using a pneumatic balloon which has a fixed maximum diameter of approximately 3 cm in order to rapture the sphincter muscles. The balloon is placed across the cardia under X-ray screening and inflated with air. A waist can be seen in the middle of the balloon when it is correctly sited and further inflation abolishes this waist. Full dilatation is maintained for about 1 min and the balloon deflated. The treatment is successful in approximately three quarters of cases and may be repeated if symptoms recur (Fig. 11.24). Surgical treatment should now be reserved for patients who have failed to respond to balloon dilatation and consists of longitudinal incision of the muscle coats around the lower esophageal sphincter (Heller's procedure). This procedure is carried out laparoscopically. This carries an appreciable risk of causing esophageal reflux so most surgeons routinely perform an antireflux procedure at the same time. A new endoscopic approach (Per-Oral Endoscopic Myotomy) is being currently evaluated. It is a technically demanding procedure and limited to specialized units.

Esophageal Spasm

Painful esophageal spasm may occur in association with generalized disorders of esophageal motility such as achalasia but is more commonly an intermittent event, the esophageal motility returning to normal between attacks. Esophageal reflux is a common etiological factor. If this is present, then treatment should initially be aimed at suppressing the reflux. Various drug therapies have been tried for the spasm itself including anticholinergics, nitrates,

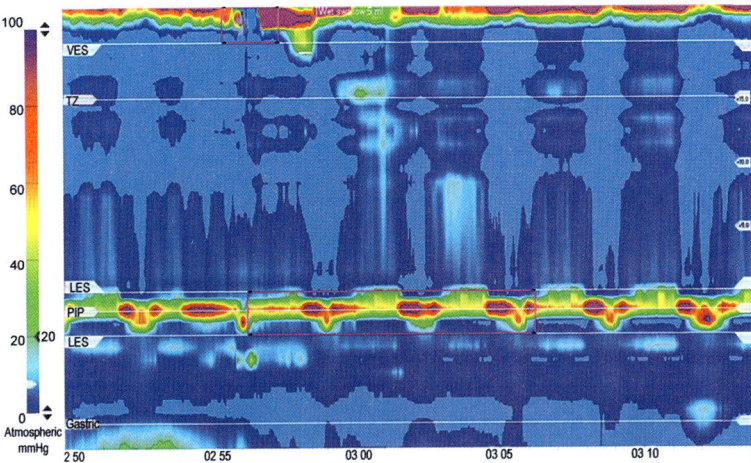

Fig. 11.23: High-resolution manometry showing type I (classical) achalasia.

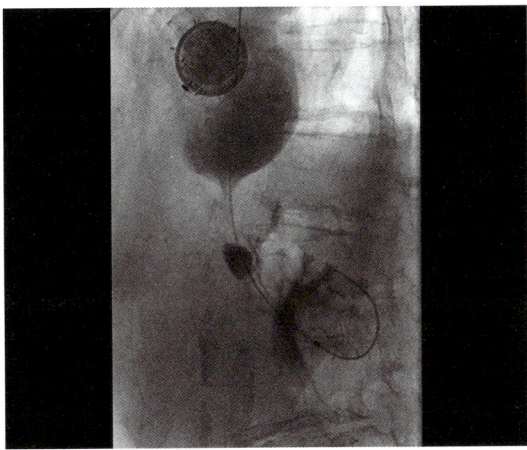

Fig. 11.24: A large pneumatic balloon is effective in treating achalasia by rupturing the circular muscles.

hydralazine and nifedipine. Of these, nifedipine 20 mg sublingually before meals is probably the most effective. Its effect lasts for approximately 60 min.

Cricopharyngeal Spasm and Pharyngeal Pouch (*See* Figs. 11.6 and 11.7)

These two conditions are closely related. A pouch occurs as a pulsion diverticulum between the upper fibers of the cricopharyngeus and the lower fibers of the inferior constrictor. As it fills with food, dysphagia results from compression of the adjacent esophagus. Regurgitation then produces relief of the dysphagia. Treatment is surgical and includes cricopharyngeal myotomy. The pouch is of secondary importance but may be excised or invaginated.

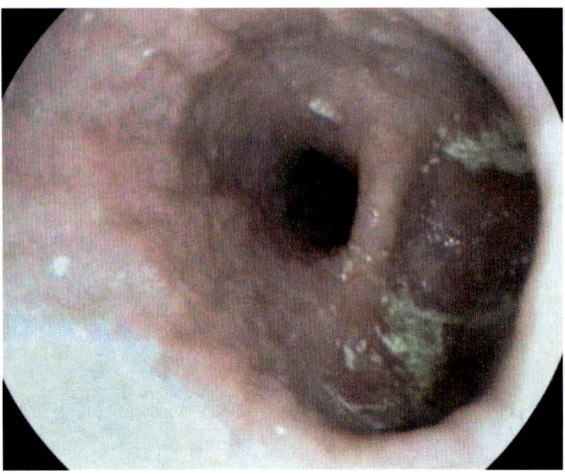

Fig. 11.25: Esophageal diverticulum.

Cricopharyngeal myotomy is also beneficial in approximately 50% of patients with cricopharyngeal spasm due to neuromuscular disorders such as motor neurone disease. Some ENT surgeons perform endoscopic stapling but there is no evidence that it is better than cricopharyngeal myotomy.

Other Forms of Esophageal Diverticula

Diverticula may also occur in the mid-esophagus as a result of traction by adjacent tuberculous mediastinal lymph nodes or as an epiphrenic diverticulum occurring as a pulsion diverticulum in the lower esophagus in association with motility disorders. Rarely, multiple tiny diverticula in the mid- or lower esophagus may also be seen in association with motility disorders. These forms of diverticula do not usually require treatment (Fig. 11.25).

Esophageal Web

Plummer-Vinson (Kelly-Patterson) syndrome has become extremely rare. It describes the association between longstanding iron deficiency and the development of atrophy and fibrous narrowing of the upper entry to the esophagus with a high risk for subsequent development of postcricoid carcinoma. The appearance of a web is best seen on barium swallow examinations but endoscopy of these patients usually fails to show any mucosal abnormality and the appearances presumably result from spasm. When a web is present, it may easily be missed unless the endoscope is passed under direct vision as it is easily broken down by passage of the endoscope. Biopsies should be taken and endoscopy repeated after a period of iron supplementation.

Schatzki Ring

This occurs in the lower esophagus, usually in association with a small hiatus hernia. It is thought to represent fibromuscular attachments running up from the diaphragm and is associated with reflux disease, suggesting that reflux is a contributory etiological factor. It only extends about 2 mm into the lumen and is usually an incidental finding on barium swallow examination but may cause bolus obstruction if unchewed meat is swallowed. It can sometimes be split by endoscopic dilatation but can be resistant to dilatation.

Hiatus Hernia

Hiatus hernia is notoriously overrated as a condition by the lay public and is often a cause of inappropriate chronic invalidity. Over 30% of asymptomatic people have a hiatus hernia. Hiatus hernias may be either sliding or rolling. Sliding hernias are commoner and are associated with symptomatic reflux in about 50%. Treatment however is aimed at the reflux and is not affected by the presence of or size of the hernia.

Rolling Hiatus Hernia and Gastric Volvulus

Rolling or para-esophageal hernias cause dysphagia rather than reflux. If large, they are invariably associated with some degree of gastric volvulus. This may be organoaxial, mesenteroaxial or a combination of the two. In mesenteroaxial volvulus, the antrum rotates upward to lie above and to the left of the fundus while in organoaxial volvulus, the greater curve rotates upward to lie above and to the right of the lesser curve. Many patients are asymptomatic but chronic discomfort, bloating, wind and embarrassingly loud borborygmi may occur. The most serious consequence is acute gastric strangulation. This presents as violent retching that tends to be unproductive, severe epigastric pain and shock. Mortality is about 50% when this occurs. Hence, surgery is often recommended whenever a large rolling hiatus hernia with associated gastric volvulus is diagnosed but many of the patients are elderly and it is unclear how high the risk of subsequent gastric strangulation is in patients with little or no symptoms (Figs. 11.26 to 11.28).

Esophageal Cancer

Natural History

Cancer of the esophagus remains a depressing disease. Figures from patients diagnosed with esophageal cancer during 2010-11 in England and Wales show that although 44% of men survive esophageal cancer for at least 1 year, only 16% survive for 5 years or more. Survival for women is slightly lower at 1 year, but similar to men at 5 years, 38% survive for 1 year or more, and 15% are predicted to survive for at least 5 years.

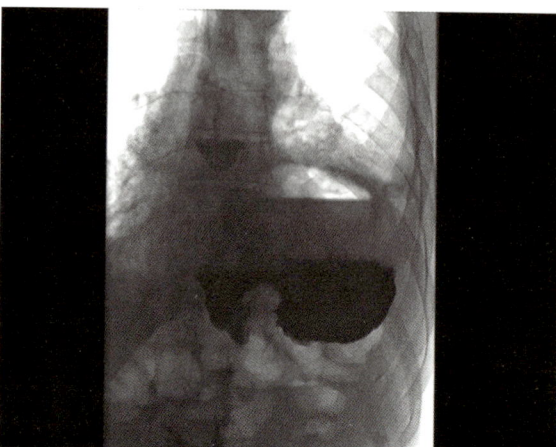

Fig. 11.26: Barium meal showing an organoaxial volvulus.

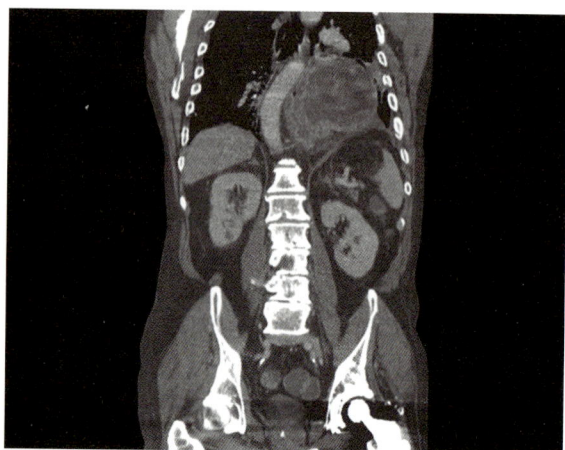

Fig. 11.27: Computed tomography shows a large diaphragmatic defect with a gastric volvulus.

Dysphagia is often very severe or total and not always easy to palliate. Even if the primary tumor can be successfully removed, secondary spread occurs in at least two thirds of patients.

In the past 30 years, there has been a remarkable change in the type of esophageal cancer encountered in the United Kingdom. Previously, squamous cell cancer (SCC) is the predominant histological type. This disease is associated with smoking and heavy alcohol intake particularly if in combination. It appears to be static or declining slightly in the United Kingdom. However, there is a remarkable increase in rates of AC which had increased by 52% between 1995 and 2010, from 6.2 to 9.4 per 100,000 males. For females, the rise in this period is smaller, with rates increasing by 32%, from 1.4 to 1.8 per 100,000 females. AC has association with obesity and reflux and

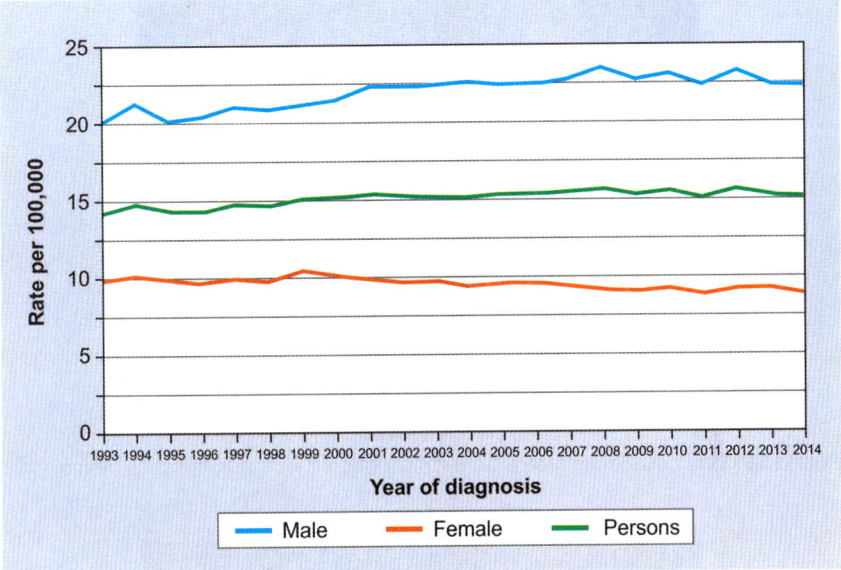

Fig. 11.28: Esophageal cancer European age-standardized incidence rates, UK, 1993–2014.
Source: Cancer Research.

Barrett's esophagus and reflects the increasing girth of United Kingdom populations. Now SCC accounts for 28%, while AC accounts for most of the rest.

The tumor may erode into other mediastinal structures resulting in esophago-bronchial fistulas with recurrent pneumonia or fistulation into the aorta with rapid exsanguination. Dysphagia, anorexia and weight loss are almost invariable but severe pain usually indicates extension of tumor outside the wall of the esophagus.

Non-metastatic manifestations include hypercalcemia and ectopic adrenocorticotropic hormone (ACTH) production but are uncommon (Figs. 11.29 to 11.32).

Management

Patients with suspected upper GI cancer would undergo an upper intestinal endoscopy. Biopsy and cytology are carried out in suspicious lesions.

Although histological differentiation from the biopsies is usually easy, immunohistochemical stainings may be required in poorly and undifferentiated cancers according to differentiate between SCC and AC of the esophagus.

Staging and Risk Assessment: Decisions on the treatment of esophageal cancer are taken on the basis of clinical staging, which should be carried

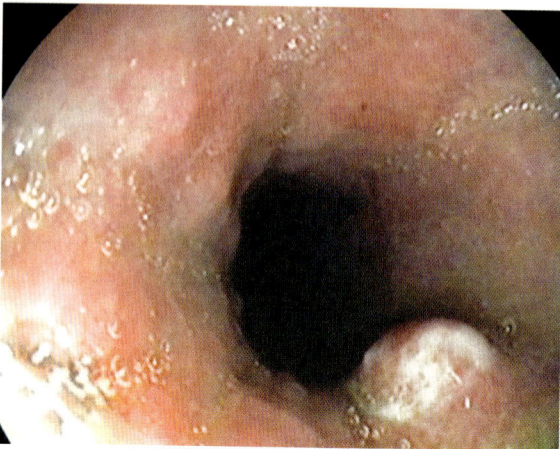

Fig. 11.29: This raised nodule in a Barrett's esophagus was an adenocarcinoma.

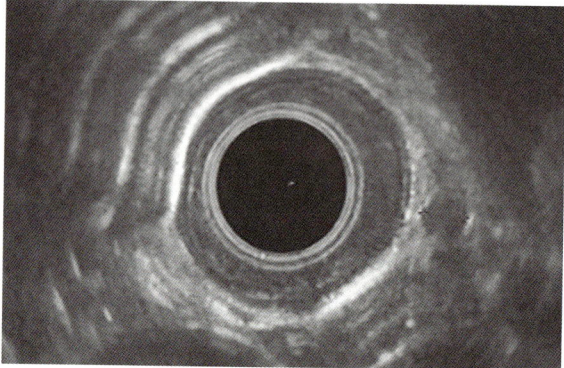

Fig. 11.30: Endoscopic ultrasound is a useful tool in esophageal cancer assessment.

out with the highest degree of accuracy possible. Staging should include a complete clinical examination and a CT scan of the neck, chest and abdomen. In candidates for surgical resection, EUS should be carried out to evaluate the tumor size, resectability and local lymph node involvement (Fig. 11.33).

^{18}F-FDG-PET scans should be carried out in patients who are candidates for esophagectomy. This involves the use of labeled fludeoxyglucose (FDG) which is taken up by cancer tissue with high metabolism and anatomically correlated with a CT scan. It would delineate smaller areas of metastatic malignancy. This tool has revolutionized staging process with improved accuracy.

In the case of esophageal SCC due to chronic tobacco and alcohol consumption, examination of oropharynx is important.

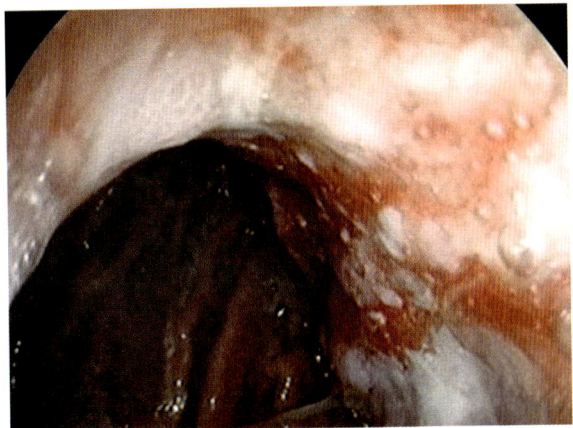

Fig. 11.31: Forward endoscopy showed minor ulceration only.

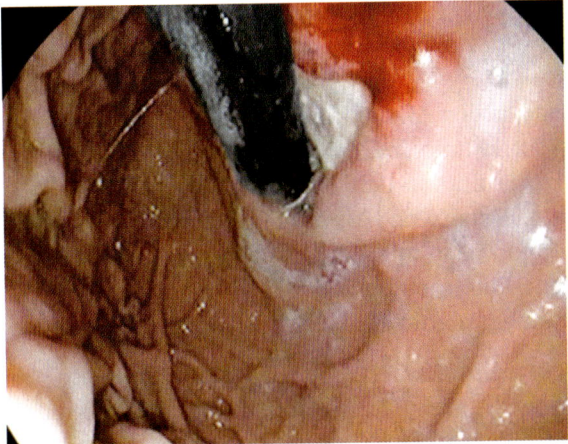

Fig. 11.32: Retroflexion of the endoscope shows an obvious cancer.

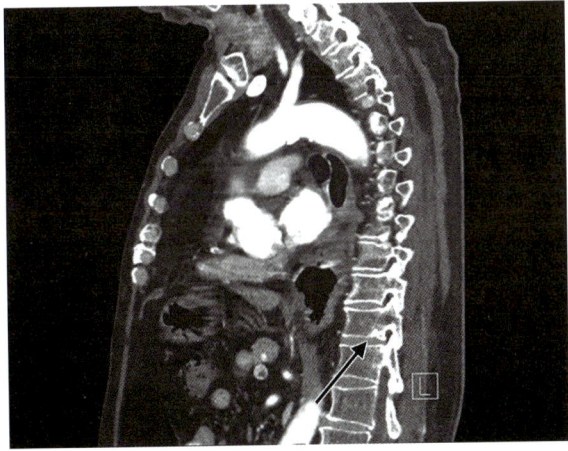

Fig. 11.33: Computed tomography shows large esophageal cancer.

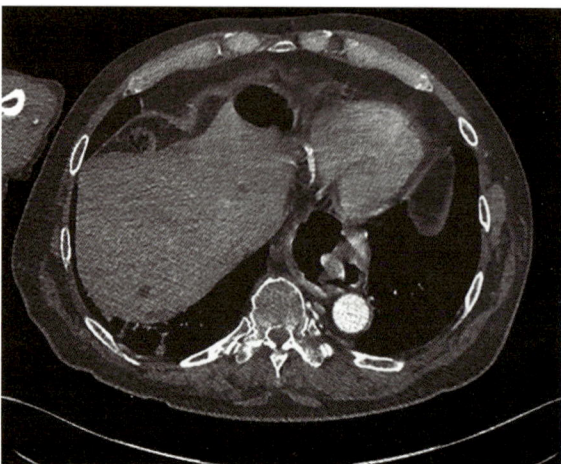

Fig. 11.34: Computed tomography showing an esophageal tumor with liver metastases.

In locally advanced ACs of the gastroesophageal junction, where there is endoscopic or radiological evidence of gastric extension of the lesion, laparoscopy can be done as part of the staging process (Fig. 11.34).

The nutritional status and history of weight loss should be assessed and nutritional support is an integral part of the medical care for patients with esophageal cancer both in the curative and in the palliative setting. Nutritional state is an important predictor of survivability of major surgery.

Management of Local Disease: Upfront interdisciplinary planning of the treatment is now the accepted standard of care for these patients. Accurate staging help the clinicians, medical oncologist and surgeons to plan therapy. Nutritional planning by dedicated dietitians with supplementary feeds is vital. If primary curative surgery is planned, then endoscopic stenting is best avoided and other routes of feeding like nasogastric feeding preferred. Surgery is the treatment of choice in limited resectable disease. In the rare patients with early disease not infiltrating beyond the lamina propria, endoscopic therapy may be possible. Usually, a transthoracic esophagectomy (Ivor-Lewis procedure) is the surgical technique of choice. Esophagectomy should be done in high volume centers, as they demonstrate a lower rate of morbidity and have better infrastructure to deal with complications following major surgery, thereby reducing mortality (Fig. 11.35).

For patients unable, because of severe comobidity or unwilling to undergo surgery, combined chemoradiotherapy is superior to radiotherapy alone. Four courses of cisplatin/5-FU combined with high fraction radiation doses are regarded as standard for therapeutic chemoradiotherapy.

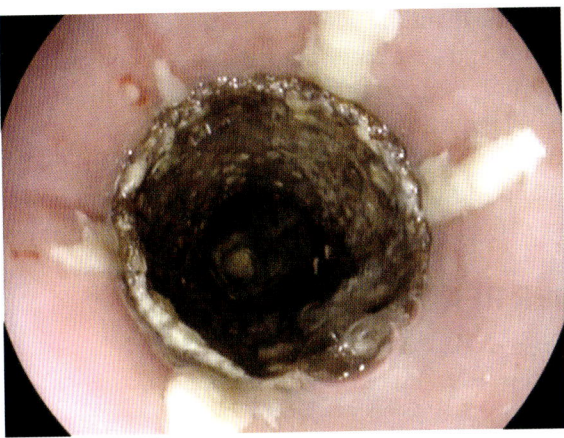

Fig. 11.35: Endoscopic stenting can improve dysphagia and greatly improve nutritional status. Nutrition is a vital part of preparation for surgery.

In patients with locally advanced esophageal cancer (cT3–T4 or cN1–3 M0), some form of preoperative (neoadjuvant) treatment is now the treatment of choice. Patients with locally advanced SCC benefit from preoperative chemotherapy with or without radiotherapy with higher rates of complete tumor resectability and better local tumor control and survival. This usually comprises weekly administration of carboplatin and paclitaxel for 5 weeks and concurrent radiotherapy followed by surgery. For patients with esophageal AC, some forms of perioperative chemotherapy or chemoradiotherapy have been shown to improve survival. Regimens tend to include a platinum and a fluoropyrimidine for a duration of 8–9 weeks in the preoperative phase (as well as 8–9 weeks in the postoperative phase, if feasible) with or without radiotherapy should be considered in locally advanced AC of the esophagus, including esophagogastric junction cancers. Occasionally, tumor may be found to achieve complete response to chemoradiotherapy but even after complete tumor response to preoperative chemoradiotherapy patients with operable AC should proceed to surgery.

Management of Advanced/Metastatic Disease: Patients with metastatic disease have a very poor prognosis. Hence, the aim of therapy is to achieve a quality of life. Discussion with patient, carers and multidisciplinary group is vital. There are different options of palliative treatment depending on the clinical situation. Single-dose brachytherapy may be a preferred option even after external RT, since it provides better long-term relief of dysphagia with fewer complications than metal stent placement. Chemotherapy is indicated for palliative treatment in selected patients, particularly for patients with AC who have a good performance status. In squamous cell esophageal cancer, the value of palliative combination chemotherapy is unproven.

Increasingly, the identification of molecular markers is playing a part. In patients with HER2-positive metastatic AC, an antibody against the receptor may be beneficial. Trastuzumab works by binding to the HER2 receptor and slowing down cell replication.

The treatment of esophageal cancer should be individualized to suit the particular patient. Although the disease carries a grave prognosis, there is some evidence of gradual improvement of survival in recent years.

■ FURTHER READING

Esophageal Cancer
1. Napier KJ, Scheerer M, Misra S. Esophageal cancer: a review of epidemiology, pathogenesis, staging workup and treatment modalities. World J Gastrointest Oncol. 2014;6(5):112-20.

CHAPTER 12

Jaundice

Lynsey Corless

■ INTRODUCTION

Jaundice is a clinical sign, for which there are multiple causes. It is a common error to immediately focus clinical attention on the liver, potentially missing the cases of hyperbilirubinemia caused by genetic or hematological conditions. Likewise, the numerous potential hepatobiliary causes of jaundice require systematic investigation to ensure that the correct diagnosis is made. A suggested approach to investigating jaundice is outlined in Figure 12.1.

Is the raised bilirubin conjugated or unconjugated?
- Purely unconjugated suggests a nonhepatic/cholestatic cause
    - Hemolysis; Gilbert's syndrome; Crigler–Najjar syndrome

If conjugated or mixed unconjugated/conjugated, consider liver and biliary disease
- Is there evidence of obstruction
    - Gallstones; malignancy; primary sclerosing cholangitis
- Is there evidence of acute illness
    - Acute viral hepatitis; bacterial infection (e.g. cholangitis or Weil's disease)
- Is there evidence of underlying chronic liver disease
    - Decompensation of cirrhosis; flare of autoimmune hepatitis or hepatitis B infection
- Is there associated pain or fever
    - Cholecystitis; cholangitis; acute portal/hepatic venous thrombosis
- Is the patient pregnant
    - Pregnancy-related liver disease

Do blood tests or imaging point to a specific diagnosis?
- For example, positive smooth muscle antibody suggesting autoimmune hepatitis, dilated biliary tree suggesting obstruction

---

Fig. 12.1: Questions to consider in the investigation of jaundice.

■ REACHING A DIAGNOSIS
Is the Hyperbilirubinemia Conjugated or Unconjugated?

This is the first critical question to ask, since a purely unconjugated hyperbilirubinemia is not associated with hepatobiliary disease, and instead points to prehepatic causes. This can be determined by sending a blood sample to biochemistry for quantification of unconjugated:conjugated bilirubin.

Unconjugated Hyperbilirubinemia

Hemolysis: Increased breakdown of red blood cells leads to increased metabolism of heme, and therefore production of unconjugated bilirubin (Fig. 12.2). Hemolysis can be confirmed by checking reticulocyte count, lactate dehydrogenase and serum haptoglobin.

The most common causes of hemolysis are sickle cell anemia, thalassemia and drug induced or de novo autoimmune hemolytic anemia. Management is dependent upon the cause.

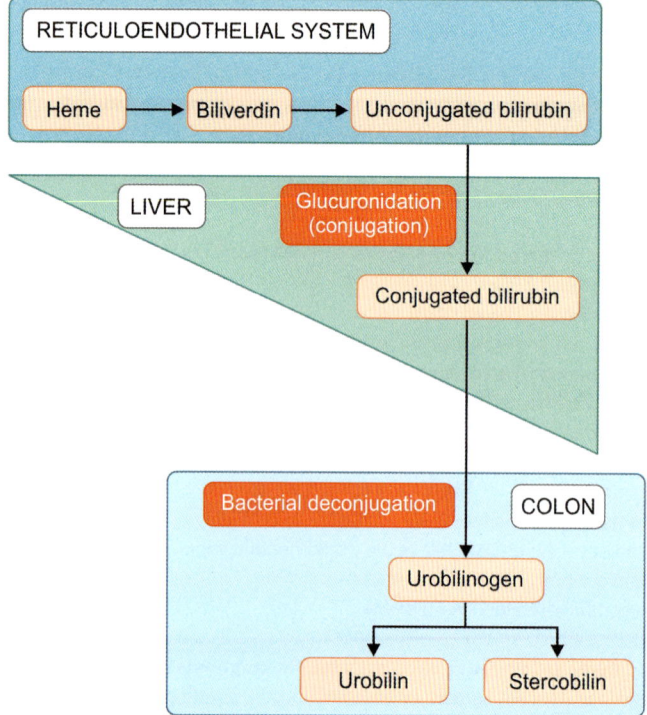

Fig. 12.2: Bilirubin metabolism. A small amount of urobilinogen is processed by the kidneys, and some is reabsorbed into the enterohepatic circulation to be re-excreted as bile.

Inherited Disorders of Bilirubin Metabolism

Gilbert's Syndrome: Gilbert's syndrome is an entirely benign disorder stemming from mutations in glucorinidation enzymes. Affected individuals tend to become jaundiced during periods of ill health, although serum bilirubin usually remains <70 μmol/L.

Gilbert's can be confidently diagnosed where:
- Raised bilirubin is unconjugated only
- Other liver function tests (LFT) are normal
- There is no evidence of hemolysis

Further investigation is not necessary, and patients can be reassured.

Crigler–Najjar Syndrome: It is rare but potentially fatal, since it is associated with major defects in conjugation enzymes. It can be inherited in an autosomal dominant or recessive fashion.

The most severe manifestation of the syndrome presents in infancy with progressive jaundice and brain damage (kernicterus).

Conjugated Hyperbilirubinemia

The investigation of conjugated or mixed hyperbilirubinemia is more complex, both because there are many more possible causes and also because there is considerable overlap in the presentation and investigative findings across different etiologies. Examples of "red herrings" include high transaminases initially suggesting hepatitis but which are also seen fairly regularly in biliary obstruction secondary to gallstones. Conversely, a high alkaline phosphatase may point to obstruction, but may actually reflect hepatic congestion as a consequence of hepatitis or cardiac failure. As discussed in Chapter 15: Abnormal Liver Biochemistry, LFT can only ever be a guide and cannot be relied upon to reveal the diagnosis in isolation.

An approach to investigation is described later, with details of specific conditions in section "Specific conditions causing jaundice".

Perform a thorough history and examination (*see* also Chapter 15: Abnormal Liver Biochemistry): In particular, enquire about exposure to infectious agents (e.g. travel, sexual contact, ingestion of undercooked food), alcohol intake, the use of drugs (illicit, over the counter, prescribed and herbal) in the past 6 months which may all point to jaundice associated with hepatitis.

Patients should be asked about associated symptoms such as pain or rigors, suggesting biliary obstruction, or features of sinister pathology including weight loss or anorexia.

Finally, medical history and family history may yield important information including evidence of autoimmune or genetic diseases, which may cause jaundice (e.g. autoimmune hepatitis or Wilson's disease).

Exclude obstruction: Radiological investigation is mandatory in investigation of jaundice, and should be performed early.

Ultrasound (US) is noninvasive, relatively inexpensive and readily available and should be requested first to allow examination of the biliary tree. Obstruction is suggested by dilatation of part or the entirety of the biliary tree (Figs. 12.3 and 12.4).

In some cases, US provides the diagnosis, but there are many situations where further imaging is required in order to exclude key differential diagnoses (Table 12.1).

Endoscopic retrograde cholangiopancreatography (ERCP) was historically used as a diagnostic tool, but has been superseded by the advent of readily available magnetic resonance cholangiopancreatography (MRCP) scanning. As a result of the invasive nature of the procedure, ERCP is associated with risks of cholangitis, perforation, pancreatitis and rarely death.

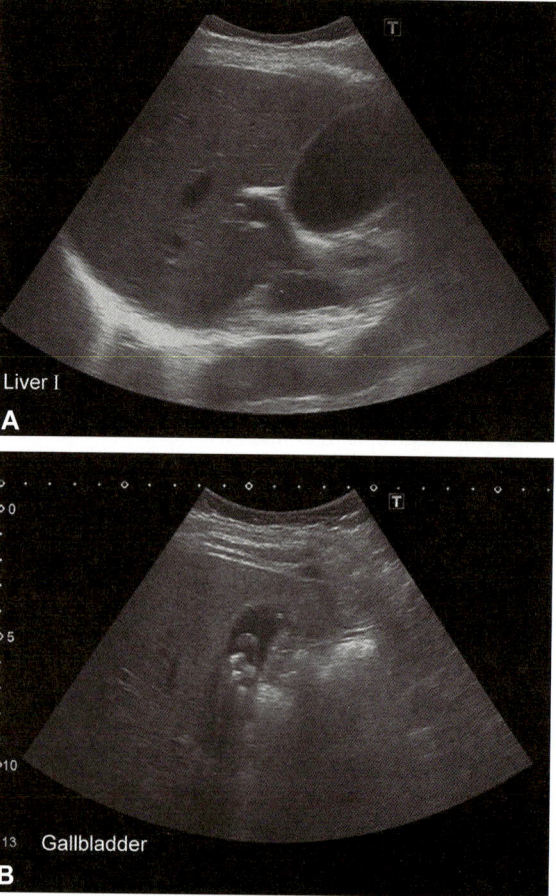

Figs. 12.3A and B: Ultrasound images of normal, gallstones and dilated biliary tree. (A) A normal liver and biliary system; (B) Gallbladder is packed with gallstones.

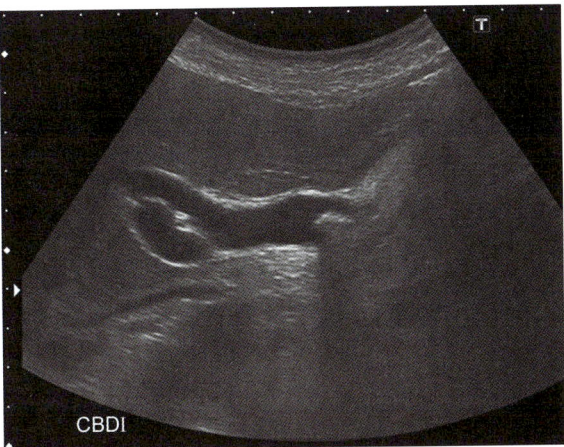

Fig. 12.3C: The common bile duct is dilated right down to the ampulla where a small stone was impacted at distal end. (CBDI: Common bile duct injury).

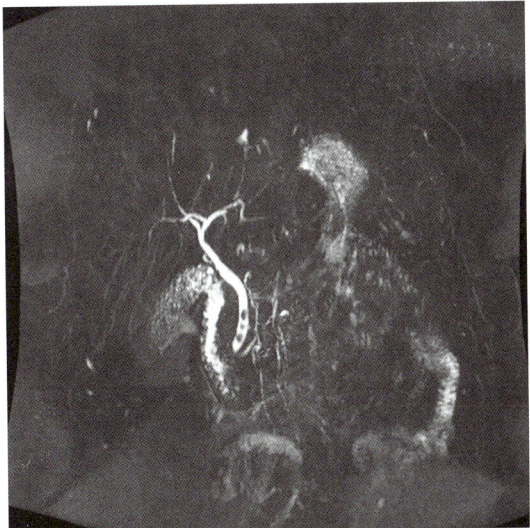

Fig. 12.4: Magnetic resonance cholangiopancreatography is an excellent method of detecting common bile duct stones.

ERCP is now primarily used for therapeutic intervention (Figs. 12.5A to C) with MRCP or computed tomography (CT) used for diagnostics. It is important to note that, while there are risks associated with ERCP, mortality is considerably higher where there is unrelieved biliary obstruction, either as a consequence, the acute infective episode or the risk of recurrent severe sepsis or pancreatitis. This is particularly true of elderly persons.

Timing of imaging can vary. While an early US is always important, urgency of subsequent investigation varies. For example, a patient with

Table 12.1: Radiological investigation of jaundice.

Findings on US	Other findings	Next investigation	Rationale
Dilated ducts with gallstones in gallbladder		ERCP*	Impacted gallstone is most likely and requires removal No further imaging is necessary
Dilated ducts and no gallstones in gallbladder	Bile ducts only with normal pancreatic duct + normal LFT	MRCP if <65 years Consider MRCP if >65 years	Gallstones are likely in younger persons. Bile duct widens physiologically with increasing age so some dilatation *may* be normal in >65 years
	Both ducts dilated + abnormal LFT	CT	Pancreatic malignancy is the most likely diagnosis
	Both ducts dilated + normal LFT	CT or MRCP	Gallstones or malignancy are possible Clinical history should dictate which modality is selected first
Normal or equivocal ducts		MRCP	Ductal gallstones may be present Normal ducts should always prompt consideration of non-obstructing pathology, i.e. intrinsic liver disease

*ERCP should also be considered in people postcholecystectomy with pain and dilated ducts. (ERCP: Endoscopic retrograde cholangiopancreatography; MRCP: Magnetic resonance cholangiopancreatography; CT: Computed tomography; LFT: Liver function tests; US: Ultrasound).

progressive jaundice and signs of sepsis will clearly require urgent investigation in order to allow relief of obstruction as soon as possible. In contrast, the person who has recovered from an episode of pain and jaundice could be discharged to await an outpatient MRCP scan.

Where there is no radiological evidence of obstruction, jaundice as a consequence of intrinsic liver disease must be considered: A full noninvasive liver screen (*see* Chapter 15: Abnormal Liver Biochemistry—Figs. 15.2 and 15.3) should be sent as early as possible.

Clues in the history that point toward the possibility of hepatic jaundice include:

- Drug use (illicit, over the counter, prescribed and herbal) in the past 6 months which may have caused a drug-induced liver injury (DILI)
- Alcohol use, potentially causing acute alcoholic hepatitis, hemolysis as a consequence of alcoholic hepatitis (Zieve's syndrome), or decompensation of chronic liver disease (CLD)
- Foreign travel or ingestion of undercooked food raising possibility of infectious disease, also examined within the sexual history

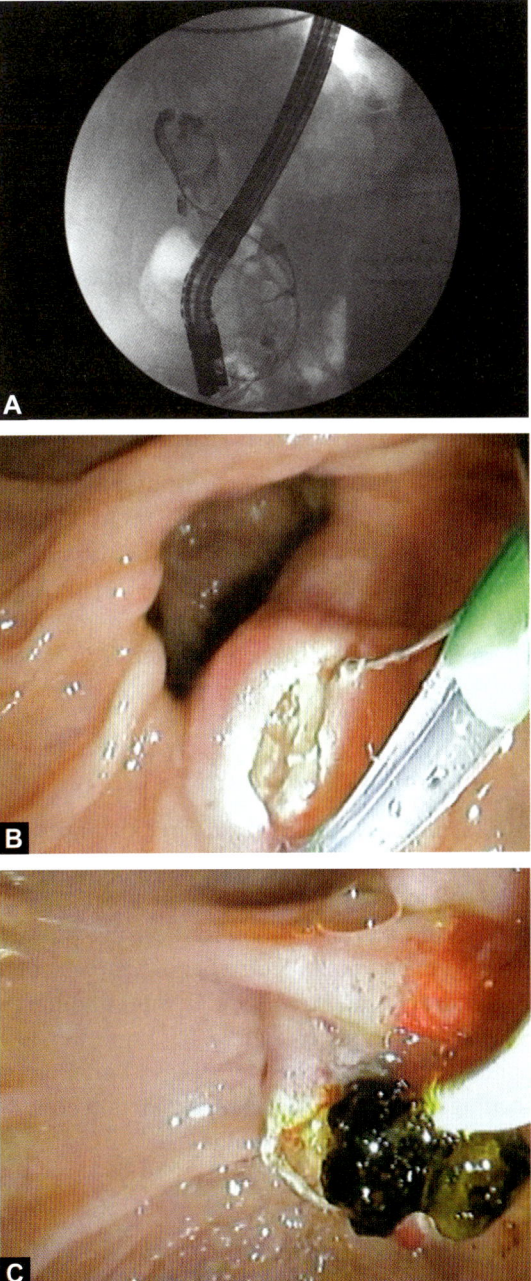

Figs. 12.5A to C: Endoscopic retrograde cholangiopancreatography in the management of gallstone disease. (A) Cholangiogram showing the common bile duct containing numerous stones; (B) There is also a periampullary diverticulum. Endoscopic sphincterotomy being performed with diathermy. There is a 1–3% chance of significant bleeding or pancreatitis, and a mortality of 0.5%; (C) A balloon being used to extract a stone from the common bile duct after sphincterotomy.

- A family history of liver disease, or a medical history of associated disorders including inflammatory bowel disease, or other autoimmune conditions.

Look for evidence of CLD, such as palmar erythema or ascites.

A systematic approach to the investigation of jaundice should result in timely diagnosis with minimal unnecessary investigation.

SPECIFIC CONDITIONS CAUSING JAUNDICE

Many of the conditions causing jaundice of hepatic origin are discussed in detail in other chapters, but are included here for illustration.

Inherited Disorders of Bilirubin Metabolism

Dubin-Johnson syndrome and the rarer Rotor syndrome are caused by defective transport of conjugated bilirubin from hepatocytes into bile. Dubin-Johnson is inherited in an autosomal recessive manner, and the gene responsible has been identified as multiple drug resistance protein 2 (ABCC2). Serum bilirubin is usually <100 µmol/L and treatment is rarely required, although a liver biopsy is often performed in order to exclude intrinsic liver disease.

Toxic Insults

Alcohol

Alcohol can cause jaundice in three main circumstances. First, prolonged excessive alcohol intake can lead to CLD which may decompensate (*see* Chapter 14: Liver Failure). Second, short-term binge drinking may cause acute alcoholic hepatitis, with or without underlying CLD (*see* Chapter 14: Liver Failure). Finally, in a very small number of people with acute alcoholic hepatitis, Zieve's syndrome can be present. In this condition, steatohepatitis is accompanied by acute hemolytic anemia. It is important to exclude Zieve's syndrome in patients with alcoholic hepatitis and anemia by checking the unconjugated:conjugated bilirubin levels to avoid unnecessary investigation. The condition settles on cessation of alcohol use.

Drugs

A full drug history is mandatory, and particular attention should be paid to the use of "supplements". Jaundice caused by the use of anabolic steroids and other muscle bulking gym supplements is increasingly common, with serum bilirubin levels of 500–600 µmol/L not uncommon. Other commonly encountered drugs causing jaundice include antibiotics (particularly coamoxiclav and flucloxacillin) and anticonvulsants.

Most cases of cholestatic DILI will resolve on drug withdrawal with no specific therapy required, although recovery can take many months. Itching can be aided by the use of ursodeoxycholic acid, cholestyramine or menthol-based topical creams. Where the presumed DILI is associated with derangement of transaminases, a biopsy is frequently performed. This will not only exclude any other potential etiology, but also demonstrate the pattern of histological injury. DILI with specific features on histology such as plasma cells, lymphocytes or interface hepatitis are frequently steroid responsive, reducing the duration of illness and risk of progressive liver damage.

Infective Causes

Viral Disease

Infection with hepatitis viruses A–E, Epstein–Barr virus and cytomegalovirus is discussed in Chapter 15: Abnormal Liver Biochemistry.

Bacterial and Parasitic Disease

Cholangitis: Cholangitis is a potentially life-threatening bacterial infection of the biliary tree, usually caused by stones in the common bile duct (CBD) or manipulation of the biliary system (e.g. ERCP or stent insertion). Less common causes of bacterial cholangitis include strictures (e.g. malignancy or primary sclerosing cholangitis—PSC ["Autoimmune Disease" section]) and biliary cysts ("Congenital Malformations of the Biliary Tree" section).

Cholangitis is suspected where Charcot's triad is present (jaundice, pain and fever). Investigations show evidence of sepsis, and often raised transaminases, alkaline phosphatase or amylase. The commonest pathogens on blood culture are *Escherichia coli, Klebsiella* and *Enterococcus* species.

Treatment focuses on antibiotic and supportive therapy, which will only be fully effective alongside relief of obstructing pathology. Examples include ERCP with duct clearance for gallstone disease (Figs. 12.3 and 12.4), or stenting/bypass of a stricture ("Autoimmune disease" and "Cholangiocarcinoma" sections).

Other Bacterial Disease

Nonviral infective causes of hepatic jaundice are relatively uncommon, but can be associated with significant morbidity. Leptospirosis (Weil's disease) is caused by infection with *Leptospira icterohemorrhagica*, most commonly by exposure to urine of rats carrying the bacterium. Jaundice is associated with features of sepsis and can be complicated by renal failure. Diagnosis is made by detection of antibodies on serological sampling. Other examples of bacterial or parasitic infections causing jaundice include secondary syphilis, Q fever (*Coxiella burnetii*) and toxoplasmosis.

Autoimmune Disease

Acute flares or progressive worsening of immune-mediated liver disease (autoimmune hepatitis, primary biliary cholangitis and PSC) can be associated with jaundice. These are fully discussed in Chapter 15: Abnormal Liver Biochemistry.

The investigation of jaundice in a patient with PSC requires careful consideration. As discussed in Chapter 15: Abnormal Liver Biochemistry, PSC is associated with destruction of both intra- and extrahepatic bile ducts. Therefore, jaundice may simply be due to progression of the underlying disease, causing worsening bile duct destruction and obstruction. On the other hand, the anatomical abnormalities of the biliary tree also increase the risk of bacterial infection, and so jaundice may be a consequence of cholangitis. Finally, progressive obstruction may be due to cholangiocarcinoma, which is considerably more common in PSC than other individuals.

Rising bilirubin in the context of PSC should always be investigated to differentiate between cholangitis, progressive disease and malignancy, but this is not always straightforward, particularly since a small cholangiocarcinoma can easily be missed on an MRI scan of already abnormal ducts. A new dominant stricture should prompt ERCP in order to facilitate stricture brushings to look for histological evidence of cholangiocarcinoma, and placement of a stent to relieve obstruction.

Vascular Causes

Congestive cardiac failure commonly causes mild derangement of liver enzymes, but occasionally jaundice can occur. US with Doppler tracing will show congestion in the hepatic veins. Treatment is aimed at improving cardiac status.

Thrombosis of the hepatic (Budd–Chiari syndrome) or portal veins can cause jaundice, often associated with sudden onset of pain and ascites. Where thrombotic disease is suspected, investigation focuses on establishing the precipitant (especially to exclude malignancy or sepsis) and possible therapeutic interventions.

Budd–Chiari Syndrome

Budd–Chiari syndrome refers to obstruction occurring anywhere between the venules of the hepatic veins within the liver to the inferior vena cava. There is usually associated prothrombotic tendency, most frequently from polycythemia rubra vera, but Budd–Chiari is also associated with protein C or S deficiency, paroxysmal nocturnal hemoglobinuria, the use of hormonal contraceptives and acute inflammatory conditions. Less frequently, it is a result of congenital venous webs or stenosis, or infection with tuberculosis or schistosomiasis.

Presentation varies from acute liver failure to decompensation of previously undiagnosed CLD, but classically manifests with pain, ascites and jaundice. The ascites has high protein content, and US with Doppler will reveal reduced hepatic venous flow. A venogram is necessary to highlight the sites and degree of obstruction. If it is due to a web or stenosis, local angioplasty or stenting can alleviate the problem. Where disease is more diffuse, stenting can still be attempted but is usually less successful. Anticoagulation is required for those with prothrombotic tendency.

Since Budd–Chiari syndrome can lead to progressive liver failure, liver transplantation is sometimes required.

Malignancy

Any hepatobiliary or pancreatic malignancy can cause jaundice. This is usually due to obstruction but in the case of hepatocellular carcinoma (Chapter 14: Liver Failure), jaundice can be a result of malignant infiltration of hepatic tissue with subsequent liver failure. This is also seen in hepatic metastases from other solid organ cancers, or infiltration of the liver in hematological malignancies such as lymphoma.

Cholangiocarcinoma

Cancers of the bile ducts are usually histologically confirmed as adenocarcinoma and can occur in any portion of the biliary tree, although the liver hilum is by far the most common site.

Although rare in the population as a whole, a number of conditions increase the risk of cholangiocarcinoma, including PSC, choledochal cysts and Caroli disease ("Congenital Malformations of the Biliary Tree" section).

Presentation is usually with obstructive jaundice, often accompanied by systemic symptoms such as weight loss or lethargy, but in some cases cholangitis is the first presentation.

Imaging reveals dilated ducts, with specific appearances dependent on tumor site. A CT scan is mandatory to fully assess local disease (e.g. vascular invasion, nodal involvement) and presence of distant metastases.

Relief of obstruction is the first priority in management. Although ERCP with placement of a plastic stent is suitable for distal tumors, it is rarely possible as most cholangiocarcinoma is situated at the liver hilum. In these circumstances, a percutaneous transhepatic cholangiogram (PTC) is performed by interventional radiology. A PTC allows indefinite percutaneous drainage by inserting a drain in the intrahepatic ducts proximal to the tumor. This allows relief of obstruction, while other staging investigations are being performed.

Where disease is operable and patients are suitable for surgery, resection has an excellent outcome. Chemotherapy can be used alongside surgery or for palliative treatment.

Carcinoma of the Gallbladder

Adenocarcinoma is the most frequent histological type of gallbladder malignancy, although squamous tumors also occur. Cancer can arise in gallbladder polyps, with those >1 cm in size considered high risk. Preventative cholecystectomy is advised in this circumstance.

Presentation of gallbladder cancer is with obstructive jaundice and disease is frequently advanced at diagnosis. Treatment will depend on patient fitness, tumor resectability and evidence of distant spread.

Carcinoma of the Pancreas

Pancreatic cancer is common in the population, and has a poor prognosis with 5-year survival under 10%. In approximately half of cases, disease is advanced and unresectable at presentation. In many others, the major and extensive surgery required for potential cure is contraindicated due to other health problems.

Most pancreatic cancer is sporadic, but approximately 5% are thought to be a late complication of chronic pancreatitis. The predominant histological type is adenocarcinoma, although neuroendocrine tumors also occur. Intraductal papillary mucinous neoplasms (IPMN) are relatively common benign tumors, which have malignant potential. This risk is particularly high in IPMN situated in the main pancreatic duct, which are therefore resected where possible. Side-branch IPMNs are usually monitored radiologically in the first instance.

Presentation and Investigation: Tumors in the head of the pancreas (Figs. 12.6A and B) more frequently present with jaundice, as the tumor abuts the pancreatic duct. In contrast, lesions in the tail only cause jaundice in approximately 10% of cases, and usually present instead with nonspecific symptoms such as weight loss, nausea or epigastric discomfort; severe pain is unusual.

Investigation of painless jaundice where malignancy is suspected should include urgent US and CT scanning. In many cases, endoscopic ultrasound (EUS, Fig. 12.7) is also utilized and has two key benefits:
- Lesions can be scrutinized in fine detail and biopsied via fine needle aspiration, allowing differentiation between malignancy, benign IPMN or a cystic lesion in challenging cases
- Structures surrounding the lesion, particularly blood vessels, can be closely inspected for evidence of invasion.

The use of EUS has significantly reduced the need for surgical exploration and also allows delivery of neoadjuvant chemotherapy, as histological typing is available prior to excision.

Surgical Management: There are number of surgical approaches for resection of pancreatic cancer, which is possible in approximately 20% of people.

Jaundice

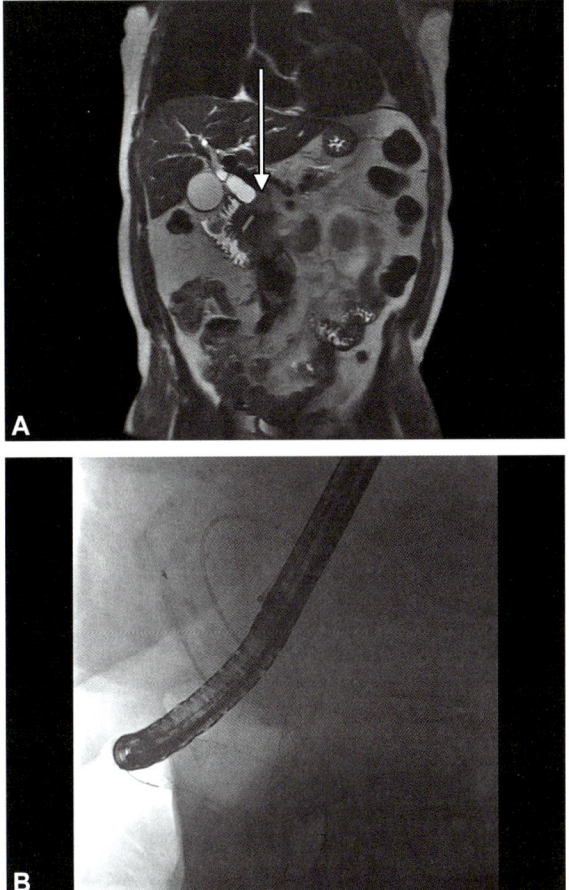

Figs. 12.6A and B: (A) Magnetic resonance imaging scan of pancreatic cancer: note the dilated common bile duct and gallbladder; (B) Pancreatic cancer causing both biliary and duodenal obstruction. Both may be palliatively stented.

The most common operation is a pancreaticoduodenectomy, known as a Whipple's procedure. Here, the head and neck of the pancreas (and often the entire gland) are removed along with the duodenum, the lower end of the CBD, the gallbladder and a portion of the lower stomach. Median survival after planned curative surgery is 12–19 months, with 5-year survival of up to 20%.

In unresectable disease, a surgical bypass can be performed, or a palliative stent can be placed, both giving improvement to quality of life.

Chemotherapy: Adjuvant treatment using gemcitabine-based regimes is the standard treatment for resected pancreatic cancer. Chemotherapy is also frequently used for palliative treatment alongside management of pain, which can be severe in later stages with the need for strong analgesia.

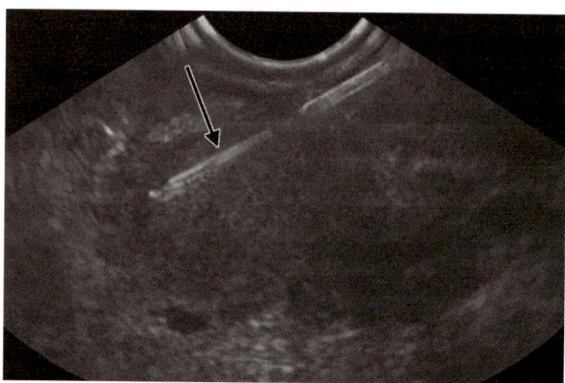

Fig. 12.7: Endoscopic ultrasound of pancreatic lesion. Note the fine needle aspiration taking place.

Pregnancy

Jaundice in pregnancy is discussed in Chapter 15: Abnormal Liver Biochemistry.

Inherited Diseases

Intrinsic liver disease as a consequence of Wilson's disease, hereditary haemochromatosis and alpha-1 antitrypsin deficiency is discussed in Chapter 15: Abnormal Liver Biochemistry.

Congenital Malformations of the Biliary Tree

Biliary Atresia

This affects approximately 1 in 10,000 births. The extent of atresia ranges from atresia of the cystic duct only to complete atresia with total absence of extrahepatic ducts. Presentation is with progressive jaundice (conjugated hyperbilirubinemia) in the neonatal period. Many cases of atresia are managed surgically in the early neonatal period with a Kasai portoenterostomy procedure, where part of the small bowel is used to create a duct to facilitate biliary drainage. Kasai procedures commonly result in progressive liver disease through childhood and most ultimately require liver transplantation.

Choledochal Cysts

Polycystic liver disease, Caroli's syndrome, congenital hepatic fibrosis and choledochal cysts are conditions that sometimes coexist, and may all be manifestations of similar developmental anomaly.

Choledochal cysts are cystic dilatations of the CBD and vary in anatomical site and size. Extensive disease presents in childhood. There is an increased risk of adenocarcinoma in affected individuals and once diagnosed, surgical excision should be undertaken.

Caroli's Syndrome

Caroli's syndrome is a rare congenital abnormality of the intrahepatic bile ducts. About one third of people will also have congenital hepatic fibrosis. Patients present with cholangitis and jaundice, and there is frequently an enlarged, tender liver on palpation. Recurrent sepsis and significantly increased risk of cholangiocarcinoma are the main complications. Management focuses on prevention and treatment of sepsis. Surgical treatments include partial hepatectomy for localized disease, or liver transplantation for diffuse disease causing portal hypertension and cirrhosis.

■ FURTHER READING

Gallstones
1. NICE Clinical Guideline. Gallstone Disease CG188. Available from: http://www.nice.org.uk/guidance/cg188 [accessed 01.12.16].

Vascular Disorders of the Liver
2. European Association for the Study of the Liver. EASL Clinical Practice Guidelines: vascular diseases of the liver. J Hepatol. 2016;64(1):179-202.

Cholangiocarcinoma
3. Khan, SA, Davidson BR, Goldin RD, et al. Guidelines for the diagnosis and treatment of cholangiocarcinoma: an update. Gut. 2012;61:1657-69.

Pancreatic Cancer
4. Pancreatic Section, British Society of Gastroenterology; Pancreatic Society of Great Britain and Ireland, Association of Upper Gastrointestinal Surgeons of Great Britain and Ireland, et al. Guidelines for the management of patients with pancreatic cancer periampullary and ampullary carcinomas. Gut. 2005;54:1-16.

CHAPTER 13

Abdominal Masses and Swelling

Her Hsin Tsai

■ INTRODUCTION

An easy availability and reliability of the modern ultrasound scanner, computed tomography and magnetic resonance imaging (MRI) has led to the widespread mistaken belief among many clinicians that technology has superseded the experienced clinical hand. Yet, a properly conducted bedside examination of the abdomen can be highly informative. Together with a careful history, a majority of gastrointestinal diagnoses may be made at the bedside. It will also direct the clinician to an efficient and expedient choice of the radiological services to employ. Patients also expect the doctor to lay an expert hand on the site of their complaints, and apart from providing useful clinical information; it helps reassure the patients that their complaints are taken seriously.

■ GENERALIZED SWELLING

The old dictum that a generalized abdominal swelling is likely to be "fat, fluid, flatus, feces or fetus" is rarely wrong. It is generally not difficult to differentiate between the five "Fs" by clinical examination alone. Gaseous distention is tympanic. Such gaseous distention may be caused by intestinal obstruction where it would usually be accompanied by abdominal pain, vomiting and presence of high pitched, tinkling, active bowel sounds. Subacute or chronic intestinal obstruction may present with attenuated or absent symptoms but the signs are usually present. In cases of gastric outlet obstruction, there may be associated succussion splash in a fasted patient and in severe cases even visible peristalsis. In paralytic ileus or pseudo-obstruction the bowel sounds may be diminished or absent. Patients with functional bowel diseases and postinfective diarrhea often complain of bloating and abdominal gaseous distention which is more apparent when standing up. This abdominal distention can vary considerably over the course of a day (Fig. 13.1).

Abdominal Masses and Swelling

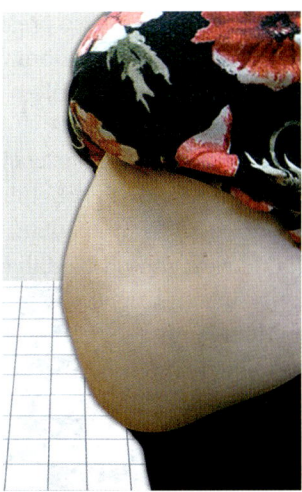

Fig. 13.1: Abdominal distention is a common complaint of the irritable bowel syndrome patient.

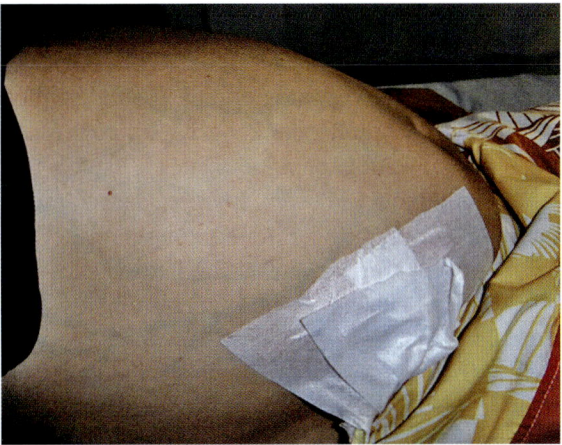

Fig. 13.2: Ascites: the dilated veins, gynecomastia and palmar erythema point to chronic liver disease as the cause.

The presence of ascites may be elicited by demonstration of shifting dullness (Fig. 13.2). This is done by first demonstrating the presence of stony dullness in the flanks which shifts to the mid-abdomen when the patient is lying on the side. It is usually necessary to have at least 2 L of fluid before ascites can be confidently demonstrated. The umbilicus may be everted and its distance from the pubis symphysis diminishes in relation to its distance from the xiphisternum. If there is a large amount of peritoneal fluid, a fluid thrill may be demonstrated. It is important to place the ulnar border of a hand across the mid-abdomen before demonstrating a fluid thrill to prevent transmission through subcutaneous fat. Fluid thrills are also present in large ovarian cysts. One discriminating sign is that aortic pulsations are transmitted through ovarian cyst but not ascites. Ovarian cysts, unless they are very large, may also be demonstrably arising from the pelvis.

Clues as to the source of the ascites are often available to the careful examiner. Examination of the ascitic fluid is also very helpful. Ascitic protein content differentiates transudates (<20 g/L) from exudates (>20 g/L). The presence of stigmata of chronic liver disease should be diligently sought: palmar erythema, spider naevi, leukonychia and signs of feminization in the male. The presence of dilated periumbilical veins (caput medusae) with the venous flow away from the umbilicus is a sign (usually late) of portal hypertension. Ascitic fluid examination typically reveals a transudate picture (<2 g/L) and if protein content is elevated, infection should be thoroughly sought, an elevated white cell count can be taken as evidence of infection. Evidence of right heart failure should alert the clinician to a possible cardiac cause. Constrictive pericarditis may also cause substantial ascites and may be suspected by a high jugular venous pressure (JVP) and a pulsus paradoxus. An echocardiogram is usually diagnostic. In tuberculous ascites, the abdominal distention is not great and has a doughy feel. The fluid is high in protein content and mycobacteria may be cultured from it. In malignant ascites, clinical clues of the primary may be present. The liver may be enlarged and nodular. The fluid typically has a high protein content and may be bloodstained. Ascitic cytology is often performed but has a low diagnostic yield. Pancreatic ascites is usually mild, with a history of acute abdominal pain and a very high amylase content in the ascitic fluid. Abdominal ultrasound and computed tomography (CT) scanning are often helpful in diagnosing the cause of ascites if doubt still exists.

Fecal loading may present as generalized abdominal swelling, often more prominent in the flanks. In untreated Hirschsprung's disease and acquired megacolon, this may be quite dramatic. To make a diagnosis, abdominal palpation and digital rectal examination usually suffice. A plain abdominal film is very helpful if fecal loading is in the proximal colon. Fecal loading may be present even in the presence of diarrhea or bowel frequency. This occurs in overflow incontinence and also quite commonly in patients with distil colitis, where the proximal constipation may actually exacerbate the disease.

■ HEPATOMEGALY

An enlarged liver is felt below the right coastal margin and roughly parallel to it. It is important to start palpation in the right iliac fossa to avoid missing a very large liver. It is also important to start palpation lateral to the rectus abdominis muscle as it may be mistaken for a liver. Other features that characterize a liver edge are movement with respiration, inability to get above the mass and dullness to percussion. A liver edge may be palpable in the absence of hepatomegaly if the diaphragm is displaced inferiorly by emphysematous lungs or fluid. However, this is rarely more than 1 or 2 cm below the costal margin. Percussion is often unhelpful as fluid is dull and a hyperinflated chest is often resonant all the way down. A Riedel's lobe may be mistaken for an enlarged liver. It is more common in women and is an anatomical variant of the right lobe. It extends down the right hypochondrium and occasionally extends to the iliac fossa. Its presence is obvious to the experienced hand but if in doubt, an ultrasound scan will easily demonstrate a Riedel's lobe.

Having felt an enlarged liver, the examiner should decide if it is smooth or nodular. The examiner should feel the liver surface and not merely its lower edge. Any parenchymal liver disease may present as a smooth hepatic enlargement. This includes chronic liver diseases like primary biliary cirrhosis, chronic active hepatitis, hematological disorders and cirrhosis from any cause. Hepatic enlargement from chronic conditions is usually non-tender. A tender smooth enlarged liver suggest acute stretching of the Glisson's capsule and may occur in acute hepatitis, right heart failure and Budd–Chiari syndrome. In acute Budd–Chiari syndrome, the pain may be considerable. In postacute or chronic Budd–Chiari, an enlarged caudate lobe is felt anteriorly. This is because the venous outflow of the caudate lobe is direct into the vena cava and not via the hepatic veins. A very large liver may extend down to the right iliac fossa. The most common cause of a very enlarged liver is alcoholic liver disease where there is fatty change. Another cause is fatty liver of pregnancy. Other conditions associated with a fatty liver include diabetes and drugs but the hepatic enlargement is rarely significant.

Simple hepatic cysts are usually small, impalpable and asymptomatic but may occasionally be large and palpable. Hydatid cysts present as asymptomatic hepatomegaly and should be suspected in patients of Mediterranean origin, Welsh or Scottish farmers. These may be easily demonstrated at ultrasound and a plain abdominal film often show rim calcification. Serology is diagnostic.

The presence of pyrexia should alert the clinician to the possibility of hepatic abscesses. Abscesses caused by pyogenic organisms are accompanied by systemic signs of weight loss, malaise, fever and right upper quadrant pain. If suspected, abdominal ultrasound may pick it up but CT is more sensitive, particularly of lesions close to the diaphragm (Figs. 13.3 and 13.4). Amebic abscess should be suspected if the patient has been to the tropics. Unlike pyogenic abscesses, pain is more pronounced and systemic features are less common. Stool cultures may suggest diagnosis and should be done even in the absence of diarrhea and aspiration of the abscess will reveal thick brown "anchovy sauce" pus.

A nodular feel to the liver usually suggests metastatic liver disease. It may be tender but this is relatively unusual. There are few other conditions that may give a nodular liver. This includes macronodular cirrhosis and the exceptionally rare syphilitic gumma.

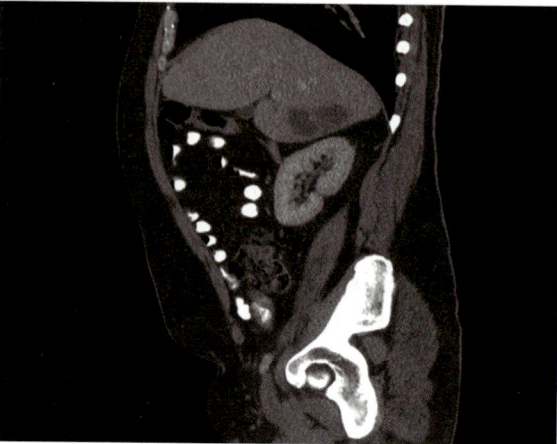

Fig. 13.3: Liver abscesses can be single or multifocal.

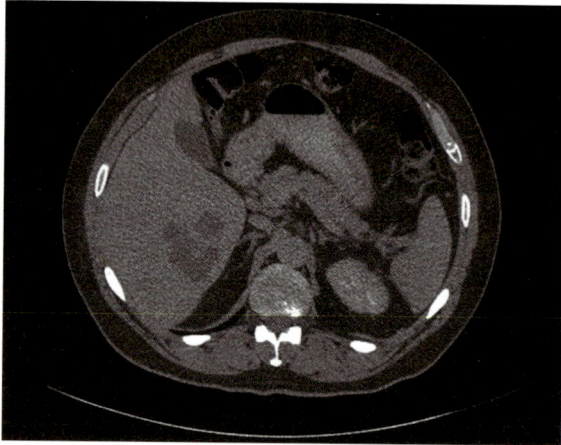

Fig. 13.4: Presence of fever or raised inflammatory markers in a patient with enlarged liver should alert the clinician of the possibility of liver abscesses. It may mimic metastatic malignancy on computed tomography.

Other masses palpable below the right costal margin include the gallbladder. The position of the normal gallbladder is usually at the tip of the ninth rib, lateral to the mid-clavicular line. The normal gallbladder, however, lies deep and is rarely palpable. As it enlarges, the fundus is displaced anteriorly, inferiorly and medially and is felt as a rounded fluid sac which is often mobile. A mucocele or empyema of the gallbladder may be felt as tender enlargement, and in the case of the latter, the patient is also septic. In the presence of jaundice, the presence of a palpable gallbladder indicates that the jaundice is not caused by gallstones but by a malignant common bile duct obstruction like a

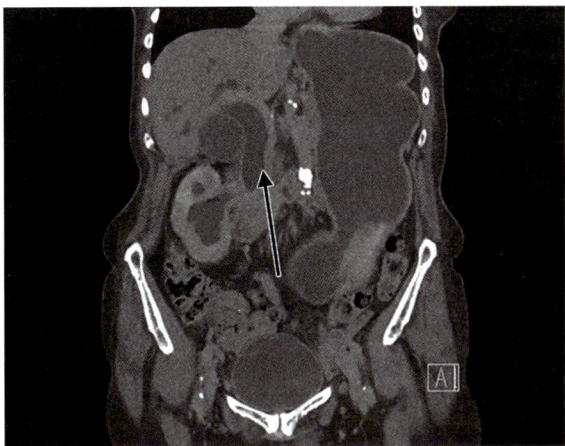

Fig. 13.5: A large ampullary tumor can obstruct the common bile duct causing it to dilate (arrow) and there is also a distended gallbladder.

head of pancreas tumor, ampullary or cholangiocarcinoma (Fig. 13.5). This is referred to as Courvoisier's law. However, its usefulness is overstated as the gallbladder is more usually impalpable in malignant biliary obstruction as the degree of gallbladder distention is rarely gross. Moreover, there are exceptions to this rule. The presence of a stone in the Hartman's pouch and common bile duct may mimic the picture but this is exceptionally rare. More common is a stone in the Hartman's pouch close to the bile ducts causing extrinsic compression on the biliary tree (Mirizzi's syndrome). It is important to realize also that the negative corollary of the law does not apply (i.e. absence of a palpable gallbladder does not indicate nonmalignant obstruction).

An abdominal ultrasound scan is the most useful investigation of a hepatic or gallbladder enlargement. The presence of dilated hepatic veins suggests right heart failure. Sometimes, clots in the hepatic veins may be visible, but Doppler ultrasound is a better tool for assessment of hepatic venous flow. Ultrasound may also detect parenchymal fatty infiltration. Elastography, in which the "stiffness" of the liver is measured, can be an indicator of liver cirrhosis. Metastases of greater than 1 cm are readily detected by ultrasonography. Computed tomography is said to detect lesions of 0.5 cm but some metastases may be radiologically isodense. However, use of different phases of intravenous contrast enhancement can be helpful in detecting and characterizing tumors.

▄ SPLENOMEGALY

A palpable spleen is at least twice its normal size, and hence always pathological. The careful examiner should be able to recognize a spleen by its characteristics.

- It is important to appreciate its position as it enlarges. The splenic tip as it becomes palpable emerges from the costal margin at the anterior axillary line. As a spleen enlarges, the tip moves inferiorly and to the right below the umbilicus and in extreme enlargement toward the right iliac fossa. Hence it is important to start palpation from the right iliac fossa if a grossly enlarged spleen is not to be missed.
- It may be possible to feel a notch, which is pathognomonic of a spleen.
- It is not possible to get above the swelling although it may be possible to get behind the swelling between the spleen and the spinal muscles in suitable subjects. The latter fact differentiates it from renal swellings. If there is still doubt whether it is a renal or splenic mass, percussion is often helpful.
- The swelling moves with respiration downward and medially. This is an important sign as it could differentiate a splenic enlargement from that of a large left lobe of liver which enlarges inferiorly.

The presence of a spleen should direct the clinician to carefully look for clues as to its etiology. Presence of anemia, purpura, etc. would suggest a hematological cause, presence of stigmata of chronic liver disease that of portal hypertension and lymphadenopathy suggests reticuloses. Chronic infections, tropical diseases and amyloidosis are other causes.

RENAL MASS

The kidneys should be palpated bimanually at the flanks. The ability to feel above the mass rules out that being the liver or the spleen. Unilateral renal masses may be due to tumor or hydronephrosis. Polycystic disease gives bilateral enlarged kidneys. There may be associated hematuria. Renal ultrasound readily discloses the diagnosis (Figs. 13.6 and 13.7).

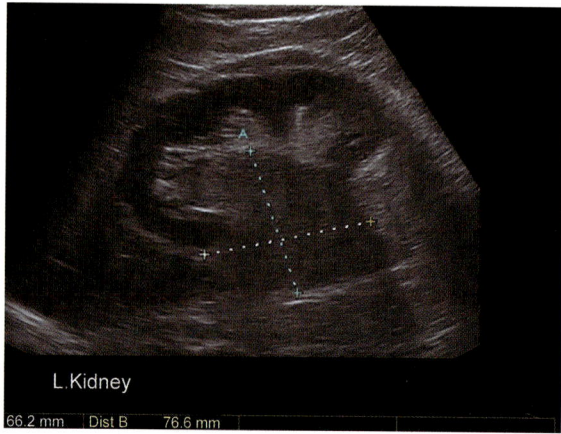

Fig. 13.6: Ultrasound easily picks up a renal mass, here a renal cell carcinoma.

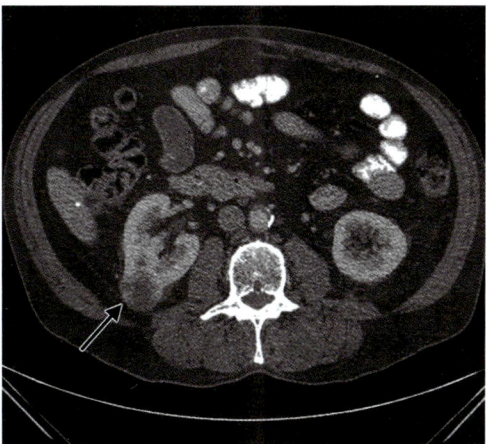

Fig. 13.7: Renal tumors are often picked up as an incidental finding on ultrasound or in this case on computed tomography scanning.

■ OTHER LOCALIZED MASSES

A central abdominal mass may be due to stomach, pancreas or abdominal aorta. A distended stomach is readily seen but often difficult to feel. A succussion splash may be elicited by rocking the abdomen sideways. It is only pathological if it occurs more than 4 h after a meal (or 2 h after fluid only). It suggests gastric outlet obstruction. Very occasionally, visible peristalsis may occur. Gastric tumors are usually not palpable unless very large.

Pancreatic lesions are also felt in the epigastrium. Pancreatic neoplasms are only palpable when very large and the patient is often emaciated and terminal. Very large pancreatic masses are usually due to postpancreatitis pseudocysts or inflammatory masses (Fig. 13.8). The pancreas lies anterior to the abdominal aorta and aortic pulsations are often transmitted.

Abdominal lymph nodes may enlarge prodigiously in lymphomas or abdominal tuberculosis and is felt as a periumbilical mass.

Abdominal aortic aneurysms are palpable as a central abdominal pulsating mass. This is often mimicked in the elderly by a tortuous aorta or merely transmitted pulsations. To demonstrate an aneurysm, the mass should be expansile, i.e. pulsating in all directions and not merely anteriorly. The presence of a flow murmur supports an aneurysm as they are often clot-laden. A tender aneurysm is an ominous sign as it suggests leakage or impending perforation (Fig. 13.9).

Suprapubic masses in a female could represent pregnancy, uterine fibroids or ovarian lesions (Fig. 13.10). In the male, it is usually a full bladder. In chronic bladder neck obstruction, this could be exceedingly large and surprisingly non-tender.

A right iliac fossa mass could represent an appendix abscess, where it follows a history of acute appendicitis. A more chronic tender mass is

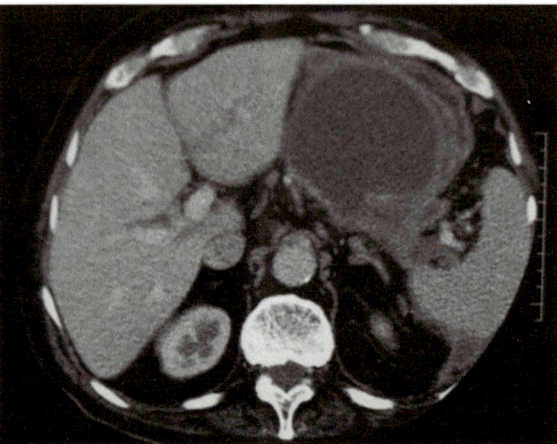

Fig. 13.8: Large pancreatic pseudocyst. Notice the stomach pushed anteriorly by the pseudocyst.

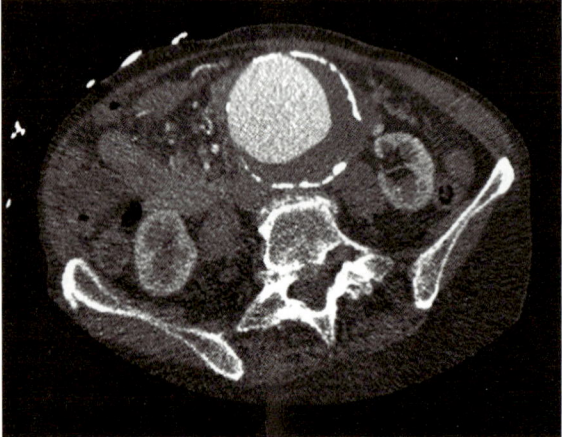

Fig. 13.9: Abdominal aortic aneurysm.

suggestive of Crohn's disease. A history of chronic abdominal pain, diarrhea or obstructive symptoms in a younger patient will suggest this diagnosis. A cecal carcinoma may be palpable if large in a thin subject. Carcinoid tumors may arise from the ilium or appendix and may enlarge to a great size. Once again, other accompanying signs (carcinoid syndrome) may provide the clue. The terminal ilium and cecum are the most common sites for abdominal tuberculosis and must be considered in patients with unexplained pyrexia or anyone from endemic areas (especially the Indian subcontinent).

It is not uncommon to be able to feel the sigmoid colon in the left iliac fossa in a thin individual. It may be tender in patients with irritable bowel or

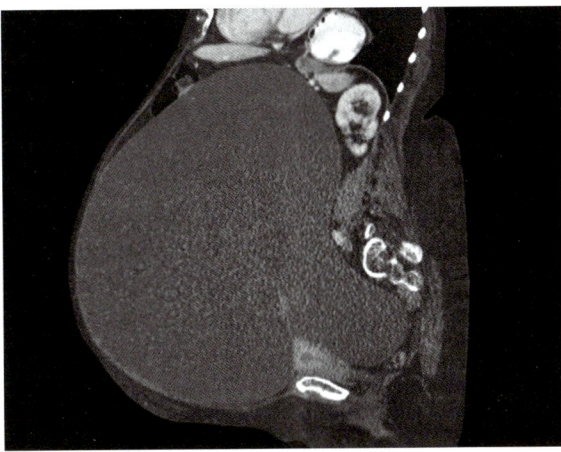

Fig. 13.10: A very large ovarian cyst on computed tomography.

diverticular disease. A mass in this region suggests an abscess, which could be diverticular in origin or due to Crohn's disease.

LIVER TUMORS

Hepatic tumors may be benign, which are of little clinical significance, or malignant. 90% of malignant tumors of the liver are metastatic in European populations but in parts of the East Africa and the Far East, primary hepatocellular carcinoma (HCC) is a very common cancer.

Hepatocellular Carcinoma (Fig. 13.11)

Primary HCC (hepatoma) is relatively rare in European populations but is the second commonest cancer in East Asia, Africa and Pacific islands. The highest incidence of HCC is in East Asia, with incidence rates in men of 35 per 100,000 population. The main etiological factors are hepatitis B and C and cirrhosis from all causes. In the tropics, the carcinogenic aflatoxin from the *Aspergillus flavus* mold which contaminates the food is another factor and may act as a cocarcinogen in patients with hepatitis B. The likelihood of HCC increases 100-fold in patients infected with the hepatitis B virus (HBV).

Carcinoma may arise from cirrhosis of any cause. In northern European countries it most commonly arises from alcoholic liver disease and hemochromatosis. There is suggestion that alcohol and iron overload may themselves be important etiological factors. Interestingly, metastatic tumor is uncommon in cirrhotic livers. There is also a significant male preponderance with a male to female ratio of 4–6:1. HCC must be

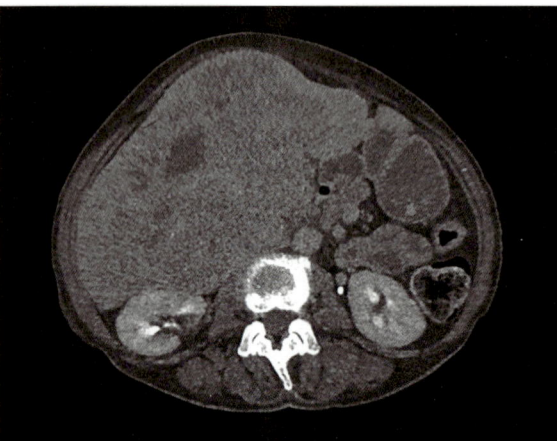

Fig. 13.11: This huge liver is caused by a primary hepatocellular carcinoma.

suspected in any patient with known cirrhosis in whom there is clinical deterioration. Increasingly, diabetic and nondiabetic nonalcoholic fatty liver disease is a major cause of cirrhosis worldwide and is increasingly an etiological factor.

The pathogenesis of HCC is still not fully determined. It is likely that inflammation, necrosis, fibrosis and ongoing regeneration that characterizes the cirrhotic liver leads to HCC development. In patients with hepatitis B, HCC can develop in livers that are not frankly cirrhotic. By contrast, in patients with hepatitis C virus (HCV), HCC invariably presents, more or less, in the setting of cirrhosis. This difference may relate to the fact that HBV is a DNA virus that integrates in the host genome, while HCV is an RNA virus that replicates in the cytoplasm and does not integrate in the host DNA.

Clinical Features

Presentation of hepatomas may be insidious and hence a high degree of clinical suspicion is warranted. In a patient with known cirrhosis with any unexplained clinical deterioration, HCC must be suspected. Increasing ascites or jaundice, palpable local lump over the liver or worsening of chronic encephalopathy are possible pointers to the development of the tumor. Particular attention should be paid to patients with hemochromatosis and HBV infection.

Weight loss, abdominal distention with pain and a low-grade pyrexia are common findings. An irregular hepatic mass may be felt and is often tender. A fiction rub due to perihepatitis and an arterial bruit are sometimes heard. Rarely, a patient may present with an acute abdomen with massive intraperitoneal hemorrhage from a raptured vessel.

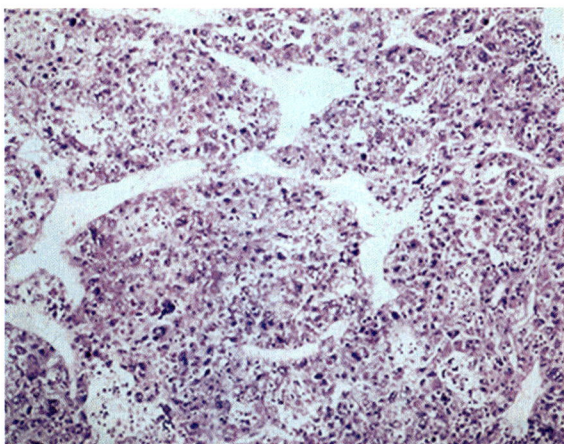
Fig. 13.12: Histological appearance of hepatocellular carcinoma.

Pathology

The tumor may be solitary or multifocal and nodular. The malignant cells resemble normal hepatocytes but are somewhat smaller with hyperchromatic nuclei arranged as finger-like projections (Fig. 13.12). An important variant is the fibrolamellar tumor where fibrosis occurs round the tumor cells. This occurs mainly in younger patients and the prognosis is considerably better.

Investigations

Serum alpha-fetoprotein is raised in 80% of cases. It is a useful screening test in a patient where hepatoma is suspected. There are a few other causes of a raised alpha-fetoprotein, such as testicular, pancreatic and ovarian tumors and hydatidiform mole, but they are rare causes. Ascitic tap reveals an often bloodstained high in protein content.

For localizing and staging of the tumor, an abdominal ultrasound is inadequate. Enhanced CT scanning is needed to localize the anatomy more clearly (*see* Fig. 13.11). MRI is probably the modality of choice as it can characterize HCC without radiation and the need for iodine containing contrast.

A liver biopsy is necessary to make a definitive diagnosis and should be performed under ultrasound control. It is particularly important to identify the group with fibrolamellar type of tumor as the prognosis is better. The combined results should be discussed in a multidisciplinary setting.

Management

Liver resection is the operation of choice for patients with tumors smaller than 5 cm in the absence of cirrhosis. These patients can often tolerate resection of up to 50% of the total liver volume. Surgical advances, better patient selection and improved postoperative care have reduced operative mortality considerably. In patients with cirrhosis, the extent of liver resection that can be tolerated is significantly more limited. In general, resection of more than two segments is contraindicated in patients with Child class B or C cirrhosis. However, among patients who do undergo successful resection, long-term survival is possible, and 5-year survival rates can be up to 50%.

The initial results of liver transplantations for HCCs were poor but with better patient selection, liver transplantation is a valid treatment and in some cases, the option of choice. Patients with established cirrhosis and either a single HCC no larger than 5 cm in diameter or as many as three HCCs no larger than 3 cm had been found to have excellent survival after transplantation. However, for patients with a large tumor the prognosis remains poor.

In patients where liver transplantation is not suitable or available, then ablative treatments are available either as palliative treatment or bridge to definitive surgery. Ethanol injection, cryotherapy or radiofrequency ablation are available, the latter now being the preferred modality.

For many patients, only palliative treatments can be offered. This may include transcatheter arterial chemoembolization (TACE). TACE is performed by an interventional radiologist who selectively cannulates the feeding artery to the tumor and delivers high local doses of chemotherapy, including doxorubicin, cisplatin or mitomycin C. To prevent systemic toxicity, the feeding artery is then occluded with gel foam or coils to prevent retrograde flow. Because most HCCs derive most of their blood flow from the hepatic artery while the rest of the liver depends on the portal blood supply, the liver is not compromised. Often impressive tumor reduction can be seen. One meta-analysis of seven randomized controlled trials with 516 patients suggested a survival advantage of chemoembolization (odds ratio for death, 0.53) compared with medical therapy. Because the treatment is reasonably well tolerated and has minimal morbidity, it can be offered to well-compensated patients with cirrhosis as a method to reduce their disease burden and to potentially extend their life.

Other Hepatic Tumors

Of the benign tumors, the most common is the hemangioma. They are usually small and single but may be multiple or large. They are mostly of the cavernous variety with true hemangiomas being rare. It is present in about 5% of autopsies and is increasingly recognized in asymptomatic subjects who undergo abdominal ultrasound or CT examination for other indications. This may cause unnecessary anxiety as hemangiomas may be indistinguishable radiologically from a primary or secondary lesion. Attempts at biopsying these lesions may lead to disastrous hemorrhage. Enhanced CT scanning usually help differentiate these vascular lesions from malignant ones. In an asymptomatic patient with no history of cirrhosis or other cancers, a follow-up scan a few months later is reassuring.

Other primary hepatic tumors are very rare. A benign adenoma is recognized in association with the pill and pregnancy. Focal nodular hyperplasia is a benign condition, characterized by an area of hypertrophy of normal liver tissue, which in rare cases may be symptomatic. Ultrasound is usually iso-echoic but can be hypo- or hyperechoic leading to concern. CT may show the lesion as a mass with a central scar. Biopsy will show normal liver tissue. Malignant hemangiosarcoma is very rare and may be associated with exposure to vinyl chloride, arsenic and anabolic steroids. Primary sarcoma is very rare except for Kaposi sarcoma in HIV-infected individuals where the liver is a common site for the tumor.

Metastatic Tumors

The liver is the most common site of blood-borne metastases. The common primary tumors are colorectal, lung, stomach, breast and pancreas. In European populations, it accounts for more than 90% of all malignant liver tumors. Diagnosis is made either as a clinical finding of an enlarged irregular, knobbly liver or radiologically by ultrasound or CT in a patient with a known primary tumor in a hunt for metastases. Prognosis is poor with the exception of resectable colorectal metastases.

HEPATIC CYSTS AND ABSCESSES

Hepatic Cysts

Cystic lesions are increasingly recognized as scanning techniques become increasingly used (Fig. 13.13). They range from small solitary asymptomatic cysts to multiple large cysts which may be part of an adult fibrocystic disease and indeed may be ends of a spectrum of the same disease entity. They are usually asymptomatic, picked up by ultrasound examination and of little clinical significance. However, some patients, particularly in the fourth and fifth decades, may experience abdominal distention and pain when these cysts enlarge. Rarely, they may cause biliary obstruction with jaundice or rapture. When symptomatic, the large cysts may be drained percutaneously and instillation of absolute alcohol may delay their recurrence. Only in exceptional circumstances surgery is required; fenestration (opening like a window) of superficial cysts can be performed laparoscopically.

Hydatid Cysts

Hydatid disease is caused by the cyst state of the tapeworm *Echinococcus granulosus*. The disease is endemic in sheep-rearing countries in the Eastern Mediterranean, Middle East, Africa, South Australia and New Zealand. It is

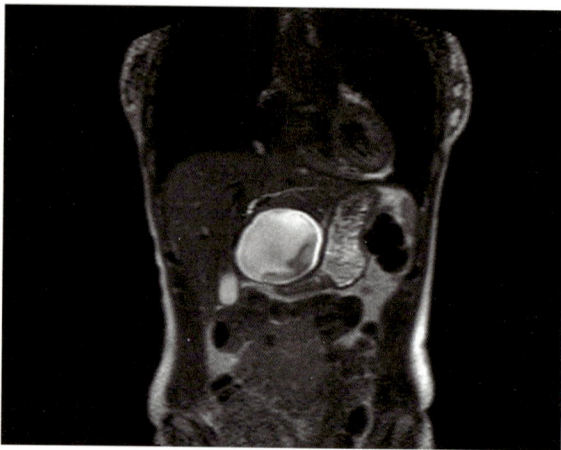

Fig. 13.13: A large simple hepatic cyst on magnetic resonance imaging. This size is likely to cause symptoms.

rare in Britain except among Welsh farmers. It is a zoonosis with the dog as primary host and man, sheep and cattle acting as intermediate hosts. Man is infected by ingesting the ova which is picked up when handling dogs or their excreta. The ova burrow into the intestinal wall and are delivered to the liver in the portal flow. The liver is the main infected organ with lungs the next likely site. Spleen bone and brain may rarely be affected.

Once in the liver, host cellular responses produce a thick ectocyst which may calcify. These cysts may be single or multiple and usually affect the inferior of the right lobe of liver. The cyst fluid is antigenic, and as the host is sensitized, leakage of the fluid may lead to anaphylaxis.

The cysts themselves are usually asymptomatic although the larger ones cause abdominal distention and discomfort. However, they become symptomatic if they rupture. This may occur intraperitoneally resulting in ascites or into the bile ducts causing jaundice. Occasionally, infection with pyogenic organisms occurs.

Diagnosis is made by characteristic ultrasound findings. Plain X-ray may show calcification. A serological complement fixation test is available but with a significant false-positive and -negative rates. Small asymptomatic cysts are best left alone. Aspiration or biopsy is contraindicated because of risk of anaphylaxis. Large solitary cysts may be surgically removed with care to shell out the entire cyst without spilling. Medical treatment with mebendazole or the less toxic albendazole may be attempted.

Pyogenic Abscess

Pyogenic liver abscesses may result from portal spread of infection, such as appendix abscesses, direct spread from adjacent infective focus or penetrating wounds, or biliary infections. The latter is increasingly common, especially in the elderly immunocompromised individuals. However, in about half of the cases, often in elderly patients, there may be no obvious source of infection. The most common infecting organisms are gram-negative cocci. *Escherichia coli* and *Streptococcus faecalis* are most often encountered. *Streptococcus milleri* is an unusual organism but also a common cause of liver abscesses. *Staphylococci* and anaerobic bacteria are increasingly encountered. *Salmonella typhi* causes a relapsing cholangitis.

The patient usually presents with swinging pyrexia, weight loss, right upper quadrant pain and in untreated cases, prostration and septic shock. With the widespread use of antibiotics, the presentation may be more subtle and insidious. There may be some right upper quadrant discomfort, cough and hepatomegaly. A high degree of clinical suspicion will aid early diagnosis. Ultrasound usually can differentiate an abscess from tumor but if in doubt, aspiration of abscess will yield pus. Culture of the abscess usually yields the offending organism unless the patient has had prior antibiotic therapy. CT scanning often provides useful additional information. Endoscopic retrograde cholangiopancreatography may be indicated if there is evidence of biliary sepsis caused by ductal stones.

Treatment is with antibiotics, guided by bacteriology. If the abscess is culture negative, a combination of a broad spectrum antibiotic with gram-negative activity, such as a cephalosporin and metronidazole should be used. Antibiotics alone are rarely sufficient and some drainage procedure should be attempted either under ultrasound or CT control. This may not be feasible if the abscesses are small and numerous. Any of the biliary obstruction must be relieved and this is best achieved by endoscopic sphincterotomy or stent insertion.

Amebic Abscess

Amebiasis is a disease of the subtropics and tropics. It is rare in European populations except those who have visited endemic areas. It may present many years after exposure. The organism *Entamoeba histolytica* exists in a free-living cystic form outside the host and when ingested passes through to the colon where it invades the mucosa forming the typical flask-shaped ulcers. From there, they invade the portal system draining into the liver.

Patients present with fever and right upper quadrant pain. The systemic features are usually less marked than pyogenic abscesses. Alcohol is said to exacerbate the pain. A tender liver is usual and the swelling may be visible in the epigastrium. Abscesses near the diaphragmatic surface may present with shoulder-tip pain and pleural effusion.

Diagnosis is made by ultrasound and serology, which is positive in over 90% of cases. Identification of amebic cysts from feces is rare. Aspiration of the cysts may yield the typical "anchovy sauce" pus. Metronidazole 800 mg 3 times a day for 10 days is the standard therapy and drainage is rarely needed.

FURTHER READING

1. Forner A, Llovet JM, Bruix J. Hepatocellular carcinoma. Lancet. 2012;379(9822):1245-55.
2. Kim RD, Reed AI, Fujita S, et al. Consensus and controversy in the management of hepatocellular carcinoma. J Am Coll Surg. 2007;205(1):108-23.
3. Kulik LM, Mulcahy MF, Omary RA, et al. Emerging approaches in hepatocellular carcinoma. J Clin Gastroenterol. 2007;41(9):839-54.

CHAPTER 14

Liver Failure

Lynsey Corless

INTRODUCTION

Liver failure encompasses a broad spectrum of severe liver disease. It is absolutely critical to differentiate between acute liver failure (ALF) and chronic liver disease (CLD), as management and prognosis are completely different.

ACUTE LIVER FAILURE

Acute liver failure is a medical emergency. It comprises abnormal liver function, coagulopathy and encephalopathy. In this circumstance, liver function is completely normal until disturbed by a specific precipitant (Fig. 14.1), often leading to massive hepatic necrosis with no time for physiological adaptation. ALF can be:
- Hyperacute (jaundice and encephalopathy within 7 days of precipitating event)
- Acute (within 8–28 days)
- Subacute (within 4–12 weeks).

Common
- Drugs, especially paracetamol
- Autoimmune hepatitis
- Hepatitis B virus (HBV)

Rare
- Infiltration (malignancy, amyloid)
- Hepatitis A virus
- Hepatitis C virus
- Ischemic hepatitis
- Wilson's disease
- Budd–Chiari
- Amanita phalloides poisoning
- Pregnancy

Fig. 14.1: Causes of acute liver failure.

Hyperacute is the most frequently encountered presentation, is most often due to paracetamol poisoning and is more readily recognized than the acute or subacute forms. Patients will usually present with vague symptoms, especially nausea, vomiting and right upper quadrant discomfort followed by development of jaundice and encephalopathy. In those with a history of paracetamol poisoning, attendance at hospital usually precedes the major symptoms and as such ALF must be actively excluded even in those who appear well. It is vitally important to recognize ALF because deterioration and death can occur rapidly if not appropriately managed.

Differentiating ALF from CLD

In many cases, the history will suggest ALF, such as recent paracetamol ingestion. Other important points in the history include recent (within 6 months) use of medications, including herbal or over the counter remedies, and whether there is a known history of liver disease (personal or family), travel, recent sexual contacts and previous and current alcohol use.

Examination should include a thorough search for stigmata of CLD, such as palmar erythema and spider naevi, which make ALF less likely, although it should be noted that ALF can occur in those with preexisting liver disease, for example secondary to paracetamol poisoning.

Finally, assess the pattern of LFT derangement and synthetic function abnormality. ALT is often well >1000 IU/mL, reflecting massive hepatocyte necrosis. This is incredibly rare in CLD, as hepatocytes are destroyed and replaced by fibrotic tissue gradually over time, and ALT is frequently normal. Coagulation is also disturbed to a greater degree in ALF versus CLD; and prothrombin time (PT) is the marker most closely reflecting prognosis (Fig. 14.2). Patients with deranged LFTs with no history of cirrhosis should not have coagulopathy, because their liver has been normal up to the advent of hepatitis, and should therefore have normal synthetic function. Abnormal clotting, even mild derangement, in this circumstance is associated with high mortality and should never be ignored.

- Prothrombin time > 50 s
- Creatinine > 300
- Hypoglycemia
- Acidosis
- Encephalopathy

Fig. 14.2: High-risk features in acute liver failure.

Approach to Management

Assessment

A detailed history, including:
- Recent health and current symptoms
- Drug history (prescribed, illicit, over the counter and herbal). Always ask about paracetamol use, remembering that even normal doses of paracetamol are potentially toxic, especially in those who are underweight or malnourished, and a high index of suspicion is required. If there has been a possible overdose, establish the amount taken and over what time period this occurred. A staggered overdose over hours or days has a much worse prognosis than a one off overdose. It is also important to know if the paracetamol was taken alongside other drugs or alcohol
- Alcohol history
- Recent possible exposure to hepatitis B or other infections (travel and sexual history)
- Family history, especially looking for possible autoimmune or Wilson's disease
- Psychiatric history, and if paracetamol overdose, whether there is on-going suicidal ideation
  Examination with a focus on:
- Vital signs should be noted, particularly blood glucose level; in ALF, the necrotic liver is unable to convert stored glycogen to glucose, and hypoglycemia is a sensitive and worrying sign of ALF
- Presence of stigmata of CLD, raising the possibility of decompensated CLD or an acute on chronic liver failure (ACLF) ("Acute on Chronic Liver Failure" section)
- Encephalopathy including grade
- A careful search for infection, the commonest cause of death in ALF
- Abdominal examination including liver size; a small liver is sometimes seen in subacute-ALF and hepatomegaly can be a sign of an infiltrative process or Budd–Chiari syndrome.

A panel of investigations is required to exclude the multiple potential etiologies, and stratify degree of liver failure including:
- LFT
- PT
- Arterial blood gas/lactate+bicarbonate
- Urea and electrolytes; maintenance of good renal function is critical in ALF
- Viral serology
  - Epstein–Barr, cytomegalovirus, varicella zoster, herpes simplex, hepatitis A, B and C

- Hepatitis B (HBV) serology should include both surface antigen (sAg) and core antibody, as sAg can take time to develop, hence cAb can be the only evidence of acute HBV. HBV serology should be performed urgently (same day result) so antiviral treatment can be initiated if required.
- Autoantibodies and immunoglobulins
- Blood and urine cultures
- Blood film for evidence of hemolysis
- Ultrasound scan (USS) and Doppler of vessels to be performed urgently
- Pregnancy test
- Consider ophthalmology assessment for Kayser–Fleischer rings to exclude Wilson's disease
- In hyperacute-ALF, a liver biopsy is rarely required, and may unnecessarily delay treatment. In subacute-ALF, a biopsy can provide useful information, for example a patient with possible autoimmune hepatitis in whom steroids may be useful.

Management

- Determine if signs of severity are present (Fig. 14.2). These signify massive liver damage and a reduced chance of spontaneous recovery, and such patients may require immediate transfer to a liver transplant unit
- If the patient is under the care of a nonspecialist team, it is advisable to discuss cases of ALF with the regional liver transplant unit, even without high risk features
- Monitor vital signs including 2 hourly BM
- Monitor encephalopathy grade 1–2 hourly; patients developing grade 3 encephalopathy should be transferred to intensive care, as coma can quickly occur
- If paracetamol overdose is suspected, prescribe N-acetyl cysteine (NAC) and continue until PT is near normal. NAC can also be useful in non-paracetamol ALF
- Intravenous fluids to ensure adequate hydration; many people with ALF are severely dehydrated and must be aggressively rehydrated to safeguard renal function. Fluid balance should be carefully monitored
- Acid suppression with oral proton pump inhibitor
- Perform PT every 8 h while rising. PT is the best measure of clinical progress, with morbidity and mortality rising as PT climbs
- Intravenous vitamin K should be given to ensure vitamin K deficiency is not contributing to the coagulopathy, especially in people who are malnourished (intake deficiency) or jaundiced (absorption deficiency). Vitamin K will not correct coagulopathy due to hepatocyte failure, so clinical progress can still be accurately monitored. However, patients should

not receive fresh-frozen plasma, because this will correct *all* coagulopathy, and the ability to monitor the trend of PT is lost
- If PT >30 s, risk of sepsis and renal failure increase significantly; therefore, a urinary catheter should be inserted and broad-spectrum antibiotics and oral antifungal prescribed.

Complications

Acute liver failure can deteriorate with alarming speed, and patients require close monitoring and early discussion with specialist services.

The major complications occurring in ALF are listed as follows:
- Renal impairment; patients with ALF are frequently severely dehydrated, and may also have sepsis. In paracetamol overdose, there is the added element of drug-induced acute tubular necrosis. Occasionally, dialysis will be required but most renal impairment will respond to early and judicious fluid management
- Infection is extremely common, and this is partly explained by the key role the liver usually plays in immune system function. Fungal sepsis is particularly concerning, and as such prophylaxis is indicated
- Cerebral edema can occur on hyperacute-ALF due to rapid changes in acid–base status increasing intracerebral pressure, especially in paracetamol overdose
- Cardiovascular collapse caused by profound vasodilatation leading to significantly lowered systemic vascular resistance.

Is a Liver Transplant Required?

There are clear established criteria to determine whether patients with ALF are eligible for liver transplantation (LT, Fig. 14.3). However, there will be

ALF secondary to paracetamol overdose
- pH <7.30 or
- INR >6.5 (PT >100 s) + serum creatinine >300 mmol/L + grade 3 or 4 encephalopathy

ALF (except paracetamol overdose)
- INR >6.5 (PT >100 s) or
- Any three of:
  - Age <10 or >40 years
  - Etiology non-A, non-B hepatitis or idiosyncratic drug reaction
  - Time from jaundice to encephalopathy >7 days
  - INR >3.5 (PT >50 s)
  - Serum bilirubin >300 µmol/L

Fig. 14.3: King's college criteria.

some patients who met these criteria but are unsuitable for other reasons. Transplantation decisions will be made in liver transplant units by the multidisciplinary team. It is important that patients are aware that this is a potential outcome of an episode of ALF.

Many patients will not require a transplant, and should make a full recovery once PT begins to fall and renal function normalizes. Both of these parameters should be monitored to ensure complete resolution before planning discharge.

CIRRHOSIS AS A CONSEQUENCE OF CHRONIC LIVER DISEASE

Pathophysiology

Cirrhosis is the end stage of a pathophysiological process taking years or decades. The most frequent scenario in CLD is a persistent inflammatory process, for example due to alcohol use or autoimmune disease, which sets up a chronic cycle of injury and repair. This results in the formation of fibrotic tissue, which is ultimately associated with structural remodeling and nodule formation in liver tissue, which is diagnostic of cirrhosis (Fig. 14.4). Regardless of initial etiology, cirrhosis heralds hepatic and systemic physiological changes, many of which are irreversible without LT.

However, it is now known that in some etiologies particularly viral hepatitis, eradication of the causative agent can result in regression of fibrosis and major improvements in hepatic function, although complete reversal of cirrhosis is not currently thought possible.

Portal Hypertension

Cirrhosis results in reduced volume of hepatocytes, and hence reduced liver synthetic functional capacity (e.g. production of albumin and coagulation factors), but the major clinical complications of cirrhosis (ascites, encephalopathy, varices and renal disease, discussed later) arise as a result of portal hypertension, a systemic adaptive response to the structural and functional

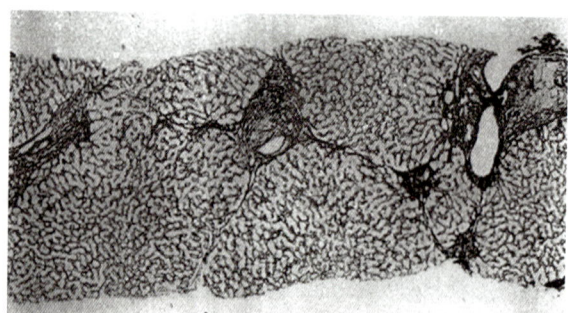

Fig. 14.4: Cirrhotic liver biopsy: fibrosis and regenerative nodules.

impairment of the cirrhotic liver. Development of portal hypertension is therefore a landmark event in the natural history of cirrhosis.

Staging of Chronic Liver Disease

Cirrhosis is frequently asymptomatic in early stages, but can be suspected clinically by the presence of one or more risk factors for liver disease (e.g. history of excess alcohol, obesity or viral hepatitis) and stigmata of CLD (Figs. 14.5A to C). These in conjunction with biochemical evidence of liver synthetic dysfunction including low albumin and raised bilirubin (*see* Chapter 15: Abnormal Liver Biochemistry) can be diagnostic. Ultrasound imaging will often show that the liver has an irregular edge and a coarse echotexture, but cannot in isolation stage severity of disease. The addition of elastography provides additional information where diagnostic doubt remains, and occasionally a liver biopsy will be required to definitively confirm or refute cirrhosis.

As cirrhosis becomes more advanced, morbidity and mortality rises, so it is important to stratify cirrhosis according to severity. The major classifications are Child's Pugh and the model of end-stage liver disease (MELD).

The Childs-Pugh score (Table 14.1) was originally developed by a surgeon who sought to determine the risk of postoperative mortality in his patients

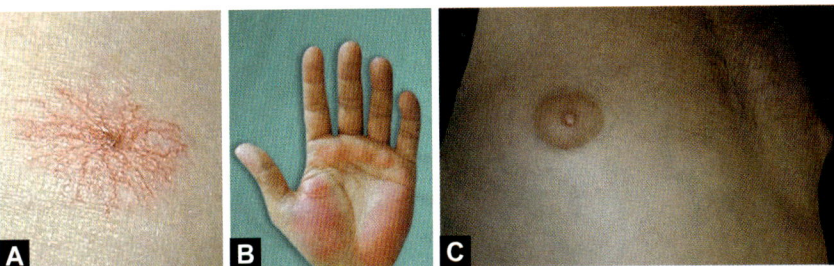

Figs. 14.5A to C: Classical stigmata of CLD include the cutaneous manifestations of: (A) Spider nevi; (B) Palmar erythema; (C) Gynecomastia. (CLD: Chronic liver disease)

Table 14.1: Child–Pugh score and associated annual mortality.			
Measure	1 Point	2 Points	3 Points
Bilirubin	<35	35–50	>50
Albumin	>35	28–35	<28
INR	<1.7	1.7–2.2	>2.2
Ascites	None	Controlled	Uncontrolled
Encephalopathy	None	Grade I/II	Grade III/IV
Points	Class	1 year (%)	2 years (%)
5–6	A	100	85
7–9	B	81	57
10–15	C	45	35

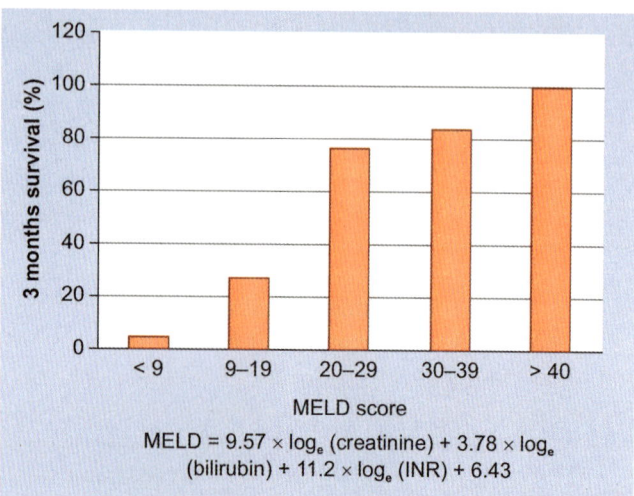

Fig. 14.6: Survival by MELD score. (MELD: Model of end-stage liver disease)

with liver disease. This is a good general guide to the stage of liver disease and can be easily calculated after clinical examination and basic blood tests are complete. It includes measures of liver synthetic and excretory function (bilirubin, coagulation and albumin) and markers of severity of portal hypertension (ascites/encephalopathy). People with Child's A disease are usually relatively well, and may not have any outward appearance of liver disease. With increasing Child's score, severity of liver disease, and subsequent risk of annual mortality rises. Those with Childs B or C disease may be suitable for consideration of liver transplantation ("LT and Transjugular Intrahepatic Portosystemic Shunt" section).

The MELD score (Fig. 14.6) is the most accurate predictor of short-term (3 months) mortality, and was developed to aid prioritization of patients awaiting LT. It is also extremely useful when estimating the likelihood of survival during an admission with decompensated liver disease, with mortality rising rapidly at scores >20. A variant of MELD incorporating serum sodium (UKELD) is additionally used in the United Kingdom, with a minimum score (49) required in most cases to meet basic eligibility for consideration of transplantation.

Decompensation of CLD

People with cirrhosis can spend long periods of time feeling well and with little outward sign of serious disease ("compensated") but can quickly decompensate, usually in response to a specific precipitant. Common precipitants are sepsis, blood loss, constipation, alcohol excess or alcoholic hepatitis (AH), portal vein thrombosis and development of hepatocellular carcinoma (HCC).

Decompensation is defined as a patient with cirrhosis presenting with acute deterioration in liver function associated with one or more of:
- Jaundice
- Increasing ascites
- Encephalopathy
- Renal impairment
- Gastrointestinal bleeding
- Signs of sepsis/hypovolemia.

Early recognition of decompensation and treatment of associated features is critical to prevent a poor outcome. Mortality of all decompensation events in the United Kingdom is estimated at 10–20%, and there is often a sense of nihilism in the management of these patients, particularly those who continue to abuse alcohol. It should never be forgotten that the outcome for patients with liver disease is greatly influenced by the attitude and early decision making of the clinical team. Seeking and treating sepsis and renal dysfunction in early stages can save lives.

Acute Kidney Injury

Decompensation is frequently due to sepsis or hypovolemia, both situations where there is an inherent risk of developing acute kidney injury (AKI). In addition, portal hypertension causes adaptive renovascular physiological changes with the aim of retaining salt and water ("Hepatorenal Syndrome" section), which significantly increases susceptibility of the kidneys to any extraneous insult. Recently, large-scale studies confirmed that previous thresholds of renal dysfunction in cirrhosis were set too high, as it is now known that absolute increases in creatinine matter, with a rise of just >26.5 µmol/L (and/or >50% from baseline) associated with higher probability of critical care transfer, longer admission and increased in-hospital and 90-day mortality. Such small rises in serum creatinine will not always flag up as abnormal on laboratory reports, especially in patients who are slim and/or malnourished where baseline serum creatinine is frequently very low. Therefore, monitoring the trend and changes in baseline function, and acting quickly to reverse an upward trend, is vitally important. At all levels of renal dysfunction, management focuses on withdrawal of diuretics and other nephrotoxic drugs, aggressive management of sepsis and volume expansion if hypoalbuminemia is present. In more advanced AKI, further measures may also be necessary, for example the use of human albumin solution (HAS) and terlipressin ("Hepatorenal Syndrome" section).

Ascites

Ascites (Figs. 14.7A and B) is the most common complication of cirrhosis, with 60% of patients developing ascites within 10 years. The pathophysiology is

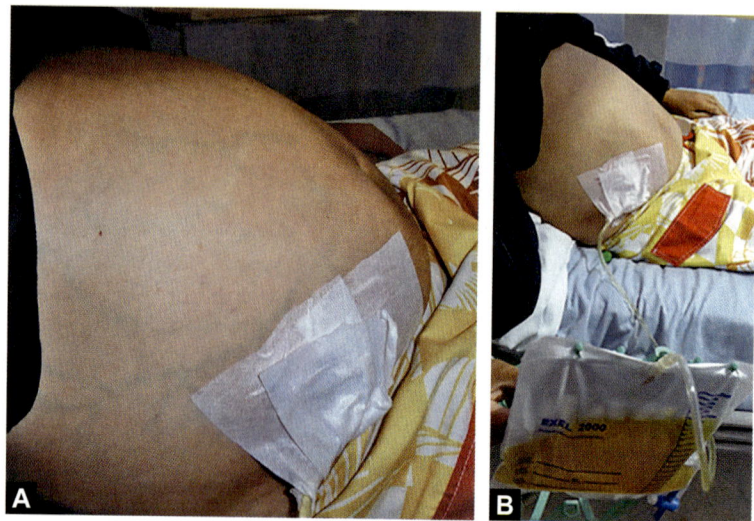

Figs. 14.7A and B: An ascitic drain in situ. (A) A drain is sited in the right iliac fossa, covered by bandaging; (B) Ascitic fluid is draining freely from the peritoneal cavity into a collection bag, where volume can be measured and replaced appropriately with intravenous albumin.

Flowchart 14.1: Development of ascites.

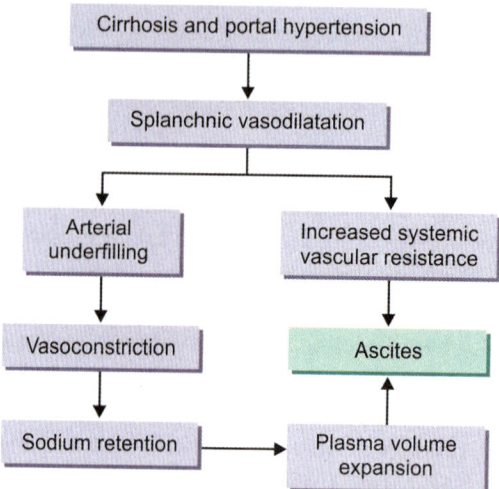

outlined in Flowchart 14.1, and is primarily due to inadequate sodium excretion, as a result of increased renal tubular sodium reabsorption; the mechanism of increased proximal tubular reabsorption is not fully understood but at the distal tubule is the consequence of secondary hyperaldosteronism. This is important as the presence of ascites indicates that there are coexisting renal physiological changes in response to cirrhosis, and this impacts mortality.

Sodium retention is accompanied by water retention, increasing total blood volume. However, hypoalbuminemia and venous stasis exacerbated by the structural abnormalities in cirrhosis promotes intra- to extravascular fluid shifts, with subsequent drop in circulating intravascular volume, and thus further renal vasoconstriction.

The onset of ascites represents advanced liver disease, with median survival following the onset of 2 years. In patients with progressive liver diseases, especially autoimmune or viral hepatitis, ascites usually heralds progressive liver failure and death. In alcohol-related and nonalcoholic fatty liver disease (ALD and NAFLD), ascites can occur earlier in the disease process, because the fibrosis is typically centered round the hepatic venules, causing venous congestion with otherwise relatively well-preserved liver parenchyma.

Ascites increases the risk of other complications, in particular spontaneous bacterial peritonitis (SBP), hyponatremia and hepatorenal syndrome (HRS). Managing ascites improves quality of life, reduces admissions and reduces risk of SBP and HRS.

Principles of Management (Table 14.2): The first episode of ascites should prompt consideration of whether LT would be a potential treatment, since ascites implies advanced liver disease is present. A diagnostic ascitic tap should be performed for cell count (to exclude SBP; a neutrophil count >250/mm^3 is diagnostic), albumin (to calculate serum ascites albumin gradient) and cytology. This will ensure that potentially treatable SBP is detected, and that the ascites can be confidently attributed to liver disease rather than an extrahepatic cause of ascites.

In recurrent ascites, or in patients with unchanged ascites plus abdominal pain or fever, it is important to exclude SBP on each occasion, and so a diagnostic tap for cell count should always be performed.

A focus on fluid balance is critical, to reduce further third space losses but avoiding exacerbation of renal impairment. Nephrotoxic drugs such as non-steroidal anti-inflammatory drugs and angiotensin-converting enzyme

Table 14.2: Grading of ascites.		
Grade	**Definition**	**Treatment**
1: Mild	Only detectable on ultrasound	None
2: Moderate	Clinically apparent	Restrict sodium
		Diuretics
3: Severe	Gross ascites	Paracentesis
		Restrict sodium
		Diuretics
		Consider TIPSS/transplant

inhibitors should be stopped. Fluid restriction is only required if sodium is <135 mmol/L, otherwise it will exacerbate hypovolemia and place additional strain on the kidneys. A suggested approach, after taking clinical assessment into consideration, would be:
- 100–115 mmol/L restrict to 750 mL/day
- 115–125 mmol/L restrict to 1000 mL/day
- 125–130 mmol/L restrict to 1500 mL/day.

Pharmacotherapy is partially dependent on the degree of renal dysfunction. Where renal sodium excretion is not yet severely impaired, sodium excretion is low relative to intake. Here the aim is to counteract renal sodium retention and achieve negative sodium balance. Dietary sodium should be reduced to 80–120 mmol sodium/day (4.6–6.9 g salt/day). Diuretics are used to increase sodium excretion; spironolactone 100 mg is the preferred first choice as it counteracts the secondary hyperaldosteronism driving the formation of ascites and can be increased to 400 mg if renal function and blood pressure allow. Furosemide 40 mg can be added daily (up to 160 mg) if spironolactone alone is not sufficient.

If there is impaired renal function or hyponatremia, diuretics will need to be reduced or avoided altogether. This usually indicates advanced cirrhosis and/or HRS and in this situation, the only definitive treatment is LT.

Large volume paracentesis (LVP) is required where the ascites is massive, and causing significant discomfort, respiratory compromise or is refractory to diuretics. LVP can cause significant fluid shifts, which can precipitate renal failure in cirrhotic patients who have preexisting renovascular disturbance. Safe LVP comprises:
- Up to date biochemistry and secure intravenous access
- Withhold diuretics while the drain is in place
- Assessment of circulating volume to ensure that the patient is not dehydrated, in which case intravenous albumin may be required preprocedure
- Insertion of the drainage catheter under aseptic conditions, ideally between the left anterior superior iliac spine and umbilicus
- Intravenous 20% albumin should be prescribed, at a rate of 100 mL per 2.5 L drained. This minimizes the risk of large fluid shifts, but care should always be taken to ensure that people are not overfilled triggering pulmonary edema; monitoring the Jugular venous pressure and respiratory rate/oxygen saturations can help avoid this
- Drains should remain in situ for no >24 h, but usually less if there is any hypovolemia or renal impairment.

If diuretics and LVP do not control ascites, more definitive management with either LT or placement of transjugular intrahepatic portosystemic shunt (TIPSS) should be considered ("Transjugular Intrahepatic Portosystemic Shunt" section).

The development of SBP is a concerning feature, since it occurs only where there is both ascites and poor liver synthetic function. As liver function deteriorates, bacterial translocation from the progressively leaky gut increases, introducing bacterial species into the peritoneal space. The presence of ascites and the impaired immune function in such patients allows infection to become established.

Diagnosis of SBP by ascitic fluid cell count and culture should prompt consideration of transplantation, as it implies poor prognosis. Where SBP is strongly suspected (remembering that in advanced cirrhosis, the systemic response to infection can be muted), treatment should commence immediately after diagnostic tap is performed. The risk of AKI and HRS in this group is very high, and close attention should be paid to fluid status.

Hepatorenal Syndrome

Hepatorenal syndrome (HRS) is a manifestation of end-stage liver failure, with a median survival for all HRS cases of just 3 months, and is a consequence of the physiological response to portal hypertension (Fig. 14.8). Splanchnic vasodilatation reduces effective arterial blood volume, leading to the activation of the sympathetic nervous system and renal vasoconstriction. This increases the sensitivity of renal blood flow to changes in mean arterial pressure. Cardiovascular changes are compounded by cirrhosis-induced cardiomyopathy, which further reduces compensatory rises in cardiac output secondary to vasodilatation.

Hepatorenal syndrome is split between type 1, the form most frequently encountered in acute decompensation, and the much more rare type 2 (Table 14.3). HRS is often managed suboptimally, with opportunities missed to prevent or improve renal function. HRS should not be confused with AKI, and can only be diagnosed after meeting strict criteria (Table 14.4). Conventionally, type 1 HRS is only diagnosed where serum creatinine has doubled to at least 221 μmol/L, but appropriate treatment should not be delayed to this point, as median survival with untreated type 1 is just 1 month and early treatment can make the difference between survival and death.

Management of HRS rests fundamentally on the rapid identification of renal dysfunction and a comprehensive exclusion of other potential causes,

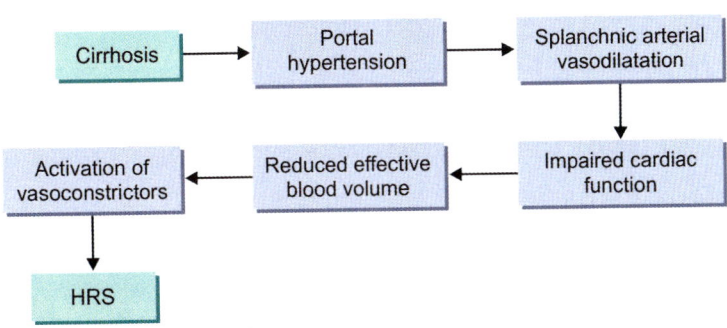

Fig. 14.8: Development of hepatorenal syndrome (HRS).

Table 14.3: Types of hepatorenal syndrome.

Type 1	Type 2
Rapidly progressive acute renal failure	Steady, moderate degree of functional renal failure
Usually occurs in acute decompensation, particularly due to sepsis	Can occur in any patient with refractory ascites
Doubling of baseline creatinine to at least >221 µmol/L	Can spontaneously develop type 1 at any time

Table 14.4: Diagnosis of hepatorenal syndrome.

Cirrhosis plus ascites
Serum creatinine > 133 µmol/L
Absence of shock
No improvement in function after 48 h volume expansion (HAS 1 g/kg/day) and withdrawal of diuretics
No nephrotoxic drugs
No intrinsic renal disease

by urinalysis and renal USS. Where there is a possibility of LT, it may be appropriate to consider renal biopsy to conclusively determine if there is coexisting renal disease, which may warrant concurrent renal transplant. Most type 1 HRS is caused by sepsis, and 30% is due to SBP alone. A thorough search for, and treatment of infection is therefore required. Fluid management is critical. Of note, 20% HAS is mandatory in the context of SBP, but in other infection, fluids should be chosen judiciously to restore euvolemia without aggravating third space losses. Terlipressin improves circulating volume by selective splanchnic vasoconstriction and is effective in 40–50% of cases, although up to 2 weeks of therapy may be required to see a full response.

Renal replacement therapy, i.e. dialysis, is not associated with improved survival and is very rarely indicated. LT is the definitive treatment of choice with a survival in this group of approximately 65%. This is considerably lower than standard liver transplant populations, as renal failure is a major predictor of poor outcome posttransplant. This cohort also has high waiting list mortality. Decisions should be made early in the treatment of HRS as to the suitability of LT in the individual, and if this is not indicated, the high probability of short-term mortality should trigger liaison with specialist palliative care services.

Encephalopathy

Encephalopathy is a neuropsychiatric disturbance secondary to cirrhosis, ranging from minimal, almost imperceptible changes in behavior through to a comatose state (Table 14.5).

It primarily arises as a consequence of poor liver parenchymal function, and can be seen in ALF as well as established CLD. In a healthy subject,

Table 14.5: Grades of encephalopathy.

Grade	Mental state
1	Mild confusion, slowing of ability to do mental tasks e.g. serial 7's
2	Drowsiness, inappropriate behavior
3	Somnolent but rousable, marked confusion
4	Coma

blood rich in substances ingested through or contained within the gastrointestinal tract enters the liver from the portal circulation prior to entering the systemic circulation. This is to ensure that any potentially harmful substance can be metabolized before reaching other organs. For example, low levels of bacteria entering the portal circulation from the gut microbiome are usually rendered harmless through the process of deamination (removal of NH3 group from the molecule) due to the action of hepatocellular enzymes. In CLD, a reduction in functional hepatocytes, coupled with increased bacterial translocation, reduces the effectiveness of this process, leading to release of ammonia into the systemic circulation. These nitrogenous compounds cross the blood–brain barrier causing neuropsychiatric disturbance.

A good history will often reveal encephalopathy, with relatives often describing very small changes in personality or troublesome forgetfulness in the early stages. Behavior becomes more obviously different as encephalopathy worsens. Clinical examination will confirm the presence of a flapping tremor (asterixis), and rapid tests of cognitive function should be performed, such as serial 7s (counting backwards in increments of 7 from 100), or drawing a 5-point star. In some situations, there is doubt as to whether cognitive disturbance is a consequence of encephalopathy or another process. In these circumstances, and electroencephalogram can be undertaken, and will show characteristic abnormalities where encephalopathy is present.

Encephalopathy can be persistent, but is more often episodic, heralding an episode of decompensation. When episodic, the usual precipitants are sepsis and constipation, both of which increase bacterial load and reduction in liver synthetic function. Treatment therefore includes:

- A search for, and treatment of, sepsis
- Relief of constipation (daily phosphate enema and regular lactulose up to 30 mL tds)
- Good nutrition ("Nutrition in CLD" section).

Those with recurrent or persistent encephalopathy, who do not respond to good nutrition and regular laxative treatment, should also receive daily rifaximin. Rifaximin is a nonabsorbed antibiotic, which reduces the levels of gut bacteria and has been shown in large clinical trials to reduce the frequency of encephalopathy-related hospital admissions. A poor response to optimal medical management should prompt consideration of liver transplant. Finally, it is critically important that those with established encephalopathy are advised that they should not drive, and should contact their national driving authority.

Variceal Bleeding

Despite great advances in endoscopic and pharmacotherapy, an episode of acute variceal bleeding is still associated with up to 20–30% mortality. This is greatly influenced by the severity of underlying liver disease, with mortality rising in accordance with Child's score.

The management of variceal bleeding is discussed in detail in Chapter 6: Gastrointestinal Bleeding and Anemia; however, there are some key points to remember:

- Bleeding will frequently lead to decompensation of liver disease, and management should therefore include close monitoring for development of renal impairment, sepsis, etc.
- Variceal bleeding is often associated with sepsis (either because the bleeding episode increases bacterial translocation, or because the bleed was triggered by a preexisting infection), and as such antibiotics are always indicated. Of note, it is the use of antibiotics, and not endoscopic therapy that has had the greatest effect in reduction in mortality in variceal bleeding in the past 2 decades
- Management should include a search for potential precipitants, either sepsis or a driver of increased portal pressure such as acute portal vein thrombosis or development of HCC
- Where bleeding is recurrent or poorly controlled, insertion of TIPSS can be lifesaving, but should be used with caution in those with advanced (Child's C) disease ("Transjugular Intrahepatic Portosystemic Shunt" section).

Surveillance

Because acute bleeding from varices is associated with such high mortality, screening and surveillance of varices is a key feature of CLD management, and there are national guidelines available for this (Further Reading). Current guidance recommends that everyone diagnosed with CLD should be offered an index gastroscopy to screen for varices. Well-compensated individuals with no varices can return on a 3 yearly basis, or annually for Child's B/C. Those with small varices who are well compensated can also return annually without the need for treatment. For all others (i.e. small varices with Child's B/C disease or anyone with moderate/large varices should be offered primary prophylaxis).

Primary prophylaxis is either beta-blocker pharmacotherapy (usually propranolol 40–160 mg bd) or obliteration of varices by repeated endoscopic ligation. Both options significantly reduce the risk of bleeding. It is important that those offered beta-blockers are on a dose sufficient to reduce heart rate by 25%. In the event of an acute bleed, beta-blockers and endoscopic ligation are used in tandem thereafter as long-term secondary prophylaxis.

Hepatocellular Carcinoma

Hepatocellular carcinoma is a late and devastating consequence of cirrhosis, with a 5-year survival of just 10%. Incidence of HCC has climbed over the past 3 decades, following the fourfold rise in cases of CLD. CLD is a consequence of repeated injury and repair to hepatic tissue, and this chronic parenchymal damage is associated with multiple genetic and epigenetic modifications, including activation of oncogenic pathways. As a result, liver cells may ultimately go through malignant transformation. In some cases, the procarcinogenic milieu of cirrhotic tissue is exacerbated by the oncogenic nature of the etiological agent itself, such as alcohol or chronic HBV infection, both classified as carcinogens.

Most HCC is either diagnosed incidentally during investigation of nonspecific symptoms such as anemia or abdominal pain, or is identified as part of a 6-monthly ultrasound surveillance program, which should be offered to all patients with cirrhosis. HCC has characteristic features on imaging, and can be diagnosed in the context of cirrhosis without the need for biopsy using magnetic resonance imaging (Fig. 14.9). Diagnosis is aided by the finding of raised serum alpha-fetoprotein levels, which is released by HCC cells.

Surgical resection is the gold standard treatment and is potentially curative, but is only available to patients with small tumors, mild or no CLD, no extrahepatic metastases and no vascular invasion. Unfortunately, most HCC patients present in advanced stages and are considered unfit for surgery. LT is considered optimal treatment for cirrhotic patients with HCC, with 5-year

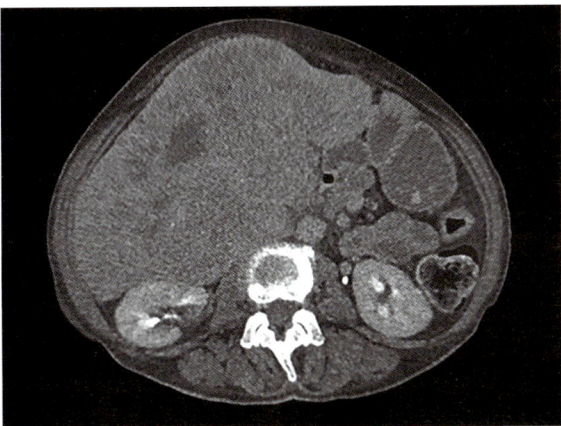

Fig. 14.9: Hepatocellular carcinoma on computed tomography.

survival of 75%; but patients must meet a number of eligibility standards with only a small overall proportion of patients meeting criteria. HCC is relatively resistant to radio- or chemotherapy, but palliative therapies are available which benefit patients with regard to quality of life and median survival. These measures include ablative therapies such as transarterial chemo-embolization (TACE) and radio-frequency ablation (RFA), and systemic chemotherapy using a multikinase inhibitor, sorafenib. These palliative options can extend median survival by a few months (sorafenib) to well over 1 year (TACE/RFA). Those for whom best supportive care is the only option have a postdiagnosis median life expectancy of only 8–12 weeks.

Acute Exacerbations of CLD

Acute Alcoholic Hepatitis (AH)

Alcoholic hepatitis can occur in the absence of cirrhosis, and up to one third of those with an episode of AH will not become cirrhotic, but as a rule these patients have some degree of underlying CLD. This group is often young, and AH is frequently associated with AKI, coagulopathy and sepsis with resultant high mortality.

Alcoholic hepatitis is triggered by an episode of heavy alcohol intake, usually over a period of weeks. Individuals usually complain of jaundice, abdominal pain and nausea. This can occur within days of the alcohol binge or a few weeks after. Hepatic damage is mediated by both direct toxic necrosis and the resultant immunological response to injury, very much like any other drug-induced liver injury.

Investigations show a typical pattern of predominantly raised bilirubin, with some rise in ALT. There is usually a leucocytosis and a degree of coagulopathy. Diagnosis is usually made on the basis of clinical history and blood tests, but where doubt remains, a liver biopsy will usually show typical features (Fig. 14.10). As patients are usually coagulopathic, biopsy may need to be performed by the transjugular route.

Optimal management comprises:
- Detailed search for sepsis, including ascitic tap
- Stop all nephrotoxic drugs given the risk of AKI
- Judicious use of intravenous fluids to replace losses and prevent AKI—renal dysfunction is common in this group and is associated with poor prognosis
- Intravenous high dose vitamins to reduce risk of Wernicke's encephalopathy
- Vitamin K (20 mg single dose or 10 mg in 3 daily doses) if PT is prolonged
- Good nutrition (including formal dietetic review)—nutrition is one of the very few interventions shown to improve prognosis in acute AH.

It is important to assess the severity of AH in order to identify those at high risk, and also those who may benefit from treatment with corticosteroids.

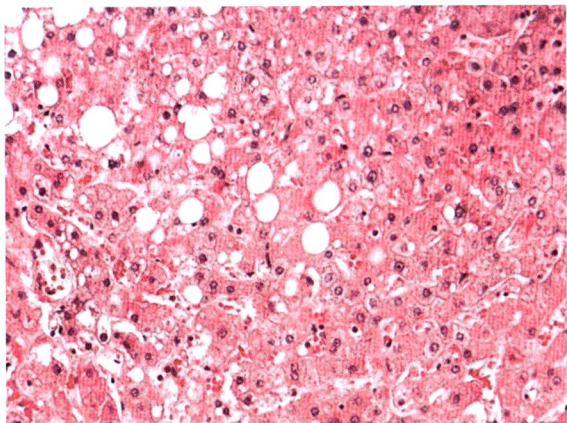

Fig. 14.10: Alcoholic hepatitis with steatosis and hepatocyte ballooning with neutrophil infiltration.

To date, there is no clear evidence that steroids significantly influence outcome but trials are ongoing and currently the use of steroids in severe AH is still advocated by most specialists.

A number of scoring systems are available online, including:

- Maddrey's discriminant function (4.6 × PT (s)-control) + (serum bilirubin (µmol/L)/17)—steroids are indicated where score is >32 and the patient does not have sepsis
- Glasgow AH score incorporating age, white cell count and hepatorenal function—>9 indicates severe disease
- MELD score—>21 indicates severe disease.

Those with severe disease should receive prednisolone 40 mg daily for 1 week, at which time response should be assessed, by comparing the pre- and posttreatment bilirubin. This can be calculated using the Lille score (*www.lillemodel.com*), but as a rule of thumb if bilirubin has not dropped by 25% after 1 week, the steroids should be stopped. Otherwise, therapy should continue for a total of 4 weeks.

After recovery, people with an episode of AH should be followed up to monitor for the development of cirrhosis.

Acute-on-Chronic Liver Failure

The concept of ACLF is a relatively new one, but on a fundamental level, it simply describes an acute decompensation of liver disease, which is associated with hepatic or other organ failure and high short-term mortality. Thus, every episode of ACLF includes decompensation, but not every decompensation is associated with ACLF.

Clinical studies have shown that the prognosis after decompensation depends on the presence or absence of ACLF, which is present in approximately 30% of decompensation events (20% at admission and 10% during hospitalization). In those with ACLF, 28-day mortality exceeds 30%, reaching 50% by 3 months. In contrast, a decompensation event not accompanied by ACLF has an estimated mortality of <2% at 28 days, and <10% at 3 months.

The excess mortality is thought to be due to up-regulated inflammatory response secondary to a specific trigger, in much the same way as infection can precipitate a systemic inflammatory response syndrome. In fact, those with ACLF often have raised inflammatory markers independent of infection. In keeping with this, sepsis is one of the key risk factors for development of ACLF (others include alcohol abuse and acute AH).

Acute-on-chronic liver failure can be precisely diagnosed by the use of an online calculator (*www.clifresearch.com/ToolsCalculators.aspx*), but routine clinical and laboratory assessment will point to the presence of organ failure in the first instance, and this should signal consideration of ACLF and therefore that the individual is at high risk of morbidity and mortality. ACLF should always be suspected in a decompensated patient where there is renal failure (creatinine >175 µmol/L), or renal dysfunction (creatinine >130 µmol/L) plus grade 3 or greater encephalopathy.

In light of the high mortality, those with ACLF should ideally be managed in a high-dependency environment, and serious consideration should be given to the possibility of LT, which is the treatment of choice.

Nutrition in CLD

Protein energy malnutrition is found in 40–80% of patients with end-stage liver failure. Malnutrition occurs for two main reasons: first, CLD is a catabolic state where people require considerably more calories than normal and second, appetite is reduced for myriad reasons (e.g. impaired digestion, presence of nausea, ascites reducing stomach volume), thereby dropping overall caloric intake.

Malnutrition increases the risk of decompensation and variceal bleeding, and nutritional intervention has been proven to improve outcomes following decompensation. Therefore, good nutritional support is the cornerstone of any decompensation event, and all patients with CLD should have a nutritional assessment, preferably by a specialist dietitian. Additionally, calcium and vitamin D supplementation is recommended for all, due to the increased risk of osteoporosis.

LT AND TRANSJUGULAR INTRAHEPATIC PORTOSYSTEMIC SHUNT

Medical therapy, including treatment of the underlying cause of cirrhosis and the resultant complications, is sometimes insufficient to maintain patients in a compensated state. Chronic liver synthetic failure or persistent clinical features of decompensation (ascites, encephalopathy, variceal bleeding and HCC) should trigger consideration of more definitive management in order to improve outcomes and quality of life. The two key interventions are TIPSS and LT.

Transjugular Intrahepatic Portosystemic Shunt

Transjugular intrahepatic portosystemic shunt (TIPSS) is used as a means of reducing portal pressure where medical management has failed to control the consequences of portal hypertension. The major indications are diuretic resistant or intolerant ascites, and intractable variceal bleeding.

The TIPSS is an invasive procedure, usually performed under general anesthesia, where a guidewire is inserted from the internal jugular vein into the right or middle hepatic vein (Fig. 14.11). From here, a needle is passed through the wall of the hepatic vein and into a branch of the portal vein. A self-expanding metal stent is then placed across this tract, creating a route (shunt) between the portal and systemic circulation which bypasses the smaller vessels within the liver, and hence much of the hepatic parenchyma. The end result is a significant reduction in portal pressure. This is associated with decompression of varices, and a major reduction in accumulation of ascites.

Ascites

Before proceeding with TIPSS as a treatment for ascites not responding to diuretics, suitability for LT should be considered for two reasons: first, the presence of ascites usually signals poor liver synthetic function which will not be improved by a shunt procedure and second, the placement of TIPSS will

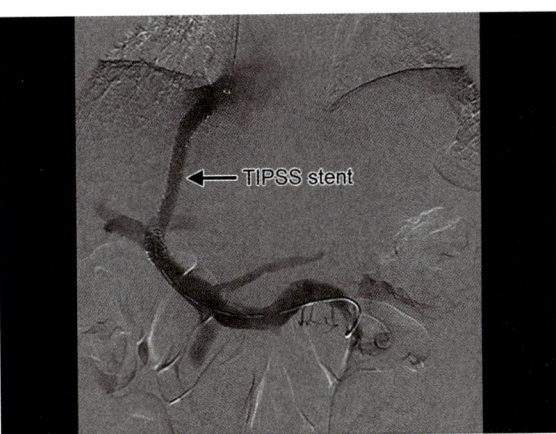

Fig. 14.11: Angiogram showing TIPSS between portal and hepatic veins. (TIPSS: Transjugular intrahepatic portosystemic shunt)
Source: Raghuram Lakshminarayan.

create technical difficulties for the surgical team if LT goes ahead at a later date.

Where transplant is not thought appropriate, TIPSS can be an excellent means to control ascites, avoiding the need for high dose diuretics (and the renal complications thereof) or frequent LVP.

Variceal Bleeding

The TIPSS has long been considered a useful salvage procedure for variceal bleeding which cannot be controlled endoscopically. In recent times, there has also been a move toward considering early TIPSS after variceal bleeding as a means of secondary prevention. There is little evidence for this approach at the current time, but the most recent guidelines for management of variceal bleeding do offer this as an option instead of repeated endoscopic ligation. In each case, the relative merits and risks of each strategy should be considered, preferably within the context of a multidisciplinary (i.e. hepatology/radiology/transplant center) team.

Clinical Considerations

The TIPSS is not suitable for every patient, and there are significant potential complications and contraindications (Fig. 14.12). In particular, creation of a shunt across the liver bypasses much of the parenchyma, increasing the risk of encephalopathy and so those with preexisting encephalopathy should not routinely be offered TIPSS. Second, shunting has major effects on hepatic and systemic blood flow, potentially worsening liver synthetic function (hence Child's C disease is usually a contraindication to TIPSS) and causing cardiac compromise.

Contraindications	Complications

• Encephalopathy
   – Objective assessment required
• Cardiac failure
• Uncontrolled sepsis
• Biliary obstruction
• Polycystic liver disease
• Child's C disease (relative)
• Pulmonary hypertension (relative)
	• Encephalopathy (20–30%)
	• Liver failure
	• Persistent cholestasis
	• Renal failure
	• Sepsis
	• Hemolysis
	• Technical issues
	   – Capsular puncture + bleeding
	   – Hemobilia
	   – Stent migration into IVC/PV
	   – Stenosis

Fig. 14.12: Complications and contraindications for TIPSS. (TIPSS: Transjugular intrahepatic portosystemic shunt)

Early post-TIPSS care includes close monitoring for signs of cardiac, renal or liver failure, bleeding and sepsis. Shunting often leads to a significant diuresis, and so renal function should be monitored, and diuretics stopped. A Doppler should be performed at 72 h to ensure patency. Thereafter, the interventional radiologists will recommend interval patency surveillance, usually at 1, 3 and 6 months by Doppler followed by a venogram at 1 year. Longer-term follow-up is dictated by the type of stent used.

Liver Transplantation

Liver transplantation is the definitive treatment of cirrhosis, with several hundred performed each year in the United Kingdom. It is by nature a limited and precious resource and as such the utmost care must be taken to select individuals who will have the greatest benefit from transplantation. Assessment of suitability for LT can be broadly divided into three main areas:
- Is the liver disease severe enough that LT is required?
- Is the individual fit enough to endure major surgery?
- Are there cofactors that influence suitability?

Assessment begins at the local hospital, with the responsible clinical team raising the question of suitability. Events that herald major landmarks in progression of liver disease, such as first decompensation, development of ascites and occurrence of SBP, should always trigger this discussion.

In the United Kingdom, there are specific criteria that must be met prior to consideration (*http://odt.nhs.uk/pdf/liver_selection_policy.pdf*). There are many patients with severe liver disease who either do not meet the minimal criteria for severity of liver disease, or who have a contraindication to LT and as such are not eligible for further assessment. Although not listed as an absolute contraindication, in the case of ALD, most specialists would not consider LT referral for those continuing to drink or who had been abstinent for <6 months. This is for two reasons. The first is that prolonged abstinence can lead to tremendous improvements in liver synthetic function, to the point where LT is no longer clinically required. The second is achieving prolonged abstinence is a sign that the individual has come to terms with the diagnosis and the key part alcohol has played in the problem. This correlates with long-term abstinence and preservation of graft function for the longest possible period.

If the local team feels that LT should be considered, patients will be referred to one of seven UK liver transplant centers, where a comprehensive assessment will take place. Once on the list, waiting time varies according to availability of organs and blood type, and patients require frequent monitoring to ensure on-going suitability and fitness for major surgery. Following a transplant, people spend approximately 1 week in hospital and then enter long-term follow-up care with both the transplant center and the local hospital. This care focuses on maintaining sufficient immune-suppression to prevent graft rejection, but at the lowest level possible to avoid complications of therapy (e.g. renal impairment and increased risk of some cancers). Liver grafts can function for many decades and graft dysfunction is now very rarely associated with morbidity and mortality. In fact, mortality in LT recipients is most frequently due to cardiovascular disease, and therefore prevention of hypertension and other cardiovascular pathophysiology is a key aspect of posttransplant care.

■ FURTHER READING

Acute Liver Failure
1. King's College Criteria for LT in ALF: O'Grady JG, Alexander GJ, Hayllar KM, et al. Early indicators of prognosis in fulminant hepatic failure. Gastroenterology. 1989; 97:439-45.

Cirrhosis
2. Angeli P, Gines P, Wong F, et al. Diagnosis and management of acute kidney injury in patients with cirrhosis: revised consensus recommendations of the International Club of Ascites. J Hepatol. 2015;62:968-74.
3. EASL: The Home of Hepatology. European Association for the study of the liver. www.easl.eu. Guidelines for Management and Surveillance of Varices
4. McPherson S, Dyson J, Austin A, et al. Response to the NCEPOD report: development of a care bundle for patients admitted with decompensated cirrhosis-the first 24 h. Frontline Gastroenterol. 2016;7(1):16-23. Epub 2014 Dec 2.
5. MELD Calculator Online. http://www.mdcalc.com/meld-score-model-for-end-stage-liver-disease-12-and-older/ [accessed 01.12.16].
6. Tripathi D, Stanley AJ, Hayes PC, et al. UK guidelines on the management of variceal haemorrhage in cirrhotic patients. Gut. 2015;1-25. Also available at: http://www.bsg.org.uk/clinical-guidelines/liver/uk-guidelines-for-the-management-of-variceal-haemorrhage-in-cirrhotic-patients.html
Management of AKI in Liver Disease
7. UKELD Calculator. http://www.odt.nhs.uk/transplantation/guidance-policies/tools/

Acute Exacerbations of CLD
8. ACLF. CLIF consortium for chronic liver failure including diagnosis of ACLF. http://www.clifresearch.com/Home.aspx [accessed 01.12.16].
9. Forrest EH, Evans CD, Stewart S, et al. Analysis of factors predictive of mortality in alcoholic hepatitis and derivation and validation of the Glasgow alcoholic hepatitis score. Gut. 2005;54:1174-9.

CHAPTER 15

Abnormal Liver Biochemistry

Lynsey Corless

■ INTRODUCTION

Abnormal liver function test (LFT) results are detected frequently on routine biochemical testing. Where there is no known previous history of liver disease, this requires further investigation.

The approach to investigation will vary according to the pattern and severity of LFT abnormality. The purpose of investigation is to identify treatable causes and avoid or reduce significant liver disease. The great majority of liver disease is caused by preventable factors (excess alcohol consumption, obesity/metabolic syndrome and chronic viral hepatitis infection). Considered investigation of abnormal LFT offers an opportunity to identify such conditions and plan treatment before irreversible liver disease is established.

There are two important caveats to remember prior to investigation: first, there are many non-hepatic causes of abnormal LFT which should be considered (Table 15.1); and second, standard liver biochemistry is a poor measure of liver functional capacity, for which further testing of liver synthetic function is required ("Assessment of Synthetic and Excretory Function" section).

■ REACHING A DIAGNOSIS

Isolated Rises of One Liver Enzyme

Transaminases (ALT and AST)

Most laboratories routinely perform either alanine amino transferase (ALT) or aspartate amino transferase (AST). AST is produced in greater quantities in skeletal/cardiac muscle than ALT, and is also raised in some cases of hypothyroidism and pernicious anemia, and is therefore less specific to the liver than ALT, although ALT can also be elevated due to non-hepatic causes.

The AST:ALT ratio can help identify the potential etiology, with a ratio of >2 favoring alcohol-related disease.

An isolated rise in ALT should first prompt retesting, since approximately 15% of these are transient and quickly return to normal. A pragmatic approach to persistently abnormal transaminases is described later and in Flowchart 15.1.

Table 15.1: Potential causes of persistently abnormal LFT.

Enzyme	Major site of activity	Likely pathophysiology	Non-hepatic causes
Alkaline phosphatase (ALP)	Bile ducts Hepatic canaliculi	Infiltration Congestion Toxic/metabolic Biliary tree disorder	Growth (adolescence) Pregnancy Bone disease Congestive cardiac disease
Alanine aminotransferase (ALT)	Hepatocyte	Hepatitis Toxic/metabolic	Celiac disease Skeletal/cardiac muscle release
Aspartate aminotransferase (AST)	Hepatocyte	Hepatitis Toxic/metabolic	Skeletal/cardiac muscle release Hemolysis
Gamma glutamyl transferase	Bile ducts	Liver disease unlikely	Cardiovascular disease Drug metabolism

(LFT: Liver function test.)

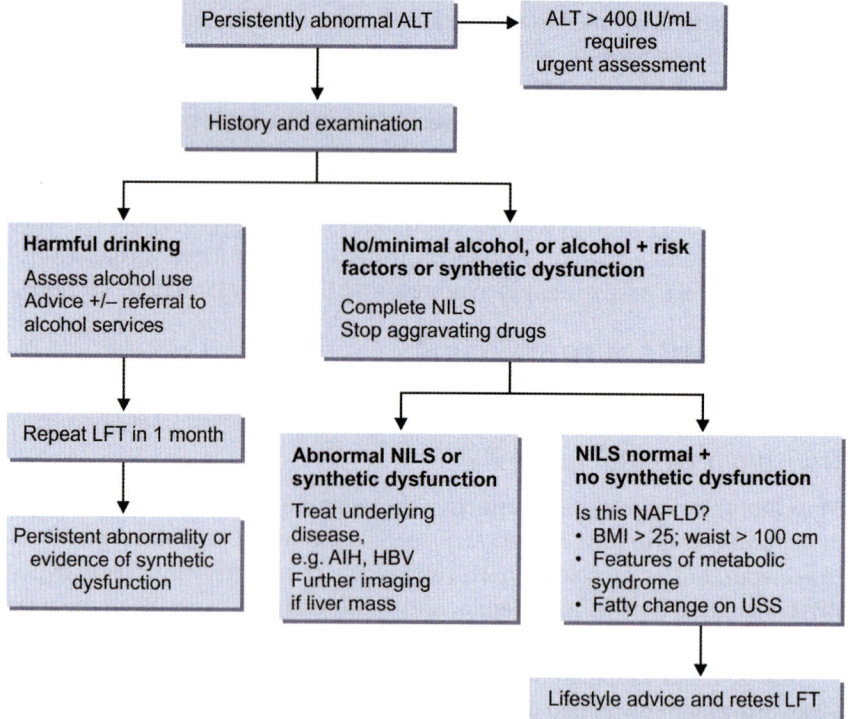

Flowchart 15.1: Approach to investigation of persistently abnormal ALT.

(AIH: Autoimmune hepatitis; ALT: Alanine amino transferase; BMI: Body mass index; HBV: Hepatitis B virus; LFT: Liver function test; NAFLD: Non-alcoholic fatty liver disease; NILS: Non-invasive liver screen; USS: Ultrasound scanning).

Abnormal Liver Biochemistry

> **Liver-directed history and examination**
>
> **History**
> - Alcohol intake
> - Drug use
>   - Prescription
>   - Over-the-counter
>   - Herbal/supplements including gym supplements
>   - Illicit (current or previous)
> - Obesity
> - Features of metabolic syndrome
>   - Hypertension, diabetes, hypercholesterolemia
> - Transfusions
> - Travel
> - Sexual contacts
>
> **Examination**
> - Jaundice
> - Stigmata of chronic liver disease
> - BMI
> - Hepato/splenomegaly

Fig. 15.1: Key features of history and examination in people with abnormal LFT. (BMI: Body mass index; LFT: Liver function test).

It is critical to determine early whether there is advanced liver disease, as this influences the speed and scope of subsequent investigation, and ultimate prognosis for the patient. A persistent rise in ALT mandates assessment of liver synthetic function ("Assessment of Synthetic and Excretory Function" section), with a focus on identification of jaundice, stigmata of chronic liver disease (CLD), and abnormal bilirubin, albumin and prothrombin time (PT) levels. Where ALT is very high (>400 IU/mL), urgent assessment is vital to exclude the possibility of acute liver failure, which is a medical emergency (*see* Chapter 14: Liver Failure).

The history and examination are included as shown in Figure 15.1.

Associated Symptoms

Examples include jaundice, itch, fatigue and altered bowel habit/stool color.

Thorough Assessment of Alcohol Use

Alcohol use should be quantified according to the type and strength of alcohol used. Information on alcohol units is widely available. Alcohol use can be categorized by relative risk (Table 15.2) and those drinking more than recommended limits should be given appropriate advice (e.g. reducing to safe levels, at least 2 alcohol-free days per week, information on local support services). It is important to recheck LFT in 1 month to ensure alcohol

Table 15.2: Alcohol intake and risk.

	Men	Women
Lower risk	Not more than 3–4 units per day on a regular basis	Not more than 2–3 units per day on a regular basis
Increasing risk	Over 3–4 units per day on a regular basis	Over 2–3 units per day on a regular basis
Higher risk	>50 units per week (or >8 units per day) on a regular basis	>35 units per week (or >6 units per day) on a regular basis

reduction has led to normalization of LFT. If this does not occur, or where there is concern of advanced liver disease, further investigation is required and alcohol cannot be assumed to be the only etiology.

Drug History

This should include all drugs, including prescribed (current or within last 6 months), illicit, over the counter medication especially paracetamol, herbal remedies and growth supplements including anabolic steroids and protein powders, which are used with increasing frequency in gyms and are becoming an increasingly frequent cause of cholestasis.

Risk Factors for Viral Hepatitis

For example, people originally from areas of high prevalence (e.g. Egypt, Southeast Asia), history of blood transfusion, medical treatment abroad, recent travel, previous or current intravenous drug use and any sexual contacts.

Presence of Comorbidities

This should focus on those explaining or contributing to abnormal LFT, e.g. cardiac failure, autoimmune disease, and inflammatory bowel disease (IBD). One of the commonest causes of abnormal ALT is non-alcoholic fatty liver disease (NAFLD), which is strongly associated with obesity and the metabolic syndrome, features of which should be actively sought (hypertension, diabetes and hypercholesterolemia).

Examination

This should include calculation of body mass index (BMI) and a search for stigmata of CLD (jaundice, palmar erythema, spider naevi, etc.)

Further investigation of abnormal ALT is mandatory unless this was associated with harmful alcohol use and has completely normalized on return to safe levels of drinking. Initial investigation of abnormal LFT is collectively referred to as a noninvasive liver screen (NILS) (Fig. 15.2). This comprises:
Abdominal ultrasound scanning (USS)
- Assess biliary tree, liver echotexture, signs of portal hypertension and the presence of liver masses

> **Noninvasive liver screen (NILS)**
>
> **Liver ultrasound scan (USS)**
> **Blood tests***
>
> - Liver autoantibodies and celiac serology
> - Immunoglobulins
> - Ferritin and transferrin saturation
> - Hepatitis virus serology (HBV cAb + sAg, HCV cAb)
> - EBV and CMV serology
> - Alpha-1 antitrypsin
> - Alpha–fetoprotein
>
> *Include ceruloplasmin in those under 50 years

Fig. 15.2: Components of the noninvasive liver screen. (CMV: Cytomegalovirus; EBV: Epstein–Barr virus; HBV cAb: Hepatitis B virus core antibody; HCV cAb: Hepatitis C virus core antibody; sAg: Surface antigen).

- In specialist care, further noninvasive assessment of liver disease is usually performed with elastography. Alongside USS, a probe is used to assess stiffness of the liver tissue, which correlates with degree of liver fibrosis. This can avoid the need for liver biopsy and provide greater information on the severity of disease. It should be noted that elastography is less reliable in the context of abdominal obesity or active hepatitis, where readings can be artificially high and as such biopsy may still be required.

Tests for autoimmune liver disease
- Autoantibodies including antinuclear antibody (ANA), smooth muscle (associated with autoimmune hepatitis (AIH)) and mitochondrial (associated with primary biliary cholangitis (PBC) when present in the typical pattern)
- Immunoglobulins; e.g. raised IgG associated with AIH, raised IgM associated with PBC, raised IgA seen in NAFLD/ALD (ALD, alcohol-related liver disease)
- Celiac serology; common cause of raised ALT and associated with autoimmune liver disease

Viral serology
- Hepatitis B (HBV) serology including core antibody (Ab) indicating previous or acute exposure and surface antigen (Ag) (evidence of chronic HBV infection if present on two occasions at least 6 months apart)
- Hepatitis C (HCV) Ab
- Epstein–Barr (EBV) serology; acute EBV is a very common cause of abnormal LFT, usually with raised ALT in isolation but can also present with jaundice
- Cytomegalovirus (CMV) serology; a much less frequent cause of abnormal LFT than EBV but where there are symptoms suggestive of viral

infection, it is prudent to exclude this, alongside other viral causes of acute hepatitis (acute HBV, EBV, varicella zoster virus (VZV) and herpes simplex virus, HSV)

Iron studies
- If raised, ferritin and transferrin saturation should be repeated in 3 months to ensure persistence as these are frequently elevated in acute phase response to infection/inflammation, prior to sending genetic studies for hereditary hemochromatosis (HH)

Alpha-1-antitrypsin
- A low level will usually prompt the laboratory to perform phenotyping. Alpha-1 antitrypsin deficiency is rarely the only cause of abnormal LFT in adults, and is more usually seen as a cofactor aggravating ALD/NAFLD. However, it is important to identify those with abnormal phenotypes as genetic testing of relatives may be appropriate.

Copper studies (serum ceruloplasmin and copper)
- These should only be performed in those <50 years old to exclude Wilson's disease as it is highly unlikely to be undiagnosed beyond this age

Alpha fetoprotein
- Abnormal alpha fetoprotein (AFP) is the hallmark of hepatocellular carcinoma (HCC), and requires urgent USS. However, it is also released by the placenta and should not be checked where there is a possibility of pregnancy. Furthermore, AFP can be mildly elevated in viral hepatitis but this should not preclude imaging to ensure there is no mass lesion.

Patients should be reviewed with the results of the NILS. Specific abnormalities should be referred to the appropriate specialist for further staging of liver disease and treatment. A persistent abnormal ALT with a negative NILS and no drug trigger suggests the presence of NAFLD. This requires action to prevent progressive liver disease ("Non-alcoholic fatty liver disease" section).

Alkaline Phosphatase

All enzymes comprising the panel of LFT are also produced in non-hepatic tissue, but this is most clinically relevant when investigating an isolated rise in ALP.

The first step is to confirm that the ALP is hepatic in origin. This can be done by checking gamma glutamyl transferase (GGT; normal GGT virtually excludes hepatic origin of ALP) and/or requesting ALP isoenzymes. The latter test is the most definitive as it entails electrophoresis to identify and quantify hepatic, bone and intestinal isoforms of ALP.

If results indicate predominantly bony isoforms of ALP, no further liver testing is required. It is important to exclude normal bone growth (i.e. in adolescents) and pregnancy, before arranging further tests of bone health (e.g. calcium, vitamin D, phosphate, etc.). X-rays of chest, skull and pelvis should also be considered to exclude Paget's disease.

ALP of Hepatic Origin: Isolated hepatic ALP should first prompt consideration of biliary disorders, as ALP is predominantly derived from the biliary tree. ALP is also frequently high in infiltrative diseases (e.g. malignancy or granulomatous disease) or as a result of hepatic congestion (cardiac failure, tricuspid regurgitation) or drug metabolism. Although these are the most likely diagnoses, it is sensible and right to perform a comprehensive history and examination (Fig. 15.1) and complete a full NILS (Fig. 15.2) in all those with raised hepatic ALP.

The NILS may reveal the diagnosis, e.g. positive antimitochondrial antibody (AMA) in typical pattern confirming PBC, or USS findings suggestive of malignancy. Any drugs thought to be causing the abnormality should be stopped. In other cases, the cause may remain elusive. The need for further investigation will be determined by a number of factors, including:

- How abnormal is the result? In the absence of symptoms, an ALP just over the normal range can be safely monitored on a 3 monthly basis without need for immediate further investigation. A persistently or significantly elevated ALP however may warrant liver biopsy ("Is a Liver Biopsy Required?" section) or further imaging to exclude biliary obstruction or infiltrative disease (e.g. sarcoidosis, amyloidosis and lymphoma)
- Is there evidence of CLD? Abnormal LFT in the context of stigmata of CLD, or associated with synthetic disturbance (raised bilirubin, prolonged PT and reduced albumin) always warrants further investigation.
- Does the patient have other illness? A good example is the person with IBD, in whom an abnormal ALP may be the result of primary sclerosing cholangitis (PSC) necessitating magnetic resonance cholangiopancreatography scan, or due to one of their IBD medications, e.g. methotrexate, potentially requiring a liver biopsy.

Gamma Glutamyl Transferase

The GGT is an inducible enzyme with a central role in drug metabolism, and is frequently raised in the absence of liver disease or significant liver damage, particularly in the context of alcohol ingestion and use of many drugs (e.g. anticonvulsants, non-steroidal anti-inflammatories and lipid lowering agents). As such, an isolated rise in GGT is not evidence of intrinsic liver disease, and does not require further investigation.

Since GGT is a poor measure of liver function, it is not routinely checked in secondary care, although it can be a useful test to help determine the source of raised alkaline phosphatase, e.g. liver or bone.

Mixed Patterns of Abnormal LFT

In most cases of abnormal LFT, a mixed pattern of abnormality is seen rather than isolated rises in one enzyme. It is usual to try to classify patterns

Table 15.3: Pattern of abnormal LFT.

Pattern	Hepatocellular	Cholestatic	Infiltrative
ALT >ALP	Common	Less common	Very rare
ALP >ALT	Rare	Common	Less common
Raised ALP with normal ALT	Very rare	Common	Common

(ALP: Alkaline phosphatase; ALT: Alanine amino transferase; LFT: Liver function test.)

of abnormal liver biochemistry as hepatocellular, cholestatic or infiltrative (Table 15.3) as these patterns can help determine the most likely etiologies and hence prioritize and rationalize investigation. Alongside the pattern, one must consider patient features including gender, age and medical history, which impact the likelihood of individual etiologies.

It should always be remembered that LFT results are poor indicators of liver function, and can be influenced by myriad non-hepatic elements. However, it is always important to seek a cause for these abnormalities in order to avoid progression of a preventable disease.

Is a Liver Biopsy Required?

Liver biopsy can be extremely useful in investigation of abnormal LFT, and is considered the gold standard for determining the etiology and stage of liver disease. Biopsy incurs risk (bleeding, perforation of other viscus and death), and although much of the risk is mitigated by performing the biopsy under USS guidance, there should always be a clear rationale for invasive investigation.

Key areas where biopsy is useful include:

Multiple Possible Etiologies

A typical example would be a female patient in middle age with IBD, who is on methotrexate treatment. Investigation has revealed a hepatocellular pattern of abnormal LFT, alongside positive ANA and an IgG at the upper limit of normal. In this circumstance, the possible etiologies include AIH, PSC and drug-induced injury, and the pattern of LFT abnormality could be seen with any of these. Each of these etiologies would require a different approach to treatment, and may influence the management of her IBD. In this situation, a biopsy is the only way to further clarify the situation so management can proceed.

Lack of Clarity on Severity of Disease

An example here would be a patient with chronic HCV genotype 3 infection and alcohol excess, with persistently raised ALT alongside low platelets, an enlarged, fatty liver on USS and a moderately high elastography reading. The low platelets could be due to marrow suppression from alcohol, or due to early portal hypertension. The moderately high elastography reading may be as a result of on-going hepatitis or because there is advanced fibrosis.

Establishing the stage of liver disease via liver biopsy is critical not only to select the appropriate HCV eradication treatment, but to determine whether this person will require long-term follow-up even if the HCV is eradicated (i.e. if they require hepatoma surveillance due to the presence of cirrhosis).

If used judiciously, liver biopsy is an excellent assessment of liver disease, which cannot yet be replaced by noninvasive means, although advances in elastography and biomarkers may reduce the need for biopsy in the years to come.

Assessment of Synthetic and Excretory Function

Measurement of liver synthetic function is crucial in order to stage disease and determine urgency of investigation and referral.

While raised ALT suggests increased turnover of hepatocytes, levels do not correlate with the degree of hepatocyte injury. Furthermore, in established cirrhosis, hepatocytes are replaced by scar tissue and as such serum levels of ALT are frequently normal, rendering the standard LFT panel of little value in this situation.

Much more useful are the markers of liver synthetic and excretory function, which form the basis of well-validated tools to stratify liver disease, including the Child's and MELD scores (*see* Chapter 14: Liver Failure).

Albumin

The liver produces albumin, and as such a low level in the context of liver disease signals reduced hepatocyte function.

Albumin can be reduced in many other circumstances (e.g. acutely in sepsis or burns; chronically in renal disease or protein losing enteropathy), which should be sought particularly where there is little other objective evidence of advanced liver disease.

Coagulation

Adequate liver reserve is required for vitamin K synthesis and function. Where this is insufficient, PT will be prolonged and even mild prolongations of PT signal significant liver damage.

Prothrombin time can be artificially prolonged in cholestasis, where dietary vitamin K cannot be absorbed. Administration of 20 mg IV vitamin K will correct any nutrition or cholestasis-induced deficiency, allowing a more accurate measurement of coagulation status. A very prolonged PT (>20 s) after vitamin K is highly unusual in CLD, and should prompt consideration of acute liver failure (*see* Chapter 14: Liver Failure).

Bilirubin

In the context of CLD, rising bilirubin indicates reduced excretory function and worsening cholestasis.

Isolated hyperbilirubinemia is not suggestive of liver disease, but rather is usually due to Gilbert's syndrome, or less commonly Dubin–Johnson syndrome. Here there is a mild elevation of unconjugated (Gilbert's) or conjugated (Dubin–Johnson) bilirubin (typically 20–40, but always <100). In presumed Gilbert's, it is prudent to check the conjugated:unconjugated bilirubin ratio to ensure that conjugated bilirubin levels are normal, and to exclude hemolysis (check reticulocyte count and haptoglobin level) alongside an USS. Cases of Dubin–Johnson will often require liver biopsy, as it is difficult to exclude intrinsic liver disease in the context of raised conjugated bilirubin.

The investigation of jaundice is described in Chapter 12: Jaundice.

Creatinine

Renal dysfunction in the context of CLD is a marker of advanced liver disease, and elevated creatinine and is discussed in Chapter 14: Liver Failure.

ABNORMAL LFT IN PREGNANCY

Investigation of abnormal LFT in pregnancy follows a different path, and is in general pursued with a greater degree of urgency, as abnormal LFT in this situation can be life threatening for mother and baby. The advice of a hepatologist and an obstetrician should always be sought.

When investigating abnormal LFT in pregnancy, it is important to consider whether the abnormality is as a result of the pregnancy, coincidental to the pregnancy or due to pregnancy complicating underlying CLD. It should also be remembered that pregnant women may have palmar erythema spider naevi, etc., and these are unlikely to be due to liver disease if not previously apparent. Note that although albumin may be reduced and ALP elevated, the transaminases and bilirubin should remain normal throughout pregnancy.

Specific examples of abnormal LFT in pregnancy include:

Hyperemesis Gravidarum

Alanine aminotransferase elevated, occasionally reaching 1000 IU/mL. Mild abnormalities of bilirubin (under 100 IU/mL) are seen. LFTs should settle completely when vomiting improves. No liver-specific treatment is required.

Intrahepatic Cholestasis of Pregnancy

This can only be diagnosed where there is on-going pruritus, usually worse on the palms and soles. It usually presents in second or third trimester and can be associated with raised ALT/AST, usually not higher than 500 IU/mL. Serum bile acids are raised. As this condition is linked with increased risk of stillbirth, obstetric teams may occasionally induce labor. Treatment with ursodeoxycholic acid may be appropriate but this should be discussed with obstetrics and hepatology.

Preeclampsia/HELLP

Patients with preeclampsia usually have deranged LFT, which is most often a minor elevation of transaminases. Where there is significant liver dysfunction, early delivery of the fetus is recommended.

The HELLP (hemolysis, elevated LFT, low platelets) tends to occur in the third trimester, and can present immediately after delivery. In 20% of cases, there is a history of preeclampsia. A transaminitis is usually seen (<500 IU/mL) and jaundice is rare (<5%). Hepatic rupture is a rare complication.

Delivery of the fetus is required. Liver function does not always improve after delivery and can worsen. Patients with HELLP are critically unwell and usually require multiorgan support.

Acute Fatty Liver of Pregnancy

Acute fatty liver of pregnancy is rapidly progressive and requires immediate delivery of the fetus to avoid fulminant hepatic failure. It presents in the third trimester, usually at 34–36 weeks. Patients complain of nausea and abdominal pain and can be jaundiced. Blood tests show ALT/AST usually <750 IU/mL, and a relatively mild coagulopathy (PT <30 s) compared to severity of illness, which includes confusion, renal impairment and hypoglycemia. Alongside delivery, treatment usually includes IV vitamin K and N-acetyl-cysteine.

Preexisting Disease

Pregnancy will place additional strain on the liver therefore any CLD can be aggravated by pregnancy.

Liver biopsy is very rarely indicated in pregnancy, and should be avoided unless on the advice of a specialist liver unit.

■ GUIDANCE ON SPECIFIC CONDITIONS

Conditions usually presenting with jaundice are discussed in Chapter 12: Jaundice.

Alcohol-related Liver Disease

Alcohol-related liver disease still accounts for the majority of CLD in the United Kingdom, and is the predominant etiology for those admitted to hospitals with decompensation, and accounts for 40–50% of UK listings for liver transplantation.

Alcohol is not harmful if used within safe limits (current recommendation is 14 or fewer units/week for women and 21 or fewer for men; 1 unit is equivalent to 10 g of pure ethanol, i.e. 25 mL of sprits, 75 mL of standard strength wine or 200 mL of standard strength beer). The strength of alcoholic beverages, particularly wine, has increased considerably over the past

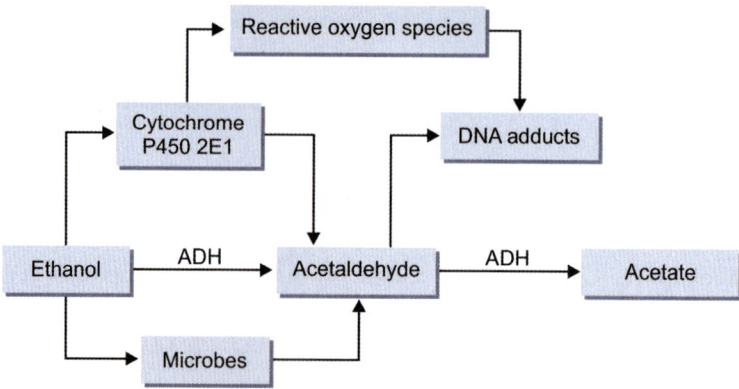

Fig. 15.3: Alcohol metabolism. (ADH: Alcohol dehydrogenase)

3 decades, and most people will underestimate the number of units they drink. It is therefore important to quantify consumption by type and strength, rather than relying on a report of "X units."

Ethanol is canonically metabolized to acetate by a number of alcohol dehydrogenase enzymes, via a toxic intermediate, acetaldehyde. In chronic or high consumption, gut microbes and cytochrome P450 2E1 (CYP2E1) also metabolize alcohol to acetaldehyde, with acetaldehyde further metabolized to acetate in the mitochondria. This results in the formation of nicotinamide adenine dinucleotide (NADH) which must be reoxidized to maintain optimal cellular chemistry. The involvement of CYP2E1 and reoxidation of NADH both result in the formation of reactive oxygen species (ROS) in mitochondria. Both acetaldehyde and ROS react destructively with cellular deoxyribonucleic acid (DNA), crating DNA adducts. DNA adducts cause further damage both directly (by incorporating into host DNA, impairing synthesis or base pair formation) and indirectly by forming adducts with proteins involved in DNA repair, or upregulating those with proinflammatory or profibrogenic properties. Once alcohol intake exceeds the capacity of the canonical metabolic pathway (Fig. 15.3), acetaldehyde begins to accumulate, and other toxic by-products are produced. This multifactorial process alongside genetic susceptibility is thought to cause the hepatic damage associated with ALD. In keeping with many liver diseases, most damage is reversible in early stages (*see* Chapter 14: Liver Failure) but chronic abuse will lead to permanent damage eventually.

Alcohol-related liver disease can present in myriad ways, from an isolated raised ALT found incidentally, admission with acute alcoholic hepatitis (*see* Chapter 14: Liver Failure) to full decompensation. There are often clues that the etiology in alcohol, for example thrombocytopenia in the absence of portal hypertension is suggestive of alcohol-induced bone marrow toxicity, as is a raised mean corpuscular volume. A low serum urea is also often seen, and there may be pointers in the history and examination such as morning nausea, Dupuytren's contracture or parotid gland enlargement. In some cases,

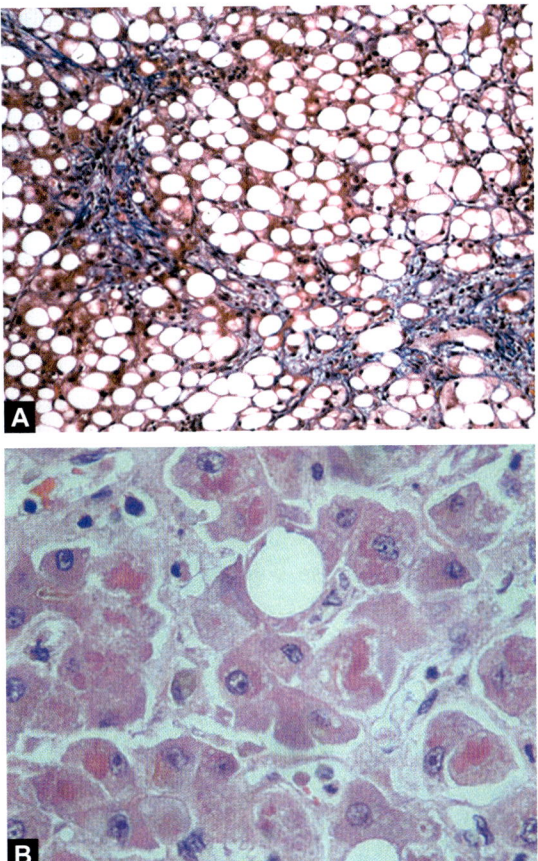

Figs. 15.4A and B: Biopsy of classical ALD. (A) Fatty liver with fibrosis is typical findings of alcoholic liver disease; (B) Mallory's hyaline are pink staining inclusion bodies found in the cytoplasm, found in alcoholic liver disease, but also in Wilson's. (ALD: Alcohol-related liver disease).

patients may be evasive about alcohol use, and if this is suspected, a liver biopsy may be required. This will frequently show Mallory's Hyaline, neutrophil infiltration and steatosis (Figs. 15.4A and B).

Management should focus on clear advice to achieve total abstinence, and this should be documented. Those drinking at very high levels are at risk of delirium tremens if alcohol is suddenly stopped, and so a program of gradual reduction is advised. This is best conducted with the support of alcohol services, who can also arrange community or residential detoxification regimes if required.

Abstinence will lead to dramatic improvements in liver function in the majority of people, even where there is cirrhosis. In cirrhosis, recovery of synthetic function can be seen up to 1 year after abstinence often resulting in recompensation to Child's A disease (*see* Chapter 14: Liver Failure).

This is one of the reasons that liver transplantation is usually only considered in those who have been abstinent for at least 6 months as well as allowing time to show on-going commitment to a life without alcohol. Those with cirrhosis should enter the appropriate HCC and variceal surveillance programs (*see* Chapter 14: Liver Failure) and should remain under the care of specialist services long-term.

Non-alcoholic Fatty Liver Disease

Non-alcoholic fatty liver disease is the most common cause of isolated rise in ALT in primary care, and is also the most common cause of what was previously referred to as cryptogenic cirrhosis. It is closely linked with obesity and the metabolic syndrome (hypertension, diabetes and hypercholesterolemia).

The usual presentation is raised ALT, with or without lesser elevation of ALP alongside fatty change on USS with an otherwise negative NILS. Most patients will be overweight/obese, or have another manifestation of the metabolic syndrome.

Non-alcoholic fatty liver disease with ALT <100 and no evidence of significant fibrosis on elastography can be considered at low risk of progression of liver disease, but the risk of cardiovascular disease and stroke is significantly increased and these should be aggressively managed. A liver biopsy should be considered where ALT is >100, or where there is suggestion of advanced fibrosis to adequately stage disease and establish degree of on-going inflammation as this will determine the need for, and frequency of, specialist follow-up. Where there is clear evidence of cirrhosis, biopsy is unnecessary but long-term follow-up including hepatoma and variceal surveillance is mandatory.

Key management strategies comprise:
- *Weight loss*: Specific targets are better than generic advice to "lose weight." Loss of 10% body weight correlates with regression of liver fibrosis and should be the ultimate target. A short-term goal of 4–7% in 3–6 months is a reasonable initial strategy. For patients with morbid obesity (BMI >45), bariatric surgery should be considered, particularly where there are other obesity-related complications.
- *Exercise*: Target of 150 min per week with the aim of achieving 60–70% of maximum heart rate for general health and >200 minutes per week for the purposes of weight loss. Examples include brisk walking, cycling and swimming.
- *Diet*: Low in saturated fat, high fructose corn syrup and processed food, high in fruit and vegetables.
- *Management of hypertension, diabetes and hypercholesterolemia*: Statins are safe in those with ALT <100 and should be continued, as they are likely to be protective in this patient population. There is some evidence that statins are beneficial in liver disease overall, although large-scale studies have not yet proved benefit.

- *Alcohol*: Alcohol intake in the context of any liver disease is likely to exacerbate and promote hepatic damage, but this appears to be particularly relevant in NAFLD where degree of fibrosis and inflammation is significantly greater in those who also drink excess alcohol. Patients should be advised to keep alcohol intake at minimal levels (<10 units/week).

Follow-up should include review of lifestyle changes, and repeat LFT at 6 monthly intervals. Of note, 70% of low risk NAFLD patients will have improvement of LFT with lifestyle measures alone.

Viral Hepatitis

About 1 in 12 people worldwide is infected with chronic HBV or HCV infection. Chronic viral hepatitis accounts for a major proportion of worldwide liver disease mortality. HBV and HCV are very different at a virological level, although both cause similar patterns of CLD once established. Effective treatments to suppress or clear viremia are available for both these infections, and those felt to be at risk should be screened and referred as a matter of course.

Hepatitis B Virus

The most common mode of HBV acquisition is perinatal transmission from infected mothers, leading to chronic infection in almost 90% of cases. In this situation, the infant is infected before the development of a mature immune system, which subsequently fails to recognize the HBV as "other." This leads to a long (20+ years) period of immune tolerance, with high levels of viremia with little hepatic damage. In the third or fourth decade, the immune system recognizes HBV as "other" and mounts a florid response, with resultant damage to hepatocytes; this period is marked by reducing levels of viremia with abnormal ALT. This phase will either result in eradication of chronic HBV infection (<10% of cases), suppression of viremia with no on-going hepatitis but on-going chronic infection (viral load persistently <2000 IU/mL plus normal ALT), or persistent active hepatitis with high viral load (viral load >2000 IU/mL or raised ALT). Only the latter definitely requires antiviral treatment. Where the pattern is not clear cut, for example in those with oscillating patterns of viral load or ALT, biopsy if frequently necessary to determine the degree of on-going inflammation and stage of fibrosis (Table 15.4). In some cases, antiviral treatment will be instituted on the basis of biopsy findings. All patients with cirrhosis and detectable viremia require antiviral therapy.

In adults, HBV is transmitted in blood and bodily fluids with an incubation period of 6–24 weeks. Acute HBV manifests with typical viral symptoms, associated with raised ALT (can reach 1500 IU/mL) and jaundice, and can be deep. In rare cases, this can result in acute liver failure (0.5%), necessitating urgent treatment and transfer to a specialist liver transplant unit.

Table 15.4: Management of chronic hepatitis B virus infection.

HBeAg	HBV DNA (IU/mL)	ALT	Comment
Positive	>2000	Normal	Immune tolerant. Consider biopsy if ALT rises
Positive	>2000	High	Likely to require treatment but consider biopsy first
Negative (HBeAb +/–)	>2000	High	Likely to require treatment. Requires biopsy. Possible pre-core mutant
Negative (HBeAb +/–)	<2000	High	May require treatment. Consider liver biopsy
Negative (HBeAb +)	<2000	Normal	Inactive carrier state

Notes: Normal ALT implies persistently normal readings. Loss of HBeAg should eventually lead to acquisition of HBeAb, but can take many months. Failure to develop HBeAb can signify the presence of a pre-core or core mutation. Here, the patient remains HBeAg+ but the gene encoding the core protein has a mutation, which prevents eAg detection on serological testing. ALT: alanine amino transferase; HBV: hepatitis B virus.

Table 15.5: Hepatitis B virus serological patterns.

	HBcAb IgM	HBcAb IgG	HBeAg	HBeAb (anti-Hbe)	HBsAg	HBsAb (anti-HBs)
Acute	+	±	+	–	±	–
Immunity	–	+	–	+	–	+
Chronic	–	+	±	±	+	–

Notes: In the immediate phase of acute infection, core IgM and HbsAg may not yet be detectable. Those who have cleared an acute infection have long-term immunity and no further treatment is required. Exceptions are reactivation of acute HBV in those undergoing immunosuppressive therapy and the phenomenon of occult HBV, with serological evidence of immunity and no detectable circulating HBV DNA, but evidence of viral replication in hepatic tissue. Diagnosis of chronic HBV requires persistence of HBsAg for 6 months. Hepatitis B core antibody (HBcAb); hepatitis B e antigen (HBeAg) and antibody (HBeAb/anti-HBe); hepatitis B surface antigen (HBsAg) and antibody (HBsAb/anti-HBs). HBV: hepatitis B virus.

In adults, a chronic infection is only established in approximately 10% of cases, and most are managed conservatively without the need for antiviral therapy. HBV can also manifest in adults as reactivation of previously cleared disease. This is because during HBV infection, viral DNA is integrated into the host genome, and persists in a covalently closed formation within the nucleus. Although serology shows cleared infection, during periods of intense immunosuppression (e.g. chemotherapy or biological treatment with monoclonal antibodies), HBV can reactivate, mirroring an acute infection. All patients undergoing such immunosuppressive therapy should be screened for HBcAb and HbsAg prior to treatment.

Management should first establish whether the infection is acute or chronic (Table 15.5), and should include advice on minimizing transmission risk (covering cuts, do not share toothbrushes, practicing safe sex). Women of childbearing potential should be advised that infection can be transmitted, particularly if the mother is HBeAg+. Obstetric units have established protocols for management, which will include administration of HBV immunoglobulin therapy at delivery for babies born of HBeAg positive mothers.

The mainstay of antiviral treatment is with oral nucleoside analogs which provide excellent viral suppression long term, and often result in seroconversion from HBeAg+ to HBeAb+ which signals improvement in prognosis and reduction in HCC risk. In these circumstances, antiviral therapy can sometimes be stopped, although with very careful monitoring to ensure there is no relapse and in the majority, oral nucleoside analog treatment is continued indefinitely. Oral therapy rarely results in eradication of the chronic infection (2%). In selected cases, treatment with pegylated interferon is advocated. This offers a greater chance of clearance and treatment is of finite duration, although it is only suitable in specific circumstances and is now only rarely used.

In chronic HBV, hepatoma surveillance is offered to all patients with cirrhosis, and non-cirrhotics with a family history of HCC. Surveillance should also be considered for those at high risk (south East Asian origin >40 years old).

Some cases of chronic HBV infection can be complicated by superinfection with hepatitis D virus (HDV). HDV is a satellite virus; this means that the virus is unable to independently complete a lifecycle, and instead relies upon HBV proteins for replication and packaging. HDV super-infection is associated with severe flares of HBV infection, and accelerates disease progression. Management focuses on suppression of HBV, which is indicated at lower HBV viremia thresholds in the context of HDV infection.

Hepatitis C Virus

Hepatitis C virus is transmitted in blood and bodily fluids, most commonly in the United Kingdom and developed countries by injecting drug use. Maternal transmission is rare (<5%). HCV is primarily an iatrogenic problem in Egypt due to a mass Schistosomiasis vaccination program using non-sterilized needles, which has left almost 20% of the population chronically infected. HCV establishes a chronic infection in up to 85% of those infected. The acute infection is usually subclinical, and patients are usually diagnosed during routine screening (e.g. at drug support services) or once CLD has been established. A raised ALT is frequently the only abnormality seen (usually <200 IU/mL), and is not always present.

Chronic HCV treatment has changed beyond recognition in recent years, with the expectation of achieving eradication of HCV in the majority

Table 15.6: Currently licensed directly acting antiviral agents (DAA) for HCV.

Class	Mechanism of action	Examples
Protease inhibitors	Block action of HCV NS3/NS4A protease	Simeprevir, Ombitasvir
NS5A inhibitors	Block action of HCV NS5A, responsible for multiple aspects of the viral lifecycle	Daclatasvir, Ledipasvir
Polymerase inhibitors	Block action of HCV NS5B polymerase	Sofosbuvir, Paritaprevir

(HCV: Hepatitis C virus.)

of cases. The potential for complete eradication is due in part to the fact that HCV is an RNA-based virus, which never integrates into the host genome, and has an entirely cytoplasmic lifecycle. There are six distinct genotypes of HCV infection, of which genotypes 1 and 3 are the most predominant in the west. Treatment varies according to genotype, but consists of combination therapy with directly acting antiviral agents (Table 15.6), with or without pegylated interferon and ribavirin. This is given for 8–24 weeks and is associated with minimal side effects. Treatment is appropriate at all stages of liver disease, although in those with decompensated cirrhosis, assessment of suitability for liver transplantation should be conducted first, since in some cases it may be better to transplant and then treat. Furthermore, there is a small risk of worsening liver function toward the end of treatment, in which case a prior decision regarding fitness for transplantation is helpful. HCV treatment is currently evolving, with almost a dozen molecules recently licensed for use, although not all options are available on the National Health Service, pending a full review by the National Institute for Clinical Excellence (NICE).

Other Agents Causing Viral Hepatitis

Hepatitis A Virus (HAV): HAV is a picornavirus with an RNA genome. Transmission is fecal-oral and it is therefore common in areas with poor sanitation. The incubation period is approximately 28 days, with those infected complaining of non-specific malaise, nausea and abdominal pain. Jaundice is present in two thirds of cases, alongside raised transaminases.

Diagnosis is made by detection of HAV IgM in the serum. It is important to check PT and renal function, as HAV can in rare cases cause acute liver failure. There is no specific management other than rest and adequate hydration, with advice to avoid alcohol in the acute period. Most patients will complain of residual lethargy for some weeks after resolution of abnormal LFT. HAV does not establish chronic infection.

Hepatitis E Virus (HEV): HEV is an RNA virus, also spread by fecal-oral transmission. It is common in areas of poor sanitation. HEV can also be transmitted through ingestion of undercooked pork or close proximity to swine, and this is thought to be the primary source of HEV in the United Kingdom.

Hepatitis E virus presents with vague symptoms similar to HAV, but jaundice is less commonly seen. ALT can be in the high hundreds. HEV is usually a mild, self-limiting illness but can cause significant decompensation of liver disease in those with cirrhosis, and can cause acute liver failure and death in pregnancy. Treatment is supportive, focusing on good hydration and rest, and HEV does not establish chronic infection.

Epstein–Barr Virus (EBV): EBV (infectious mononucleosis) is a very common cause of abnormal LFT. The most frequent presentation is typical viral illness symptoms with a high ALT, but it can also present with a predominantly cholestatic pattern; in these individuals, jaundice can persist for many weeks causing very troublesome itch and anorexia.

Epstein-Barr virus is diagnosed by detection of positive EBV IgM (monospot test). Treatment is supportive, with symptoms usually settling within a few weeks. EBV IgM should disappear within 6 months, accompanied by detection of EBV IgG confirming seroconversion. It is prudent to ensure that full seroconversion has occurred especially in the immunosuppressed (e.g. posttransplant), in whom persistent EBV can be a sign of lymphoproliferative disease.

Other: CMV, HSV and VZV can all cause a viral hepatitis very similar in presentation to EBV. HSV and VZV can also rarely cause acute liver failure.

Although treatment is simply supportive, serological tests should be performed to confirm the diagnosis, and an alternative explanation should be sought where serology is negative. It is also important to ensure that there are no features suggestive of significant acute liver injury, which would mandate hospital admission and close monitoring.

Autoimmune Liver Diseases

In keeping with other autoimmune disease, immune-mediated liver diseases are more commonly seen in those of female gender, and can be associated with major shifts in hormones (e.g. post pregnancy, menopause). Although this is the typical presentation, autoimmune disease affects many men and younger people, and should always be specifically excluded in those with abnormal LFT.

Primary Biliary Cholangitis

Primary biliary cholangitis was recently renamed having previously been known as primary biliary cirrhosis. The name change reflects that the spectrum of liver disease is broad, and in fact the majority of patients do not develop cirrhosis.

Immune-mediated destruction of the bile ducts causes persistent inflammation (cholangitis), which can result in progressive scarring and duct destruction, with consequent detrimental effects on liver function. Due to the site of damage, portal hypertension can develop early in disease, before the advent of major liver synthetic dysfunction.

In the majority of cases, patients present with vague symptoms such as fatigue or itch, and are found to have an abnormal ALP, frequently in isolation but raised ALT can also be seen. A NILS will usually show a positive AMA in the typical (M2, M4 or M9) pattern and the presence of positive AMA with abnormal ALP is sufficient to diagnose PBC. In total, 10% of people will have AMA negative PBC, in which case only a liver biopsy is diagnostic. A number of patients with completely normal LFT will have a detectable AMA in typical pattern on testing for another condition. In this circumstance, people should be advised that they have a very high (>95%) chance of developing PBC and should have periodic LFT monitoring and referral when these are abnormal. Some centers would advocate treatment in those who have yet to develop abnormal LFT, although this is not currently widespread practice.

Treatment is with a bile acid analog, ursodeoxycholic acid, given long term at a dose of 13–16 mg/kg. This is associated with reduced risk of disease progression, and is well tolerated. A minority of patients will develop cirrhosis and should be managed appropriately.

Autoimmune Hepatitis

Presentation of AIH is protean, from isolated abnormality of ALT, to decompensated cirrhosis. A further small but significant minority will present acutely with jaundice or acute liver failure.

There is often a history of other immune disease, either in the patient of a close relative, and a history of non-specific symptoms, in particular fatigue, can often be elicited. Where the patient has abnormal LFT and the NILS shows positive smooth muscle antibody (SMA) with or without raised IgG levels, the diagnosis is straightforward, although a liver biopsy should always be performed prior to starting therapy to fully stage underlying disease, as this has implications for follow-up. AIH is not always associated with SMA positivity, and in these cases, diagnostic algorithms can be used, such as those produced by the British Society of Gastroenterology. Again, most cases will require liver biopsy prior to committing the patient to long-term medical treatment.

Therapy is immunosuppressive and initially corticosteroids are used at 0.5–1 mg/kg, depending on protocol. Corticosteroids should lead to a rapid reduction in ALT and IgG and steroid-sparing treatment should then commence alongside prednisolone, usually with azathioprine at a dose of 1 mg/kg. Alternatives where azathioprine is contraindicated or not tolerated include 6-mercaptopurine, mycophenolate mofetil or more powerful agents including tacrolimus. Once the steroid-sparing agent has been instituted, steroid should be gradually weaned to 5–10 mg daily. Dual therapy should continue until ALT and IgG have been persistently normal for at least 1 year prior to considering steroid withdrawal. It is the best practice to repeat the liver biopsy to confirm histological remission prior to withdrawal.

Those presenting with acute liver failure are likely to require urgent liver biopsy, intravenous steroid therapy, and discussion with a liver transplant unit in case transplantation becomes necessary.

Long-term treatment should be with azathioprine or alternative and this should not be stopped without biopsy and an understanding that withdrawal of immunosuppression can lead to major flare of disease. For this reason, many patients will remain on treatment indefinitely. Those with cirrhosis should be managed accordingly.

Primary Sclerosing Cholangitis

Primary sclerosing cholangitis (PSC) is a rare autoimmune condition causing destruction of intra- and extrahepatic bile ducts, leading to characteristic "pruned" appearances of the biliary tree on imaging (Fig. 15.5).

There is usually a history of IBD (the majority of those with PSC have IBD, but only a fraction of IBD develop PSC). Even where IBD is not previously diagnosed, annual colonoscopy is recommended, both to seek out IBD and because the risk of colorectal cancer in PSC is considerably increased.

Liver failure tests are predominantly cholestatic and patients may also have jaundice. Serum antibodies may be positive (ANA or antineutrophil cytoplasmic antibody). Magnetic resonance imaging of the liver and biliary tree is often diagnostic, with biopsy used to stage disease. Clinical presentation relates to the pattern of bile duct injury. Where there is stricturing of large bile ducts (dominant stricture), the appearance is that of classical biliary obstruction with jaundice and dilatation of the proximal biliary tree,

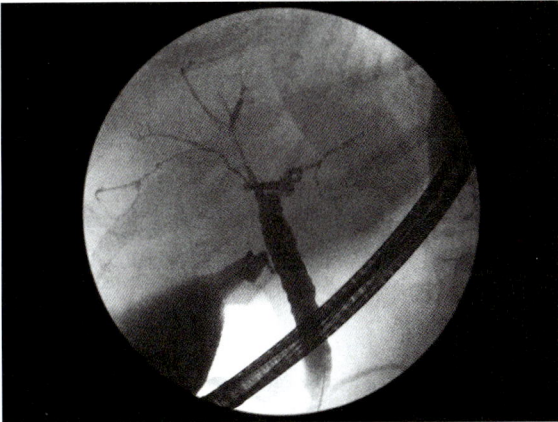

Fig. 15.5: Characteristic ERCP appearances of primary sclerosing cholangitis showing beading of secondary and tertiary ducts. (ERCP: Endoscopic retrograde cholangiopancreatography).

with or without cholangitis. In predominantly small duct disease, presentation is more insidious, with episodes of recurrent cholangitis or abnormal LFT with or without jaundice. In keeping with other cholestatic disease, patients with PSC can become deficient in fat-soluble vitamins and can have more marked nutritional compromise than other liver diseases. There is a very high risk of cholangiocarcinoma, and the very abnormal appearances of the biliary tree can make it difficult to exclude small cholangiocarcinoma on imaging. Any sudden deterioration in a patent with PSC should warrant urgent LFT, screen for cholangitis and imaging, to exclude a new dominant stricture, which may be amenable to treatment with endoscopic retrograde cholangiopancreatography (*see* Chapter 12: Jaundice), or cholangiocarcinoma. Advanced PSC can be treated with liver transplantation, and it is not infrequent to find a small cholangiocarcinoma in the explanted liver.

Inherited Liver Diseases

Hereditary Hemochromatosis

Hereditary hemochromatosis is an inherited disorder of very variable penetrance, leading to iron accumulation in red cells and susceptible organs (liver, pituitary, heart and pancreas). The most frequent mutations, C282Y and H63D, are point mutations in proteins, which usually control intestinal intake of iron but are structurally damaged by mutation allowing unchecked iron absorption and subsequent deposition.

A high serum ferritin raises the possibility of HH, but as ferritin is an acute phase protein, raised levels should be repeated and confirmed to be associated with elevated transferrin saturation (>45%) prior to genetic testing. Raised levels can also be seen in alcohol misuse and diabetes, although usually <1000 IU/mL. Liver biopsy is usually only recommended where ferritin is over 1000 or there are other signs of CLD.

All patients with HH should be investigated for other end organ damage (diabetes mellitus, cardiomyopathy and pituitary function) and most will complain of arthralgia as iron is also deposited in the joints.

There is no requirement for a low iron diet, although vitamin C supplements should be avoided as these boost intestinal iron absorption.

Removal of excess iron by venesection should be commenced at the time of diagnosis, with the aim to reduce ferritin to <50 IU/mL and to maintain transferrin saturation <50%. Initially, this will be required weekly, but once stabilized most patients require venesection 3–4 monthly.

Genetic screening should be offered to siblings, parents and children and this can usually be arranged by the local clinical genetics service.

Wilson's Disease

Wilson is an exceptionally rare disorder of copper metabolism, and often manifests in people with previous psychiatric or neurological history.

It is extremely uncommon for Wilson's to present in those >40, and copper studies should not form part of the NILS in older age groups. Ceruloplasmin and copper are unreliable in the context of acute inflammation/infection and an abnormal result should first be repeated. Furthermore, ceruloplasmin is not always abnormal even in people with proven Wilson's. Therefore, if Wilson's disease is strongly suspected, it should be comprehensively excluded, usually with slit lamp ophthalmologic examination and 24-h urinary copper measurement.

Presentation is variable, from isolated abnormal ALT to fulminant hepatic failure. It can also rarely present with hemolysis and jaundice and the index of suspicion should be high in younger people with neuropsychiatric history.

Treatment is with chelation therapy (D-penicillamine) and families should be offered genetic screening.

Alpha-1 Antitrypsin Deficiency

Alpha-1 antitrypsin deficiency (A-1AT) is an inhibitor of neutrophil elastase, and deficiency can allow unchecked inflammation in the lungs, and accumulation of abnormal A-1AT in the liver. Overall A-1AT affects 1 in 3000 people in the United Kingdom, but both copies of the abnormal Z protein (PiZZ) must be inherited for clinically apparent disease, which results in A1-AT levels approximately 15% of normal. Other abnormal phenotypes (PiMS, PiMZ and PiSZ) lead to reduction of 40–60% but this does not cause liver disease in isolation and lung disease is usually avoided in those who do not smoke. A-1AT rarely causes clinically significant liver disease in isolation, but it can be a cofactor in CLD of other etiologies. There is no specific management of A-1AT other than avoidance of alcohol and cigarette smoking.

■ SUMMARY

The goal of investigation of abnormal LFT should always be to identify treatable conditions, and to prevent or slow progression of liver disease. Most cases of cirrhosis are a consequence of entirely preventable disease (e.g. alcohol excess, obesity and viral hepatitis) and early identification and intervention in these illnesses is an opportunity to avoid the development of advanced liver disease and the sequelae.

■ FURTHER READING

1. British Society of Gastroenterology Guidelines for Management of Autoimmune Hepatitis Gleeson D, Heneghan MA. Gut 2011. Available from: http://www.bsg.org.uk/clinical-guidelines/liver/guidelines-for-the-management-of-autoimmune-hepatitis.html.

2. European Association for the Study of the Liver (EASL) Clinical Practice Guidelines for all liver diseases. Available from: www.easl.eu.
3. NICE Guidelines on Management of Chronic Viral Hepatitis HBV https://www.nice.org.uk/guidance/cg165.
4. NICE Guidelines on Management of Non-alcoholic Fatty Liver Disease https://www.nice.org.uk/guidance/ng49/chapter/Recommendations.

CHAPTER 16

Enteral and Parenteral Nutrition

Her Hsin Tsai

■ INTRODUCTION

It is the primary function of the gastrointestinal (GI) tract to deliver nutrition to the host. The human GI tract has considerable capacity and redundancy, hence even after major surgical resection, the tract can absorb enough nutrients to support the individual. So whenever possible, nutrition should be delivered through the GI tract.

■ IS THE PATIENT AT RISK OF MALNUTRITION?

Malnutrition is common in hospitalized patients and a large number of patients visiting the GI clinic. It may be subtle, an individual who is septic and infected would be in a severe catabolic state, may look well or even large but may well be malnourished. As they are anorexic or inadequately fed or starved awaiting surgery, the patient will rapidly become malnourished. A healthy individual on a weight reducing diet would lose similar amount of weight and still be well nourished.

In general, any individual who:
- Has a body mass index (BMI) of <18.5 kg/m^2
- Has unintentional weight loss >10% within the last 3–6 months
- Has a BMI of <20 kg/m^2 and unintentional weight loss >5% within the last 3–6 months would be considered to be malnourished.

Any individual who has not eaten for 5 days or more or in a catabolic state or has compromised absorption would be at high risk of being malnourished.

Assessment of Nutritional Status

There are several checklists now extent to assess nutritional status. All patients admitted to hospital or in GI clinics who may be at risk should have some form of formal assessment. Use of such a checklist would reduce risk of missing the patients who at risk of malnutrition. One such checklist is given in Figure 16.1.

History:
1. Weight change
   a. Baseline weight kg
   b. Change in past 6 months, ___ kg (gain/loss), ___ % loss
   c. Change in past 2 weeks kg (gain/loss)
2. Dietary intake change
   a. None/increased/decreased
   b. Duration of change weeks
   c. Type of change (if decreased)
      • Suboptimal solids/full liquids/hypocaloric liquids/starvation
3. Gastrointestinal symptoms (persisting for at least 2 weeks)
   a. None/nausea/vomiting/diarrhea/anorexia
4. Functional capacity
   a. No dysfunction/dysfunction
   b. Duration of dysfunction (if present) ___ weeks
   c. Type of dysfunction (if present)
      • Working suboptimally/ambulatory but not working/bedridden
5. Disease
   a. Primary diagnosis ___
   b. Related metabolic demand
      • None/low/moderate/high

Physical exam (none, mild, moderate, severe):
1. Loss of subcutaneous fat. ___
2. Muscle wasting (quadriceps, deltoids) ___
3. Ankle edema ___
4. Sacral edema, ___
5. Ascites ___

Subjective global assessment rating:
A = Well Nourished
B = Mild-Moderate Malnutrition
C = Severe Malnutrition

Fig. 16.1: Typical nutritional assessment form.

Laboratory assessments include full blood count and biochemistry screen which should be extended to include serum magnesium and glucose.

■ DOES THE PATIENT HAVE DYSPHAGIA?

If it is established that the patient has or is at risk of nutritional compromise, then the next step is to consider how to re-establish enteral nutrition. This depends on the cause of the problem. For a significant number admitted to GI wards, the problem is dysphagia. Clues of dysphagia particularly in the frail elderly may be subtle. This may include difficult, painful chewing or swallowing which may result from oral problems like pharyngitis, glossitis and ill-fitting dentures. Regurgitation of undigested food, difficulty controlling food or liquid in the mouth and drooling may suggest a neurological or pharyngeal cause as does a hoarse voice or coughing or choking before, during or after swallowing. True esophageal dysphagia or odynophagia particularly a progressive dysphagia suggest malignant disease or achalasia. Tumors of the cardia and *linitis plastica* may also present with dysphagia.

If the diagnosis has not been established, then an urgent endoscopy should be performed. Patients with a risk of aspiration should have their swallowing formally assessed. If it is deemed that the patient is unsafe for oral nutrition, then nasogastric feeding with a fine bore feeding tube should be placed. This is preferably performed under radiological screening or at least confirmatory X-ray that the tip of the tube is in the stomach. In patients subject to regurgitation, tube placement into the duodenum is preferable. In patients like those with obstructing ear, nose and throat (ENT) malignancies undergoing radiotherapy, the need for feeding may be quite prolonged then a gastrostomy tube placement is appropriate. Even in patients who had esophageal or major gastric surgery or Whipple's procedures, early enteral nutrition improves wound healing and recovery. Hence, tube feeding in the postoperative period is welcome. This is usually placed at the end of the operation.

Many patients with esophageal cancer are now offered chemoradiotherapy either prior to surgery (neoadjuvant) or as palliative procedure will need good nutrition during this treatment. Hence, a removable metal stent is placed to allow oral feeding. These stents can allow patients to eat almost normally. They may get blocked but this is easily unblocked with a fizzy beverage. Biodegradable stents are also available which slowly dissolve and do not require removing (Figs. 16.2A and B).

In patients whose swallowing problems are likely to be prolonged or permanent, a percutaneous endoscopic gastrostomy (PEG) could be placed. This is a simple procedure but should be offered only after careful consideration by a multidisciplinary team with the patient's welfare being paramount. This may involve a "best interest" discussion in patients unable to give consent. The procedure should be performed only if the patients underlying prognosis for survival is likely to be good and not in patients who are on end-of-life care.

■ IS THE PATIENT AT RISK OF REFEEDING SYNDROME?

Refeeding syndrome was said to be first observed that many starved prisoner of war camp soldiers died after being liberally fed on emancipation. Interestingly, history also relates that during the retreat from Russia, Napoleon's starved *Grande Armee* on reaching Vilnius on the Baltic half of

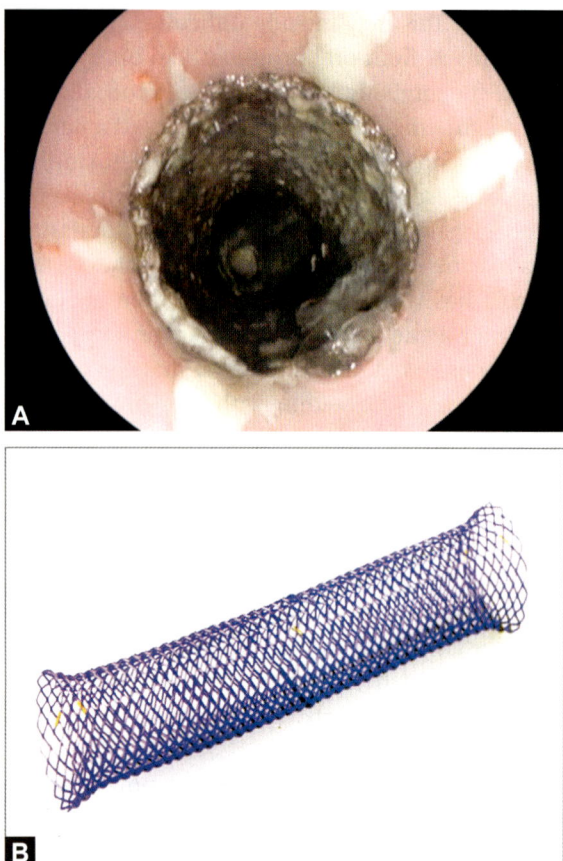

Figs. 16.2A and B: Available stents. (A) Metal; (B) Biodegradable.

the remaining men died even though there was shelter and plentiful food became first available. It was said that the men gorged themselves to death but it was likely that refeeding syndrome is at least partly responsible.

Refeeding syndrome occurs when after prolonged fast, food triggers a massive shift of electrolytes from the intravascular into the intracellular compartment leading to development of fluid and electrolyte disorders, especially hypophosphatemia which may lead to neurological, cardiac or neuromuscular complications. During the prolonged fast, the body's fuel source switches from ingested carbohydrates and fat to tissue fatty acids and starts breaking down muscle amino acids as the main energy sources. Many intracellular minerals become severely depleted during this period, although serum levels may be maintained and insulin levels are suppressed.

During refeeding, insulin secretion rebounds in response to increased blood sugar, resulting in increased glycogen, fat and protein synthesis. This process requires phosphates, magnesium and potassium which are already depleted and the stores rapidly become used up. Intracellular movement of electrolytes occurs along with a fall in the serum electrolytes, including phosphate and magnesium. This may lead to severe hypokalemia, hypomagnesemia and hypophosphatemia causing cardiac arrhythmias, confusion, convulsions and coma or heart failure resulting in possible death.

The National Institute of Clinical Excellence (NICE) has produced a simple checklist to identify those at risk of refeeding syndrome.

Criteria for Determining People at High Risk of Developing Refeeding Problems

Patient has one or more of the following:
- BMI <16 kg/m^2
- Unintentional weight loss >15% within the last 3–6 months
- Little or no nutritional intake for >10 days
- Low levels of potassium, phosphate or magnesium prior to feeding

Or patient has two or more of the following:
- BMI <18.5 kg/m^2
- Unintentional weight loss >10% within the last 3–6 months
- Little or no nutritional intake for >5 days
- A history of alcohol abuse or drugs including insulin, chemotherapy, antacids or diuretics.

The appropriate care of patients at risk of refeeding syndrome involves measured reintroduction of feeds and careful monitoring. It is best to start nutrition support at a maximum of 10 kcal/kg/day, increasing levels slowly to meet or exceed full needs by 4–7 days. In severe cases like anorexia nervosa patients with BMI <14 kg/m^2 or negligible intake for >15 days monitoring cardiac rhythm continually is recommended in these people and any others who already have or develop any cardiac arrhythmias. Oral thiamine and a balanced multivitamin/trace element supplement once daily is given.

Daily monitoring of electrolytes, and prompt correction of electrolytes is required. Usually, oral supplementation of potassium, phosphate and magnesium suffices but IV correction may be required especially in patients where there is a delay on oral refeeding.

■ TYPES OF FEEDS

Frail patients, or those with dysphagia, liver failure or refeeding of anorexics or in any patient that is tube fed will require a liquid feed of some description (Fig. 16.3). A feed should be selected for the specific needs of the patient. There are three components to think about when selecting a feed: nitrogen source, energy source and micronutrients.

Nitrogen Source

There are many proprietary feeds available and they are broadly divided into whole protein (polymeric) or elemental, where the protein is hydrolyzed into

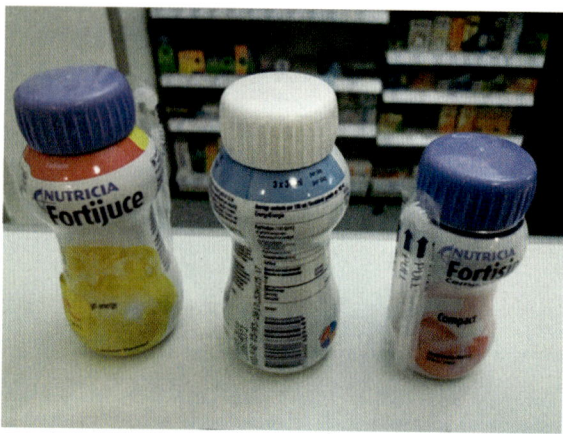

Fig. 16.3: A variety of commercial feeds are available with variable combinations of nutrients.

amino acids or short peptides. This is on the assumption that such feeds are better absorbed. There is really no evidence of this. Such elemental feeds are unpalatable and expensive. However, in Crohn's disease, there may be a role as trials of elemental diets show that they are at least as good as steroids without the adverse reactions of the corticosteroid. However, even polymeric liquid diets have an effect in Crohn's disease and it is likely that the absence of fiber in especially stricturing Crohn's alleviates the symptoms of the disease. Hence for the most part, for almost all patients, whole protein feeds is preferred.

In patients with liver failure, avoidance of aromatic amino acids has been advocated. This is achieved by giving supplementary branched-chain amino acid enriched formula feeds. However, clinical trials have failed to demonstrate evidence of its benefit. In encephalopathic patients, it may seem sensible to restrict ammonia generation from protein metabolism. However, protein restriction is usually unnecessary and may be unhelpful. It is better to prevent encephalopathy with liberal use of lactulose and neomycin or rifaximin. A high calorific intake of carbohydrates reduces protein metabolism and improves nutrition without contributing to ammonia generation. In end-stage liver disease, the liver has lost some of its capacity to synthesize and metabolize protein, glycogen and lipids, hence continuous feeding via a pump is superior to episodic feeding.

Calorie Source

For the most part, carbohydrates in the form of glucose polymers are offered. This should make up the bulk of the calories of the feed. Fat has a higher energy density and is in many feeds make up 30% of the energy provision. Short-chain fatty acids are better absorbed but are quite unpalatable, so most feeds contain long chain or medium chain fatty acids. In Crohn's disease, there is some evidence that feeds with primarily medium chain fatty acids are superior.

Micronutrients

Most proprietary feed contain adequate amounts of vitamins and minerals. However in specific situations like refeeding syndrome, liver disease and alcoholism, additional oral supplementation is required. These patients may be deprived of micronutrients for several weeks. Alcohol is a surprisingly high energy density (7 kcal/g compared to 4 kcal/g of carbohydrates), and alcoholics may depend on it for their energy source resulting in nitrogen and micronutrient deficiency. Hence, it is usual to give parenteral micronutrients, particularly thiamine to prevent Wernike's encephalopathy.

Tube fed patients may safely be discharged home if there is continuous care available to a nursing home. Intermittent feeding via PEG tubes is simple and needs little maintenance. Continuous PEG feeding using a pump can also be uncomplicated. Periodic checks of the tube and site and occasional checks of electrolytes are helpful in monitoring progress. Nasogastric tubes, however, are prone to displacement unless well secure. A bridle can prevent inadvertent displacement and is be reasonably comfortable.

PARENTERAL NUTRITION

Parenteral nutrition carries a considerable risk and expense, so should be avoided if possible but may be offered to patients who have:
- Inadequate or unsafe oral and/or enteral nutritional intake
- A non-functional, inaccessible or perforated (leaking) GI tract.

Parenteral nutrition can be given via a dedicated peripherally inserted central catheter or a dedicated centrally placed central venous catheter. This can also be given via a peripheral venous catheter if the patient only needs short-term parenteral nutrition (<14 days). This is also a valid method while awaiting dedicated central line insertion. For longer periods, a tunneling subclavian line is recommended (>30 days).

Continuous administration of parenteral nutrition is the preferred method of infusion in severely ill people who require parenteral nutrition with a gradual change from continuous to cyclical delivery should be considered in patients requiring parenteral nutrition for >2 weeks. Decision is based on clinical situation.

A typical total parenteral nutrition (TPN) requires water (30–40 mL/kg/day), energy (30–45 kcal/kg/day, depending on energy expenditure), amino acids (1.0–2.0 g/kg/day, depending on the degree of catabolism), essential fatty acids, vitamins and minerals. So a typical feed would normally be about 2 L/day of the standard solution with carbohydrate in the form of a 25% dextrose solution, but the amount and concentration depend on other factors, such as metabolic needs and the proportion of caloric needs that are supplied by lipids. Lipid emulsions are often added to supply essential fatty acids and triglycerides; 20–30% of total calories are usually supplied as lipids. Nitrogen is usually in the form of amino acids although patients with hepatic impairment may require the more expensive human albumin solution. Other essential electrolytes and minerals and trace of micronutrients make up the feed. Various formulations exist but broadly follow this mix. Additional vitamins are unusually administered separately. The emulsifier used is usually lecithin which is degraded by the body. Parenteral nutrition should be introduced progressively and closely monitored, usually starting at no >50% of estimated needs for the first 24–48 h. This is for the prevention of refeeding syndrome. Parenteral nutrition can be withdrawn once adequate oral or enteral nutrition is tolerated and nutritional status is stable. Withdrawal should be planned stepwise with a daily review of the patient's progress.

Complications of parenteral nutrition can be serious. This includes the complications around the insertion of the central line like bleeding and pneumothorax. Bleeding in this situation may be severe in liver patients with coagulopathy. Placement under radiological control and use of ultrasound to locate the subclavian vein has greatly reduced these complications.

The most important and serious complication during intravenous feed is line infection. Line sepsis carries a significant mortality rate of 15%. The main way of preventing this is to follow a clear protocol in attaching and detaching of feeds, handing of lines and use of bacterial filters. Feeding lines should be dedicated for feeding and not be used for drugs administration or transfusion of blood. Giving the care to dedicated teams has been shown to reduce infection rate. Line occlusion with clots and embolism may occur.

Other complications include fatty liver disease. This is common in TPN patients after prolonged use with >50% developing it. Usually manifests as elevated transaminase and alkaline phosphatase levels. However, severe cholestatic jaundice and liver failure can occasionally occur. It is thought that the fatty acid content may be responsible. Gallbladder disease is also prevalent due to unbuffered bile in the GI tract. Gallstones and cholecystitis are not uncommon.

For the majority of patients, there is an expectation that the gut may recover sufficiently to adequately digest and absorb enough to sustain adequate nutrition. However, patients with intestinal failure due to major resection for example in intestinal infarction may require lifelong TPN or at least until viable small bowel transplant if available.

■ FURTHER READING

1. NICE. Nutrition support for adults: oral nutrition support, enteral tube feeding and parenteral nutrition. Clinical guideline [CG32]. 2006.

Index

Page numbers followed by *f* refer to figure, and *t* refer to table

A

Abdomen
  acute 55, 58, 71
  non-gaseous 10
  obstructed 67
Abdominis muscle 336
Abscess 347
  amebic 349
  anorectal 201
  appendix 73
  crypt 110*f*
  formation 87
  ischiorectal 202*f*
  mesocolic 87
  perianal 194
  pyogenic 348
Acalculous cholecystitis 76
Acarbose 285
Achalasia 295, 298*f*, 307
  early 307*f*
  late 307*f*
Acid glycoprotein, serum 147
Acquired immunodeficiency syndrome 160
Adalimumab 150
Addison's disease 118, 260, 268
Adenocarcinoma 6*f*
  esophageal 295
  intraepithelial mucous 194
  mucinous 198
Adenoma 48
  adrenal 247
  duodenal 5*f*
  high-risk 253
  tubulovillous 250*f*
Adenomyomatosis 8, 52
Adenylcyclase, colonic 118

Adequate lateral pressure 231*f*
Adhesions 90
Adrenocorticotropic hormone,
    intravenous injection of 261
Aerophagia 274
Afferent loop obstruction syndrome 281, 283
Alanine aminotransferase 375, 376, 382
Albumin 358, 383
Alcohol 326, 385, 389
  assessment of 377
  consumption 267, 375
  dehydrogenase 386*f*
  excess 397
  metabolism 386*f*
Alpha chain disease 121, 172
Alpha-fetoprotein
  abnormal 380
  serum 345
Amebiasis, chronic 163
Ameboma 163
Amenorrhea 269
Ammonia generation 404
Ampicillin 105
Ampulla of Vater 234
Amylase 80
  serum 64
Amyloidosis
  intestinal 172
  primary 172
Anal fissures, acute 197
Anal mucosa, normal 194
Anchovy sauce 337
Anemia 115, 172, 205, 212, 286, 366
  hemolytic 320
  pernicious 375
Angiodysplasia 192, 208, 211*f*, 235
Angiodysplastic lesions 235

Angiogram 371*f*
Angiography 211, 221*f*, 222*f*
Angioplasty, coronary 219
Anorectal problems 191
Anorexia 256, 267, 313
   nervosa 269
Antacids 189, 301
   therapy 291
Antibiotics 76, 150
   broad-spectrum 74
Antibody, antinuclear 379
Anticholinergics 189
Antidiarrheal drugs 134, 166
Anti-helicobacter therapy 31
Antineutrophil antibodies, serum 239
Antireflux surgery 302
Antral gastritis 37
Aortic aneurysm 69
   abdominal 69, 341, 342*f*
   large abdominal 224*f*
   ruptured abdominal 94
Aortoenteric fistulae 223
Aphthoid 106
   ulcers 113
Appendicectomy 73
Appendicitis 59
   acute 70, 73
   diagnosis of 75
   management of 75
Appetite
   complex neurohormonal control of 266*f*
   physiology of 265
   stimulates 266
Argon plasma coagulation 235, 236*f*
Arrhythmias, cardiac 403
Arteries, inferior mesenteric 52
Arthritis 112
   rheumatoid 238
Ascariasis 164
Ascaris lumbricoides 166
Ascites 208, 335*f*, 356, 359, 371
   development of 360
   grading of 361*t*
   malignant 336
   pancreatic 174
Ascitic fluid 174, 336, 360*f*
Aspartate aminotransferase 375, 376

Aspergillus flavus 343
Aspirin 214
Autoimmune disease 327, 328
Autoimmune pancreatitis, computed tomography of 174*f*
Azathioprine 78, 134, 153, 307

B

Bacillus cereus 162
Back pain 94
Bacteria flora, colonic 127
Bacterial disease 327
Bacterial fermentation 274
Bacterial overgrowth 125
Bacterial peritonitis, spontaneous 361
Balloon tamponade 229
Balsalazide 134
Bariatric surgery 90, 279, 281, 282
   four main types of 280*f*
Barium
   enema 111, 192
   meal 312*f*
Barrett's esophagus 289, 303, 304*f*, 313, 314*f*
Barrett's mucosa 295
Barrett's visible dysplasia 304*f*
Basal cell carcinomas 194
B-cell lymphoma 47
Behçet's disease 112, 238
Behçet's syndrome 238
Belching 32, 274, 277
Bicarbonate concentration 124
Bile acid
   deconjugation of 125
   diarrhea 180
Bile duct dilation, intrahepatic 61
Bile salt
   diarrhea 118, 284
   handling, abnormal 25
   malabsorption 104
Biliary atresia 332
Biliary colic, attacks of 75
Biliary duct stones 9*f*
Biliary gastritis 6*f*
Biliary reflux
   following previous gastric surgery 258
   gastritis 41

Index

Biliary tract disease 77
Biliary tree 327
    congenital malformations of 332
    dilation 174*f*
Biliopancreatic diversion 272, 280, 280*f*
Biliopancreatic loop 283
Bilirubin 358, 383
    conjugated 326
    metabolism 320*f*
        inherited disorders of 321, 326
Biological therapy 122, 150
Biopsy 197
    esophageal 299*f*
    multiple 43
    rectal 104, 109
Bismuth subsalicylate 166
Blatchford score 205, 207, 207*t*
Bleeding 191, 209, 234, 239
    acute 366
    colonic 235
    hemorrhoids 196*f*
    life-threatening 227
    peptic ulcer 213
    rectal 115, 199
Blind loop 125
Bloating 23*f*, 26, 32, 276, 277
Blood
    electrolytes 269
    peripheral 169
    pressure 206
        labile 79
        systolic 207
    spotting 191
    testing, occult 106
    transfusion, history of 378
    urea 207
    vessels 108*f*
Body mass index 376, 377*f*, 378
Boerhaave's syndrome 81, 219
Bone
    densitometry 170
    disease, metabolic 147
    growth, normal 380
Bowel
    cancer 240
    disease 129
    ischemic loop of 58
    loop
        ischemic 71
        large 92
    obstruction, large 66*f*, 94*f*
    wall, infarction of 68*f*
Bowen's disease 194
Brachytherapy, single-dose 317
Bradycardia 269
Bradykinin 179
Brain tumors 247
Breath, shortness of 55
Bristol stool chart 182, 183*f*
Bronze diabetes 173
Budd-Chiari syndrome 328
Budesonide 159
Bulimia 270

C

Calcified vascular atheroma 18
Calcium 380
    channel blockers 189
    serum 19
Campylobacter 103, 161
    enteritis 108
    infection 160
    jejuni 102, 162
Cancer 132, 141
    classic apple-core appearance of 298*f*
    colonic 114*f*
    colorectal 1, 3, 91, 131, 132, 142*t*, 240, 242*f*
    esophageal 311, 313*f*, 314*f*
    higher risk of 243
    ovarian 3
    pancreatic 330, 331, 331*f*
    renal 20*f*
        cell 20*f*
    second synchronous 252
    sigmoid 250*f*
    stomach 44*f*
Candida septicemia 305
Capsule endoscopy 209, 211
Caput medusae 336
Carbohydrate 402, 404
    absorption 285
    fermentation of 275
    handling 276
    meal 285

Carbon dioxide 275
Carboplatin, administration of 317
Carcinoembryonic antigen 252
Carcinoid 254
   syndrome 117, 179, 342
   tumors 254
Carcinoma 43f, 90, 106
   cecal 90
   colonic 86, 113
   epidermoid 198
   gallbladder 330
   hepatocellular 343, 345, 345f, 367, 367f
   invasive 250f
   large bowel 89, 91
   medullary 180
   pancreas 330
   renal cell 340f
   small intestine 233
   stomach 41
Cardiac failure, congestive 328
Cardinal signs 59
Caroli's disease 329
Caroli's syndrome 332, 333
Catecholamines 179
Celecoxib 214
Celiac antibodies 24
Celiac disease 3, 104, 120, 120f, 168, 168f, 212
   diagnosis of 169
Central nervous system 121
Central venous pressure 79
Cerebrovascular accident 188
Chagas disease 188, 307
Charcot's triad 61, 327
Chemoembolization
   transarterial 368
   transcatheter arterial 346
Chemoradiotherapy, therapeutic 316
Chemotherapy 198, 331
   adjuvant 45
   neoadjuvant 44, 251
Child-Pugh score 357t
Chlorpromazine 264
Cholangiocarcinoma 327, 329
   risk of 329
Cholangitis 51, 77, 327, 393
   ascending 77
   primary biliary 328, 393
   suppurative 77
Cholecystectomy 51
   laparoscopic 51
Cholecystitis 51, 74
   acute 60, 61f, 75, 77
   gangrenous 77f
Choledochal cysts 329, 332
Cholera 117, 178
   management of 179
Chymotrypsin, 124
Ciprofloxacin 171
Cirrhosis 147, 356
   complications of 356
   hepatic 226
   plus ascites 364
   presence of 383
Cirrhotic liver 357
Clostridium difficile 105, 162
   colitis 162, 163f
   infection 150, 160
   toxin 105
Clostridium perfringens 162
Coagulation disorders 239
Coccygodynia 201
Colectomy, types of 140
Colic, esophageal 290
Colitis 148, 157
   chronic low-grade 135
   collagenous 22, 103, 157
   cystica profunda 199
   eosinophilic 159f
   ischemic 157
   lymphocytic 157
   microscopic 157
   ulcerative 2f, 3, 87, 106, 107f-111f, 113f, 127, 128f, 129, 130f, 253
   worse 133
Colon
   cancer 213f, 240, 252
      sporadic 248f
      staging of 251
   eosinophilic infiltration of 16f
Colonic disease 105, 146, 153
Colonic transit study 187f
Colonoscopy 142f, 210, 237f
   virtual 111
Colorectal cancer, risk of 141

Index

Columnar cells, mucin-producing 11*f*
Common bile duct 52, 175*f*, 323*f*
   injury 323*f*
   stones 323*f*
   tumor obstructing lower end of 12*f*
Computed tomography 114*f*, 250*f*, 262*f*, 268*f*, 324
   aortic angiogram 69*f*
   colography 111*f*
   scanning 12*f*, 341*f*
      abdominal 43
Condylomata
   acuminata 194
   lata 194, 198
Connective tissue disorders 85
Constipation 25, 98, 182, 185, 188, 188*t*, 189*t*
   causes of 188
   predominant irritable bowel syndrome 185
Corpus gastritis 37
Corticosteroids 78, 133, 149
Corticotropin-releasing hormone 265
Cotrimoxazole 171
Courvoisier's law 61
Coxiella burnetii 327
Cramps, abdominal 285
C-reactive protein 2, 59, 104
Creatinine 384
Cricopharyngeal spasm 309
Crigler-Najjar syndrome 321
Crohn's disease 1, 2, 2*f*, 14, 14*f*, 20, 25, 74, 87, 90, 104, 110*f*, 111*f*, 112, 113*f*, 118, 122, 127, 128*f*, 142-144, 145*f*, 148, 151*f*, 153, 157, 177, 192, 194, 197, 202, 203*f*, 204, 233, 235, 238, 342, 404
   classic hallmarks of 146*f*
   colonic 150
   diagnosis of 15*f*
   management of 149
   natural history of 148*f*
   perianal 156
   prevalence of 143
   specific complications of 154
Cronkhite-Canada syndrome 255
Cruveilhier-Baumgarten syndrome 227
Cryptosporidium 103, 161

Cullen's sign 57, 62
Curling's ulcers 35, 219
Cyanosis 299
Cystic fundic polyps 48
Cysts 163, 164
   hepatic 347
Cytochromes 98
Cytomegalovirus 305, 327, 353, 379
   biopsies 292*f*
   inclusion body 306*f*
   serology 379

D

Degos disease 239
Deoxyribonucleic acid 386
Dermatitis herpetiformis 169
Dermatomyositis 238
Desmoid tumors 247
Diabetes 173, 378, 388
   mellitus 188
Diarrhea 3, 17, 25, 26, 102, 104, 105, 109, 112, 112*f*, 117, 127, 173, 179, 276, 281, 284
   bloody 157
   chronic 106
   infective 103, 108, 160
   inflammatory infective 103
   large volume 117
   nocturnal 104
   non-bloody 259
   non-inflammatory infective 103
   predominance of 24
   secretory 178, 179
   watery 117, 118, 159, 180
Diclofenac 214
Dietary therapy 152
Dieulafoy's lesion 220, 221*f*, 222*f*
Digoxin 105
Directly acting oral anticoagulants 208
Distension, abdominal 65, 276, 335*f*
Diuretics 78
Diverticular disease 18, 63
Diverticulitis 18, 63, 85, 87, 88
Diverticulosis 235
Diverticulum, esophageal 310, 310*f*
Domperidone 302
Dopaminergic antagonists 264

Drug 258, 326
  efficacy 135
  history 378
  therapy 149, 229, 306, 308
Dubin-Johnson syndrome 326, 384
Dumping syndrome 284
  frequency of 281
Duodenal
  biopsies, endoscopic 171
  disease 3
  Jejunal flexure 95
  obstruction 258, 331*f*
  perforation 83
  ulcer
    acutely bleeding 215
    management of 29
    multiple 5
    perforated 84
    posterior 3
Duodenitis 7, 31
Duodenum 10
Dupuytren's contracture 386
Dysentery, amebic 163
Dyspepsia,
  functional 32, 33
  non-ulcer 32
Dysphagia 283, 292, 293, 308, 309, 312, 313, 400, 403
  esophageal 293
  oropharyngeal 293
Dysplasia 132, 141
  high-grade 141, 304*f*
Dyspnea 299

E

Eating disorders 265
Echinococcus granulosus 347
Ectopic pregnancy 70
  rupture of 69, 70
Ehlers-Danlos syndrome 239
Electrolytes 80
Emergency laparotomy 71
Empyema 71, 75, 338
Encephalopathy 356, 359, 364, 371
  grades of 365*t*
  hepatic 229
Endocrine disease 118
Endocrinological disorders 188
Endometriosis 20
Endometriotic cyst, spontaneous
  rupture of 70
Endomysial antibodies 120
Endoscopic therapy 216, 217, 229
Entamoeba coli 103
Entamoeba histolytica 161, 163, 349
Enteritis, eosinophilic 16*f*
Enterobiasis 165
Enterobius vermicularis 165, 165*f*, 195, 201, 201*f*
Enteroenteric anastomosis 281
Enteroscopy 211
Enzyme 376
  concentration 124
  hepatic 259
Eosinophil infiltrates 299*f*
Eosinophilic enterocolitis, diagnosis of 16*f*
Epilepsy 98
Episiotomy 193
Epithelioid cells 117*f*
Epithelium 120
Epstein-Barr
  serology 379
  virus 327, 379, 393
Erythema nodosum 147, 162
Erythrocyte sedimentation rate 2, 104
Erythromycin 105, 167
Escherichia coli 103, 327, 349
Esophageal
  cancer
    advanced 317
    large 315*f*
    treatment of 318
  candidiasis, extensive 305
  disease, antigen-mediated 306
  eosinophilia, causes of 306
  mucosa, transformed 295
  perforation, prognosis of 82
  sphincter, lower 288, 289, 301, 307*f*, 308
  stricture, balloon dilation of 305*f*
  ulcer, benign 296*f*
Esophagectomy 316
Esophagitis 300
  eosinophilic 298, 299*f*, 305
  infective 305

Index

Esophagogastric junction cancers 317
Esophagus 288
    ulcerated peptic stricture of 296*f*
Ethanol 386
Extrahepatic ducts 332

F

Fat
    intolerance 32
    malabsorption 173
Fatigue 284
Fatty acids, short-chain 274, 404
Fatty diarrhea 118
Fatty liver 385, 387*f*
    disease 406
        non-alcoholic 361, 376, 378, 380, 388
Fecal blood loss 252
Fecal calprotectin 2*f*, 104
    level of 24
Fecal incontinence 193, 200
Fecal peritonitis 88
Fecal transplant 162
Fever 327
Fibromuscular ring 297
Fibrosis 174*f*, 356*f*, 387*f*
    tissue 195
Fissure, anal 188, 197
Fistula 154, 194
    anorectal 202
    formation 87
Fitz-Hugh-Curtis' syndrome 70
Flexible sigmoidoscopy 105
Flucloxacillin 326
Fludeoxyglucose 314
Fluid and electrolyte replacement 179
Food poisoning 161, 257
    causes of 162*t*
Forceps delivery 193
Fragile superficial capillaries 238*f*
Fundic gland polyps 49*f*
Fungal infection 198

G

Gallbladder 8, 52, 71, 324, 331*f*, 338
    adenomyomatosis of 8
    cancer 330
    disease 7
    distension 339
    fossa 65*f*
    palpable 61
    ultrasound scan of 61*f*
    wall 61
Gallstone 7, 9, 50, 52, 56, 61, 75, 76, 147, 281, 282, 282*f*, 324
    development 283
    disease 282
        management of 325*f*
    formation of 51, 282
    medical management of 52
    related disease 78, 80
Gamma glutamyl transferase 376, 380, 381
Ganglioneuroblastoma 178
Gas production, causes of 23
Gastointestinal bleeding 213
Gastrectomy
    partial 286
    vertical sleeve 272
Gastric
    acid 286
    adenocarcinoma 43*f*
    antral vascular ectasia 36, 36*f*
    band 272
        laparoscopic adjustable 280*f*
        placement 279
    bypass 280
    cancer 38, 41, 44*f*, 45, 267
        early 45
        large 42*f*
        management of 43
        treatment of 45
    carcinoma 258
    dilatation, risk of 270
    disease 3
    distension, acute 281
    emptying study 260
    erosions 219
    inhibitory polypeptide 285
    lymphoma 45, 46*f*-48*f*, 223, 223*f*
    malignancies 45
    metaplasia 31, 32
    mucosa, eosinophilic infiltration of 39
    mucosal inflammation 36

neoplasm 83
operations 279
   numbers of 279
outlet obstruction 261
parietal cells 30*f*
pathology 261
perforation 83
polyps 48
scanning 260
ulcer
   benign 35
   margin, histology of 28*f*
   perforated 83
   risk of 36
varices 231, 232*f*
volvulus 18*f*, 311, 312*f*
Gastrin 30*f*, 33
   acetylcholine 30*f*
   producing tumor 5
   secreting pancreatic tumor 117
Gastrinoma 6
   duodenal 6
Gastritis 36, 36*f*, 37*t*, 38, 39, 262
   acute 37
   alcoholic 257, 258
   atrophic 40
   chronic 37
   eosinophilic 40
   granulomatous 39, 40
   helicobacter-associated 40
   hypertrophic 39
   infectious 39
   lymphocytic 40
   severe 38*f*
   viral 257
Gastroenteritis
   eosinophilic 158
   viral 168
Gastroenterology 258
Gastroesophageal
   junction 279, 288, 316
   reflux disease 300, 306
   tumor 298*f*
   varices 227
Gastrointestinal
   abdominal pain, upper 4
   bleeding 205, 359, 366
      severe 205
      upper 192

disorders, upper 288
disturbance 55
endoscopy, upper 209
infection 256
motility 265
stromal tumor 50, 50*f*, 222, 222*f*
tissue 158
tract 264, 365
   function of 399
   primary function of 183
   spontaneous perforation of 80
Gastroparesis, diabetic 258, 260*f*
Gastropathy, portal hypertensive 233
Gastropexy, vertical band 280
Gastroplasty, vertical banded 280*f*
Genetic syndromes 242
Ghrelin 265
Giant cell granulomas 117*f*
Giardia 102, 103
   lamblia 121, 161, 166
      infestation 163
Giardiasis 163, 170
Gilbert's syndrome 321, 384
Globus hystericus 292
Glomerulus 62
Glottis 81
Glucose
   isotope of 45
   tolerance tests 173
Glyceryl trinitrate 197, 229
Glycocholate breath test 126
Glycoprotein 252
Granulomas 111*f*
Granulomata, non-caseating 106, 146, 146*f*
Granulomatous disease 381
Grey Turner's sign 57
Gynecomastia 335*f*, 357*f*

H

Hartmann's pouch 339
Hartmann's procedure 93
Head
   injury 188
   tumor, pancreatic 12*f*
Headaches 284
Heart disease, ischemic 36, 229
Heartburn 33, 288

Index

Helicobacter pylori 4, 26, 28, 30, 37, 38, 38*f*, 219, 281
    diseases, putative pathogenesis of 29*f*
    eradication 29
    infection 27, 31, 37, 47, 48*f*, 213, 214
Heller's procedure 308
Hemangiomas 346
Hematemesis 209
Hematochezia 205
Hematoma 69*f*
    perianal 195
Hemochromatosis 173, 343
    hereditary 380, 396
Hemoglobin 207
Hemolysis 320
Hemorrhage 208
    acute 213*f*
    recent 206, 206*t*
    spontaneous 108*f*
Hemorrhoids 195, 196*f*
    thrombosed 188
Henoch-Schonlein purpura 239
Hepatic
    cyst, simple 337, 348*f*
    fibrosis, congenital 332, 333
    mass, irregular 344
    venous flow, assessment of 339
Hepatitis
    A 353
        virus 392
    acute 258
        alcoholic 368, 386
    alcoholic 358, 369*f*
    autoimmune 321, 328, 376, 379, 394
    B 343, 353, 354, 379
        core antibody 390
        surface antigen 390
        virus 344, 376, 379, 389, 390*t*, 391
    C 353, 379
        virus 344, 379, 391, 392
    chronic 147
    D virus 391
        infection 391
    E virus 392
    evidence of 259
    viral 357, 378, 389, 392, 397
Hepatocellular carcinoma
    development of 358
    primary 343, 344*f*

Hepatoma 343, 344
Hepatorenal syndrome 359, 361, 363
    development of 363*f*
    diagnosis of 364*t*
    types of 364*t*
Hereditary colorectal cancer syndrome 246
Hernia 90
    hiatus 17*f*, 219, 288, 311
    internal 281, 282
    para-esophageal 311
    umbilical 91*f*
Herpes simplex virus 305
High jugular venous pressure 336
Hinchey classification 63
Hirschsprung's disease 188, 189, 336
Histamine 179
    H2 antagonists 301
    receptor 30*f*, 264
Hormonal signals, peripheral 265
Hormone
    adrenocorticotropic 313
    metabolic 273
    production of 265
Howell-Jolly bodies 120
Human immunodeficiency virus infection 305
Human papillomavirus, types of 197
Hydatid cysts 347
Hydrogen production 274
Hyperbilirubinemia 319, 384
    conjugated 320, 321
    unconjugated 320
Hypercalcemia 19, 188, 258, 261
Hypercholesterolemia 378, 388
Hyperemesis gravidarum 258, 384
Hyperglycemia 266
Hyperlipidemia syndromes 19
Hyperparathyroidism 188
Hyperplasia
    crypt 120
    lymphoid 73
Hypertension 98, 378, 386, 388
    management of 388
    portal 225*f*, 226
Hyperthyroidism 261
Hypoalbuminemia 361
Hypochlorhydria 117

Hypokalemia 188
Hypolactasia 164, 167, 170
Hyponatremia 361
Hypophosphatemia 403
Hypotension, postural 260
Hypothalamus 266
Hypothyroidism 188
Hypovolemia 359
    signs of 359
Hypoxemia, severe 78

I

Ibuprofen 214
Ileal disease, terminal 153
Ileitis 148
Ileocecal valve 107*f*
Ileocolitis 148
Iliac fossa 336, 341
Immune disease, history of 394
Indomethacin 214
Infarction 68
    intestinal 67
Infectious disease 324
Infective diarrhea
    causes of 160
    consequences of 160
Infertility 70
Infiltrative lymphoma cells, proliferation of 47*f*
Inflammation
    chronic 106
    severe 163*f*
    sigmoid 16*f*
Inflammatory bowel disease 1, 56, 87, 103, 136*f*, 192, 213, 235, 244
Infliximab 150
Interleukin 160
Intestinal
    bacterial overgrowth, small 125, 177
    cancers, range of 270
    disease 12, 120, 126
    infarction 17
    ischemia 96
    obstruction 65, 88, 89, 96, 262
        diagnosis of 65, 92
    peptide, vasoactive 178, 179
Intestine
    contractions of 12
    small 164, 178
    vasculitis of 238
Intra-abdominal pathology 64, 96
Intraductal
    epithelial neoplasms, malignant 11*f*
    papillary mucinous neoplasm 330
Intrahepatic ducts, dilated 12*f*, 13*f*
Intrathoracic pressure 256
Iron
    deficiency 286
    replacement therapy, simple 286
Irritable bowel syndrome 1, 2*f*, 3, 21, 24, 104, 184, 192, 276, 335, 335*f*
    postinfective 23
Ischemia 67
    intestinal 53
    mesenteric 17, 52

J

Jaundice 208, 319, 319*f*, 326, 327, 332, 359, 378
    degree of 7
    radiological investigation of 324*t*
Jugular venous pressure 362

K

Kasai portoenterostomy procedure 332
Kelly-Patterson syndrome 310
Kernicterus 321
Ketoprofen 214
Kidney 340
    injury 359

L

Labyrinthitis 258
Lactulose syrup 126
Lamina propria
    colonic 146*f*
    edematous 254
    mononuclear cells 169
Lansoprazole 105
Lanugo hair 269
Lanz incision 75*f*
Laparotomy, second-look 86
Large bowel obstruction, management of 93
Leptospira icterohemorrhagica 327

Index

Leukemia 197
Leukocytes 133
Leukoplakia 198
Leukotriene receptor antagonist 159
Lichen planus 198
Linitis plastica 41, 42*f*, 401
    infiltrative gastric cancer of 262*f*
Lipoma, esophageal 297*f*
Liver
    abscesses 338*f*
        causes of 349
    biochemistry, abnormal 375, 382
    biopsy 345, 382
        cirrhotic 356*f*
    disease 227, 228, 358, 375, 384
        alcohol-related 385, 386, 387*f*
        autoimmune 379, 393
        chronic 324, 335*f*, 351, 356, 357, 357*f*, 377
        history of 352
        inherited 396
        severity of 358
        signs of 208
        stage of 358
    enzyme 375
    failure 351, 361
        acute 351, 351*f*, 352*f*, 355
        acute-on-chronic 369
        chronic 353
        encompasses 351
    function test 324, 376, 377*f*, 382
        abnormal 7, 147, 375
    metastases 44*f*, 316*f*
    resection 345
    screen, noninvasive 376, 378
    synthetic function 362
    transplantation 333, 355, 373
    tumors 343
Local disease, management of 316
Lymph nodes
    abdominal 341
    enlarged 223*f*
Lymphangiectasia, intestinal 121
Lymphocytes 120
    intraepithelial 168
Lymphoid tissue, mucosa-associated 47, 48*f*
Lymphoma 90, 253
    intestinal 121, 169, 171, 172
    mediterranean 172
    primary 172
Lynch's syndromes 247, 248

M

Macroamylasemia 62
Maddrey's discriminant function 369
Magnetic resonance
    cholangiopancreatography 323*f*, 324
    enteroclysis 121, 155*f*
    enterography 3
    imaging 13*f*, 14*f*, 113*f*, 203*f*
Malabsorption
    causes of 121
    severe 172
Malignant disease
    exclusion of 267
    occult 19
Mallory's hyaline 387*f*
Mallory-Weiss tear 209, 219, 220*f*
Mallory-Weiss type 220
Malnutrition, risk of 399
Mass
    abdominal 334
    appendix 73
    central abdominal 341
    lower abdominal 58
    pancreatic 341
    renal 340
    suprapubic 341
Mast cell stabilizer 159
McBurney's point 59
Mebendazole 348
Meckel's diverticulitis 74
Meckel's diverticulum 209, 210
Melanomas 194, 198
Melanosis coli 115*f*
Meloxicam 214
Memory T-lymphocytes, migration of 135
Ménétrier's disease 39
Menetrier's hypertrophic gastritis 262
Meniere's disease 258
Menopause 393
Mesalazine 150
Mesenteric artery syndrome 52, 263

Metabolic disease 19
    exclusion of 268
Metabolic disorders 188
Metabolic syndrome 375, 388
Metaplasia 132, 303
    intestinal 38
Metastatic disease, management of 317
Metformin 105
Metoclopramide 209
Metronidazole 150
Micronutrient 405
    deficiencies 286
Mirizzi's syndrome 7, 339
Mononucleosis, infectious 393
Monospot test 393
Motor neuron disease 293, 310
Motor neuropathy 98
Mucocele 75, 338
Mucosa
    colonic 137*f*
    rectal 103, 106
Murphy's sign 60
Muscle
    antibody, smooth 394
    hyperplasia, smooth 254
    involvement 172
Muscular tear 82
Myasthenia gravis 293
Mycobacterium
    avium-intracellulare 39
    bovis 167
    tuberculosis 167
Myocardial infarction, acute 81
Myotomy, per-oral endoscopic 308

N

N-acetyl cysteine 354
Naproxen 214
Nasogastric tubes 405
National Institute of Clinical Excellence 21, 152
Nausea 32, 65, 256, 257, 259
    causes of 257, 258
    neurophysiology of 256
    painless 257
N-benzoyl-l-tyrosyl-p-amino-benzoic acid 124

Necrosis
    develops, pancreatic 78
    pancreatic 79
Neoplasms, pancreatic 341
Neoplastic disease 20
Nephrotoxic drugs 364
Nervous system, sympathetic 363
Neural tissues 178
Neurokinin 256
Neurological disease 293
Neurological disorders 188
Neuromuscular disease, primary 293
Neuropathy, diabetic autonomic 188
Neutrophil 103
    infiltration 369*f*
Neutrophilia 67
Nitrogen 274
    source 403
Nodules, regenerative 356*f*
Nonsteroidal anti-inflammatory
    agents 56, 213
    drugs 4, 189
Non-variceal upper gastrointestinal bleeding, causes of 219
Nosocomial infection 162
Nutritional status, assessment of 399

O

Oat cell carcinoma 178
Obesity 270, 279, 357, 375, 397
    surgery
        endoscopic appearance of 284*f*
        gastrointestinal complications of 279
Obstruction, relief of 329
Octaplas 228
Octreotide 51, 286
    scan 34*f*
Odynophagia 288, 291, 305
Ogilvie's syndrome 66, 92
Olsalazine 134
Opiate analgesia 76
Opioids 189
Oral mesalazine 136
Oral metronidazole 162
Oral ulcer 112, 145*f*
Osteomalacia 147

Index

Osteopenia 147
Osteoporosis 147
Ovarian cyst, torsion of 70
Oxygen therapy 79

P

Paddy fields 164
Paget's disease 194, 195, 198, 380
Pain 192, 327
    abdominal 2, 14, 19, 20, 22, 55, 58, 65, 73, 98, 172, 173, 257, 281
    agonizing 67
    anal 192
    biliary colic 7
    cardiac 290
    chest 55, 81
    chronic abdominal 1, 21
    epigastric 32, 72
    esophageal 288
    functional 1
    management of 331
    organic 1
    periodic 27
    rectal 201
    recurrent abdominal 21
    upper abdominal 72
Palmar erythema 335*f*, 357*f*, 378
Pancolitis 133
Pancreas 6, 178
    atrophic 175*f*
    computed tomography of 123*f*
    intraductal papillary mucinous neoplasm of 11*f*
    magnetic resonance imaging of 124*f*
Pancreatic cancer, magnetic resonance imaging scan of 331*f*
Pancreatic disease 10, 122, 124
    benign 124
    malignant 124
Pancreatic duct 175*f*, 234
    dilated 13*f*, 175*f*
Pancreatic function tests 123
Pancreatic imaging 123
Pancreatic insufficiency 104
Pancreatic lesion 10
    endoscopic ultrasound of 332*f*
Pancreatic malignancy 329

Pancreatitis 51
    acute 56, 61, 62, 62*f*, 77, 80
    alcohol-related 78
    autoimmune 173
    azathioprine-induced 11*f*
    chronic 13*f*, 123*f*, 124*f*, 174*f*, 177
    severe 78
Pangastritis 37
Para-aminobenzoic acid 124
Paracentesis, large volume 362
Parasites 163
Parasitic disease 327
Parathyroid 6
Parenteral nutrition 405
Parietal cell 30
    function 30*f*
Parkinson's disease 188
Parotid gland 386
Peg solution 263
Pelvic
    abscess 87, 192
    computed tomography scan 43
    esophageal stricture 304
    floor dysfunction 187
    pain 20, 70, 192
    peritonitis, acute 71
    ulcer 35, 74
        disease 37, 208, 214
Peptide secreting tumors 178
    management of 179
Percutaneous transhepatic cholangiogram 12*f*, 329
Perianal disease 148, 156, 156*f*, 203*f*
Pericholangitis 147
Peritoneal
    cavity 85
    irritation, signs of 76
Peritonitis 65
    feculent 87
    lower abdominal 85
    purulent 87
Petersen's hernia 90
Peutz-Jeghers polyps 254
Peutz-Jeghers syndrome 233
Pharyngeal pouch 294*f*, 309
Phosphatase, alkaline 376, 380, 382
Phosphate 380, 403
Phrenic dyssynergia 23, 276*f*

Pigment lesions 234
Pinworm 165
Piperacillin 229
Piroxicam 214
Plasma
    cortisol 261
    potassium 261
    viscosity 2
Plexus hematoma, external 197
Plummer-Vinson syndrome 310
Pneumatic balloon, large 309*f*
Pneumatosis 117*f*, 237*f*
    coli 237
        computed tomography of 237*f*
        management of 237
    cystoides intestinalis 116*f*
    intestinalis 68*f*
Pneumomediastinum 82*f*
Pneumoperitoneum 64*f*, 65*f*
Polya gastrectomy 125
Polyarteritis 96
    nodosa 238
Polycystic liver disease 332
Polycythemia rubra vera 328
Polyethylene glycol 15, 186
Polymyositis 293
Polyp 244
    adenomatous 242
    benign 90
    classic adenomatous 243*f*
    colonic 254
    colorectal 240
    dysplastic 245*f*
    hamartomatous 254
    hyperplastic 244, 254
    juvenile 254
    metaplastic 254
    numbers of 244
Polypeptide, pancreatic 265
Polypoidal
    esophageal tumor 297*f*
    lesions, management of 52
Polyposis
    coli, adenomatous 246
    familial adenomatous 48, 246
    syndromes 48, 49*f*
Porphyria 19, 98
    intermittent 56, 98

Portal hypertension 208, 356
    clinical features of 227
    development of 357
    etiology of 225
    pathogenesis of 225
    presinusoidal 225
    sinusoidal 226
Portal pressure, normal 225
Portal vein thrombosis 225
    diagnosis of 226
Portal venous gas 67
Positron-emission tomography scan 45
Potassium 403
    serum 285
Prader-Willi syndrome 265
Preeclampsia 385
Pregnancy, intrahepatic cholestasis of 384
Prochlorperazine 264
Procidentia 199
Proctalgia 201
    fugax 192
Proctitis 139
    ulcerative 192
Prolactinoma 6
Prophylactic antiemetics 259
Prostaglandin inhibitors 133
Protein energy malnutrition 370
Prothrombin 259
    time 352
Proton 30
    pump 30
        inhibitors 30, 282, 289, 302
Pruritus 195
    ani 195, 200
Pseudoachalasia 308
    barium swallow of 298*f*
    phenomenon of 297
Pseudocyst 174
    large pancreatic 342*f*
Pseudomembranous colitis 87, 105, 160
Pseudo-obstruction 92
Psychology 22
Psychosis 98
Puborectalis straightens 184*f*
Pus cells 103
Pyloric stenosis 258
Pyoderma gangrenosum 131*f*

Pyrexia 61
    presence of 337

R

Radiation proctitis 116*f*, 238, 238*f*
Rapid dehydration, causes of 56
Reactive oxygen species 386
Rectal mucosa, normal 106
Red blood cells 320
Refeeding syndrome, risk of 401
Reflux
    disease, endoscopy of 290*f*
    esophagitis 300
    gastritis, alkaline 39
Reiter's syndrome 162
Renal artery, lower border of 96
Renal disease 356
    intrinsic 364
Renal dysfunction 384
Renal impairment 359, 374
Retinal pigment epithelium, congenital hypertrophy of 246
Retrograde cholangiopancreatography, endoscopic 324, 325*f*, 395*f*
Reye's syndrome 259
Rheumatoid disease 173
Ribavirin 392
Rockall score 206*f*, 206*t*
Rokitansky-Aschoff sinuses 8
Roundworm 164
Roux-en-Y
    gastric bypass 272, 280, 280*f*
    reconstructions 286
    type operations 281

S

Saliva, outpouring of 35
Salmonella 103, 161, 162
    infection 160
    osteomyelitis 161
    septicemia 161
    typhi 349
Salpingitis, acute 70
Sarcoidosis 40
Schatzki ring 297, 311
Schistosome 164
Schistosomiasis 164
    haematobium 164

    japonicum 164, 166
    mansoni 164
Sclerosing cholangitis, primary 129, 132*f*, 245, 395, 395*f*
Sclerosis, multiple 188
Sclerosus et atrophicus 198
Selective serotonin reuptake inhibitors 26
Sepsis, signs of 359
Serious organic diseases 21
Sertoli cell tumors 255
Sexual abuse 192
Sexually transmitted disease 194, 197
Shigella 103, 161
    dysentery 167
Shock, absence of 364
Sickle cell anemia 320
Sigmoidoscopy, rigid 105
Sjögrens' syndrome 173, 289
Skin disease, chronic ulcerating 130
Small bowel 90, 121
    bacterial overgrowth 284
    infarction 68*f*
    obstruction 58, 66*f*, 89*f*, 154*f*
        causes of 89, 90
        management of 92
    perforation 84, 85*t*
Snail track ulcers 106
Sodium
    cromoglycate 159
    hydroxide, pellet of 105
    retention 361
Solitary rectal ulcer syndrome 189, 190*f*, 198, 199*f*
Spasm, esophageal 292*f*, 308
Spider naevi 208, 357*f*, 378
Spinal cord lesion 188
Spleen, palpable 339
Splenic atrophy 169
Splenic flexure 158
Sporadic colon cancer, pathogenesis of 247
Squamous carcinoma in situ 194
Squamous cell
    cancer 312
    esophageal cancer 317
Staphylococcus aureus 162
Steatorrhea 103, 120, 118, 122, 125, 173
    necessitates 122

Steatosis 147, 369*f*
Stenosis, stomal 283
Stercoral perforation 86
Steroid 153
    budesonide 150
Stomach, fundus of 221*f*
Streptococcus faecalis 349
Streptococcus milleri 349
Stroke 188
Strongyloides 121
    stercoralis 166
Strongyloidiasis 164, 170
Sulfasalazine 133, 150
Swallowing 288
Swelling
    abdominal 334
    generalized 334
    parotid 208
Sydney classification 36
Syphilis 197, 198
Systemic lupus erythematosus 238

T

Tachycardia 98
Tapeworm 347
Tazobactam 229
T-cell lymphoma 169
Telangiectasia
    hemorrhagic 234
    hereditary hemorrhagic 234
Telangiectatic lesions 115
Tenesmus 193
Thalassemia 320
Theophylline 105
Thiazide diuretics 105
Thiersch procedure 199
Thiopurine S-methyltransferase 134
Thoracic cavity 82
Thumbprinting, classical sign of 96
Thyroid 178
    capillary carcinoma of 247
Thyrotoxicosis 118, 258
Tissue transglutaminase 120
Toxic albendazole 348
Toxic alkaloids 227
Toxic gluten 169
Toxic megacolon 138

Transjugular intrahepatic portosystemic shunt 362, 370, 371, 371*f*
    complications of 372*f*
    contraindications of 372*f*
Traveler's diarrhea 161
    causes of 161*t*
Trichophagia 262
Trichotillomania 262
Trichuris 165
    trichiuria 166
Triosorbon 152
Tropheryma whippelii 171
Tropical sprue 170
Trypanosoma cruzi 308
Tubeless function tests 124
Tuberculosis 197
    gastrointestinal 122, 167
    intestinal 167
Tumors
    anal 198
    benign 295
    duodenal 233*f*
    esophageal 316*f*
    hepatic 346
    metastatic 347
    necrosis factor 122, 135
    neuroendocrine 34*f*
    obstructing 188
    ovarian 255
    pancreatic 10, 13*f*
    renal 341*f*
    testicular 255
Turcot syndrome 247
Turner's sign 62
Two-stage ileoanal pouch operation 141*f*

U

Ulcer 56
    colonic 235
    deep
        excavated 210*f*
        fissuring 15*f*, 110*f*
    disease 32*f*
        duodenal 4, 38, 213
    duodenal 5*f*, 26, 215*f*
    endoscopic appearance of 215*t*
    genital 112, 238
    pre-pyloric 4*f*

serpiginous 145*f*
solitary 235
stomal 281
Ultrasound 324
    endoscopic 44, 175*f*, 224*f*, 308
    scanning 376
Umbilicus 336
Uremia 258
Urinary retention, acute 58
Uveitis 112

V

Vagus nerve releasing acetylcholine 30*f*
Variceal bleeding 229, 366, 371, 372
    management of 227, 366
Varicella zoster 353
Varices 231
    portosystemic 227
Vascular bowel disease 56
Vascular occlusion, mesenteric 96
Vedolizumab 135, 150
Veins
    hepatic 371*f*
    periumbilical 336
Veno-occlusive disease 227
Venous thrombosis 68, 112
Verner-Morrison's syndrome 117
Vibrio cholerae 162, 178
Vibrio parahaemolyticus 162
Villous adenoma 250*f*
Villous atrophy 120, 168
Vipoma 117
Viral disease 327
Viral hepatitis infection, chronic 375
Vitamin
    B12
        deficiency 125
        malabsorption 125
    D 380
    K 383

Volvulus 15
    organoaxial 312*f*
    sigmoid 17*f*
Vomiting 65, 98, 256, 257, 259, 283
    causes of 257, 258
    drug therapy of 264
    epidemics of 259
    neurophysiology of 256
    psychogenic 263
    self-induced 270
    severe 258
von Willebrand's disease 240

W

Warts
    anal 197
    genital 198
Watermelon stomach 36*f*
Weil's disease 327
Whipple's disease 121, 171
Whipple's procedure 331
Whipworm 165
White blood count 59
Wilkie's syndrome 263, 263*f*
Wilson's disease 259, 321, 396

Y

Yersinia
    enteritis 162
    enterocolitica 167
    infection 74

Z

Zieve's syndrome 324, 326
Zollinger-Ellison syndrome 31, 33, 34*f*, 49, 117
    diagnosis of 5, 34
    management of 34